Pearson's Massage Therapy Exam Review

Fifth Edition

JANE S. GAROFANO, PhD, LMT, NCTMB

Owner/Director
JSG School of Massage Therapy
Northvale, New Jersey

Retired Professor of Biological Sciences
Bergen Community College
Paramus, New Jersey

Owner
SPA j
Northvale, New Jersey

PEARSON

Boston Columbus Indianapolis New York San Francisco Upper Saddle River

Amsterdam Cape Town Dubai London Madrid Milan Munich Paris Montreal Toronto

Delhi Mexico City São Paulo Sydney Hong Kong Seoul Singapore Taipei Tokyo

Publisher: Julie Levin Alexander
Assistant to Publisher: Regina Bruno
Editor in Chief: Mark Cohen
Executive Editor: John Goucher
Assistant Editor: Nicole Ragonese
Project Manager: Pat Brown
Creative Director: Jayne Conte
Designer: Karen Noferi

Production Editor: Suganya Karuppasamy
Director of Marketing: David Gesell
Marketing Manager: Katrin Beacom
Media Project Manager: Lorena Cerisano
Cover Art: wavebreakmedia ltd/Shutterstock
Composition: Element LLC
Printer/Binder: LSC Communications
Cover Printer: LSC Communications

Photo Credits: Cover: wavebreakmedia ltd/Shutterstock Images; Part 2: mythja/Shutterstock.com; Part 3: Pearson Education; Part 4: Phil Date/Shutterstock.com; Part 5: khz/Shutterstock.com; Part 6: dny3d/Shutterstock.com.

Notice: The author[s] and the publisher of this volume have taken care that the information and technical recommendations contained herein are based on research and expert consultation and are accurate and compatible with the standards generally accepted at the time of publication. Nevertheless, as new information becomes available, changes in clinical and technical practices become necessary. The reader is advised to carefully consult manufacturers' instructions and information material for all supplies and equipment before use and to consult with a healthcare professional as necessary. This advice is especially important when using new supplies or equipment for clinical purposes. The author[s] and publisher disclaim all responsibility for any liability, loss, injury, or damage incurred as a consequence, directly or indirectly, of the use and application of any of the contents of this volume.

Pearson® is a registered trademark of Pearson plc.

Pearson Education Ltd., *London*
Pearson Education Australia Pty. Limited, *Sydney*
Pearson Education Singapore, Pte. Ltd.
Pearson Education North Asia Ltd., *Hong Kong*
Pearson Education Canada, Ltd., *Toronto*

Pearson Educación de Mexico, S.A. de C.V.
Pearson Education—Japan, *Tokyo*
Pearson Education Malaysia, Pte. Ltd.
Pearson Education, Upper Saddle River, New Jersey

Library of Congress Cataloging-in-Publication Data
Garofano, Jane Schultz.
   Pearson's massage therapy exam review / Jane S. Garofano.
 — 5th ed., rev.
      p. ; cm.
Massage therapy exam review
Rev. ed. of: Success! in massage therapy / Jane S. Garofano. 4th ed., rev. c2009.
Includes bibliographical references and index.
   ISBN-13: 978-0-13-274190-3
   ISBN-10: 0-13-274190-3
I. Garofano, Jane Schultz. Success! in massage therapy. II. Title. III.
   Title: Massage therapy exam review.
   [DNLM: 1. Massage—Examination Questions. WB 18.2]
      615.8'22—dc23   2011037945

7 2021

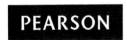

ISBN-13: 978-0-13-274190-3
ISBN-10: 0-13-274190-3

Dedication

This book is dedicated to Sienna, my chocolate Lab, who stayed by my side keeping me company and waiting for a massage!

Contents

About the Author

Jane S. Garofano, Ph.D., LMT, NCTMB graduated from NYU Medical Center, N.Y., where she studied physiology. Following her time at NYU she taught Anatomy and Physiology at Bergen Community College in Paramus, N.J., for 28 years. In 1995 Dr. Garofano studied massage therapy and became nationally certified.

Dr. Garofano has been the owner, director, and head instructor at the JSG School of Massage located in Northvale, N.J., for the past fifteen years. This institution is approved by the NJ Department of Education and Workforce Development. In addition she is a member of the AMTA Council of Schools, as well as a Lypossage™ Master Trainer and a Certified Pet Massage Therapist. The curriculum used by Dr. Garofano at her school combines PowerPoint with instructional home massage videos, both of which are incorporated into the new 5th edition of *Pearson's Massage Therapy Exam Review*. As an educator for over 40 years, Dr. Garofano is still greatly involved in improving Massage Therapy through teaching, writing and developing relationships with Volunteer Organizations. She is involved with Englewood hospital and Massage Envy, encouraging her students and graduates to find their place in this growing field of massage therapy. Dr. Garofano owns a Spa in Northvale, N.J., which offers a complete menu of massage modalities rounding out her dedication to massage as a career.

She currently lives in Tuxedo Park, N.Y., with her family, pets, wildlife, and nature.

Preface

Since Massage Therapy has become an important health care profession, more emphasis has been placed on the validation at the state and national level. And since the national exam is intended to better qualify massage therapists, this is a review book that appeals to massage therapists with various learning styles and provides a tool for that diversity of massage therapy graduates who choose to study online or use a book to qualify for national certification or licensure. This book offers many ways to study Anatomy and Physiology and Massage theory and application including easy to follow outlines, charts, figures, tables and 1,000 NCTMB and MBLEx type questions with answers and rationales and online practice tests. Practice tests, videos and PowerPoints will be available to students at www.myhealthprofessionskit.com.

This book has been used for over 10 years at Dr. Garofano's school, JSG School of Massage Therapy in New Jersey. It is used as a text, testing, and review book for the NCTMB exam. With a pass rate of 90–100% first time, Dr. Garofano and her students agree that without this simple but comprehensive review book, they would not have passed. Instructors can use it as a testing tool in preparation for the certifying exams by using questions directly from the book.

The 5th edition of Pearson's Massage Therapy Exam Review has been designed and revised according to the guidelines of the National Certification for Therapeutic Massage and Bodywork (NCTMB) exam, which is administered throughout the United States, Canada, and Puerto Rico, as well as the MBLEx exam developed by The Federation of State Massage Therapy Boards. This book contains each part as it is outlined in the NCTMB and MBLEx content outline so that the student can use this book to study section by section as it pertains to the exam of choice. This book enables the applicant to review relevant material while becoming familiar with the types of questions given on the exams. Each question has one correct answer and a brief rationale. The questions are divided into five parts that cover all the areas of Therapeutic Massage and Bodywork and correlate to the NCTMB exam content areas outlined in the *NCTMB Candidate Handbook*. Students are able to select the Therapeutic Massage and Bodywork exam (NCETMB) or the Therapeutic Massage exam (NCETM). The content is divided into Human Anatomy, Physiology, and Kinesiology; Pathology and Pharmacology; Therapeutic Massage Bodywork, Assessment and Application; and Professional Standards, Ethics, and Business and Legal Practices.

The review material and questions are also relevant for the MBLEx licensing exam and the content is divided into Anatomy and Physiology, Kinesiology, Pathology, Benefits and Techniques, Client Assessment, History and Modalities, Ethics, Laws, and Guidelines for Professional Practice.

The following is the most recent revision of the NCETMB, NCETM licensing exam content and the MBLEx candidate handbooks.

NCETMB, NCETM, and MBLEx Licensure Content Outline

I. <u>Kinesiology and Musculo-skeletal Anatomy and Physiology (19–24%)</u> (MBLEx 11%)

    A. Anatomical position and terminology (e.g., planes; directions)

    B. Muscles and muscle groups
        1. Tendons and attachment sites
        2. Actions and functions
        3. Types of contractions
        4. Agonist/antagonist and synergistic relationships

    C. Bones and bony landmarks

    D. Joints
        1. Types
        2. Locations
        3. Names
        4. Structure
        5. Function

    E. Fascia

    F. Muscle physiology

II. <u>Systemic Anatomy and Physiology (13–18%)</u> (MBLEx 14%)

    A. Integumentary

    B. Nervous

    C. Endocrine

    D. Cardiovascular

    E. Lymphatic

    F. Urinary

    G. Respiratory

    H. Digestive

    I. Reproductive

III. <u>Pathology, Contraindications and Cautionary Sites (14–19%)</u> (MBLEx 13%)

    A. Contraindications

    B. Endangerment/Cautionary Sites

    C. Soft tissue injury

    D. General pathology

IV. <u>Professional Standards (11–15%)</u> (MBLEx 13%)

    A. Law
        1. State and local credentialing requirements
        2. Business types/legal entities (e.g., independent contractor, employee, etc...)
        3. Scope of practice

        4. Active and passive range of motion assessments

        5. Functional assessment of lifestyle (activities, occupation, etc...)

  *C. <u>Basic Modality literacy</u> (familiarity with other modalities)

        1. Trigger point/neuromuscular therapy

        2. Stretching (proprioceptive neuromuscular facilitation, active isolated stretching, etc...)

        3. Myofascial release technique

        4. Muscle energy (e.g., positional release/straincounterstrain, etc...)

        5. Reflexology

        6. Seated technique

        7. Manual lymph drainage

        8. Hot stones

        9. Craniosacral technique

       10. Structural integration

       11. Reiki

       12. Shiatsu

       13. Acupressure

       14. Aromatherapy

       15. Thai massage

       16. Sports massage

VI. <u>MBLEx only</u> Massage History Culture/Modalities (History 5%)

  A. History of massage and bodywork

  B. Skill sets used in massage/bodywork

  C. Massage/bodywork modalities

VII. <u>MBLEx only</u> Guidelines for Professional Practice (Guidelines 10%)

  A. Equipment use

  B. Therapist hygiene

  C. Sanitation

  D. Safety practices

     1. Facility, client, therapist

  E. Therapist care

     1. Body mechanics

  F. Draping

  G. Business practices

     1. Business and strategic planning

     2. Office management

     3. Marketing

     4. Hiring/interview

     5. Documentation and record keeping

*not in NCETM

TIPS ON USING THIS REVIEW BOOK

Review all content chapters first before attempting questions. The charts, tables and figures are study friendly for easier review. Use caution with questions that contain words like *always, except, never, most appropriate* and other words that qualify a question. Watch out for words that put limitations on a potential answer. Be sure to read the entire question completely at least two times and then formulate the correct answer in your head before you take a look at the multiple choice answers. If you look at the choices of answers before you understand the question entirely, you may be led into choosing a wrong answer. There are four possible answers to each question. Two of the answers can often be eliminated right after reading the question through two times. Once these two answers are eliminated, you only need to decide the "best possible answer" between the two remaining choices. Check the answer and rationale. Go back to the chapter in this book to review rationale if needed.

The last section of the review book contains three comprehensive simulated exams consisting of two 160 questions for the NCETMB and NCETM exams and one 125 question exam for the MBLEx exam selected from the previous bank of questions and answers. They are organized according to the NCETMB, NCETM, and MBLEx content percentages. There are three comprehensive tests and three additional tests available for the NCETMB, NCETM and MBLEx exams. All these tests are 160 questions, stop at 125 questions for MBLEx exam. The exam is given by an electronic testing system; it includes six computerized practice tests, each of which should be completed in the 2 hour, 30- or 40-minute periods provided at the testing center. There are also 8 additional practice tests available at www.myhealthprofessionkit.com.

To help review the hands-on technique, a full body Swedish massage video is available online to demonstrate the visual aspect with a narrative description. A PowerPoint presentation for instructors is also online to assist in reviewing the content of the book. These materials will also be available to students and instructors at www.myhealthprofessionskit.com.

Introduction

The 5th edition of Pearson's Massage Therapy Exam Review is a complete exam preparation system that combines relevant exam-style questions with online-style content review and interactive technology.

This format provides you with the best preparation for your exam!

- Build your experience and exam confidence!
- Practice with realistic exam-style questions, answers, and rationales.
- Enhance your review with state-of-the-art technology that offers more practice.

WHAT'S NEW TO THIS EDITION

- Online Learning Center
- Information section
- PowerPoint presentation of content
- Full body massage video

These materials will be available to students at www.myhealthprofessionskit.com.

ABOUT THIS BOOK

- **Content Review:** This book has been designed to help the student review massage therapy and bodywork together with a content review and 1,000 multiple-choice questions, organized by the topics covered on the NCETMB, NCETM and MBLEx exams. Working through these questions and studying the content review will help you assess your strengths and weaknesses in each topic of study. The Anatomy and Physiology and Massage and Bodywork review is presented in five parts, easy-to-follow chart and table formats including labeled figures.

Part 1: Concentrates on Medical Terminology, organization of the body and body systems; Integument, Skeletal, Muscle, Nerves, Cardiovascular, Lymphatic, Respiratory, Digestive, Endocrine, Urinary, and Reproductive System.

Part 2: Describes Pathology in general, Etiology, Disease risk factors, Stress-related and terminal illnesses with an explanation and examples of pathology of each system. This part also covers the Pharmacology of Analgesics, Medications, Herbs and Supplements.

Part 3: Discusses the History of Massage dating over 5000 years ago to the present Western contemporary massage. Massage and Bodywork Assessment is defined and covered in methods including visual palpation, energies assessment areas and somatic holding patterns. Important in this part is the outline of indications, benefits and contraindications of massage.

Part 4: Relates to the Bodywork Application of Therapeutic Massage which describes the seven strokes, joint movement, stretching, draping, lubricant applications, body mechanics and routine procedures. CPR and First Aid are defined with procedures including RICE. The application of Hydrotherapy and Aromatherapy discuss their importance and how they work and benefit massage. Finally, Western and Eastern Modalities are outlined defining the different strokes and pressure used.

Part 5: Includes the definitions and Code of Ethics of Massage and Bodywork. Important are the ethical and therapeutic relationships between the client and massage therapist. Standards of Practice and Professionalism emphasis client privacy, the HIPPA law, and Scope of Practice and discrimination. All legal parameters, tax information, insurance, business plan and records and types of employment relate the business aspect of massage therapy.

Part 6: Covers the Comprehensive simulated exams and answers of the NCTMB, NCTM, and MBLEx. These test questions are chosen from the questions previously given in the book.

Included are the appendices: A—State Massage Licensing Laws, B—Massage and Bodywork Organizations, Glossary, References and Index.

The questions, correct answers and rationales are included after each content part.

- **Practice Exams:** Three comprehensive simulated practice tests are included at the end of the book. The exams represent the percentage content contained in the NCETMB, NCETM, and MBLEx exams.

  These tests will give you a chance to experience the NCETMB, the NCETM or the MBLEx exam before you actually have to take it. Two hours and thirty or forty minutes are allowed for examination time.
- Materials will be available to students and instructors at www.myhealthprofessionskit. com. Online students will find, eight practice tests with an optimal timer and a glossary to help you learn definitions of key terms. Correct answers follow questions. You will receive immediate feedback to identify your strengths and weaknesses in each topic covered.

LICENSURE AND BOARD CERTIFICATION

The National Certification Board for Therapeutic Massage and Bodywork (NCBTMB) is a nationally recognized credentialing body formed to set standards for those who practice therapeutic massage and bodywork.

The NCBTMB developed and adopted the Standards of Practice to provide a clear statement of the expectations of professional conduct and level of practice in the following areas: Professionalism, Legal and Ethical Requirements, Confidentiality, Business Practices, Client Assessment and Treatment Plans and Anatomy, Physiology and Pathology.

The NCETM/NCETMB is a 160-question massage test created and overseen by the National Certification Board for Therapeutic Massage and Bodywork. The test questions are written and based upon a sample study done of massage practitioners every five years. This ensures that the questions stay up to date with current massage therapy laws and practices. The National Massage Certification Exam is used to measure the skills and knowledge acquired by the massage student in their approved massage school or course work. An approved school or course consists of at least 500 hours of didactic massage training. This includes 100 hours of in classroom training in anatomy and physiology, 200 hours of training on massage theory and application and 2 hours of massage ethics. The remainder of the required massage course hours are to be completed in related fields such as pathology, business practices and complimentary alternative medicine (CAM for the NCETMB).

The breakdown of the massage content on the NCETM and the NCETMB is as follows:

- Kinesiology and musculoskeletal anatomy and physiology 19–24%
- Systemic anatomy and physiology 13-18%
- Pathology, contraindications and cautionary sites 14–19%
- Professional standards 11–15%
- Massage therapy theory, evaluation and techniques 30–37%

*NCTMB ONLY—Basic modality literacy (other modalities)

To contact the Board of Certification for a *NCTMB Candidate Handbook*, please call or write to:

National Certification Board for Therapeutic Massage and Bodywork
1901 S. Meyers Road
Suite 240
Oakbrook Terrace, IL 60181
1-800-296-0664 or 630-627-8000
www.ncbtmb.com

LICENSING

The MBLEx (Massage and Bodywork Licensing Examination) is governed by the Federation of State Massage Therapy Boards (FSMTB). It is designed to provide a standard examination for students of Massage for entry-level professional scope of practice in gaining licensure.

The MBLEx exam has eight concentrated areas of content: Client Assessment and Treatment plans (17%), Benefits and Effects of Techniques (17%), Pathology (13%), Massage History (5%), Business Ethics (13%), Kinesiology (11%), Anatomy and Physiology (14%), and Guidelines for Professional Practice (10%).

To be qualified to take the MBLEx you must first find out if your state accepts this exam as part of your licensing requirements. To contact the FSMTB for a handbook:

Call or write to:
Federation of State Massage Therapy Board
7111 West 151 Street
Suite 356
Overland Park, KS 66223
866-962-3926
www.fsmtb.org/mblex

EDUCATION/TRAINING PROCESS

- Candidates must have graduated with at least 500 in-class hours of formal training at an accredited school of Massage and/or Bodywork.
- The formal training must be from a state-approved training institute.

- Proof of graduation from a formal training program in the form of an official school transcript and a notarized copy of the Diploma or Certificate of Completion.

ABOUT THE EXAM

The exam is given on an electronic testing system, EXPro, which does not use paper-and-pencil answer sheets. Instead, exam questions and options are displayed on a touch-sensitive screen. A computer memory card records the responses and automatically times the exam. EXPro lets users change their answers, skip questions, and mark questions for later review. The exam will be scored upon completion, so results are immediately available, as either "pass" or "fail."

The exam does not cover any specific method of massage and/or bodywork in depth. Instead, it covers the knowledge and skills that are common among all massage and/or bodywork disciplines. It also covers the basic approaches of Western and non-Western massage and/or bodywork.

STUDY TIPS

Review Materials Choose review materials that contain the information you need to study. Before the exam, the best study preparation would be to use this question-and-answer review to identify your strengths and weaknesses. The references will direct you to additional resources for more in-depth study.

Before attempting the questions, study the review part of the book. A thorough knowledge of anatomy and physiology is essential, particularly of the bones, muscles, blood vessels, and nerves. Many methods of therapeutic massage and bodywork are important and included, as well as prominent people who are associated with the methods. Review draping techniques and personal hygiene. Be familiar with the ailments, injuries, and diseases that can benefit from therapeutic massage and how to treat them along with any first aid needed. It is also necessary to have an understanding of ethical and business philosophies, history and modalities. A knowledge of the meridians and other bodywork is essential for the NCETMB and MBLEx.

We believe that you will find the questions, explanations, and format of the text to be of great assistance to you during your review. We wish you luck on the exam of your choice.

Take Practice Tests Practice as much as possible, using the questions in this book. These questions were designed to follow the format of questions that appear on the exam you will take, so the more you practice with these questions, the better prepared you will be on test day.

The simulated practice tests in the book and online at www.myhealthprofessionskit.com will give you a chance to experience the exam before you actually have to take it and will also let you know how you're doing and where you need to do better.

Practice under test-like conditions; that is, in a quiet room, with no books or notes to help you, and with a clock telling you when to stop. Try to come as close as you can to duplicating the actual test situation.

TAKING THE EXAMINATION

Prepare Physically When taking the exam, you need to work efficiently in the time allowed. If your body is tired or under stress, you might not think as clearly or perform as well as you usually do. If you can, avoid staying up all night. Get some sleep so that you can wake up rested and alert. The best advice is to eat a light, well-balanced meal before a test.

Materials Be sure to take photo ID all other required identification materials, registration forms, and any other items required by the testing organization or center. Read information and instructions supplied by the testing organizations thoroughly to be sure you have all necessary materials before the day of the exam.

Read Test Directions Read the exam directions thoroughly! Read each set of directions completely before starting a new section of questions.

Selecting the Right Answer Keep in mind that only one answer is correct. First read the stem of the question with *each* possible choice provided and eliminate choices that are obviously incorrect. Be cautious about choosing the first answer that *might* be correct; all possibilities should be considered before the final choice is made; the best answer should be selected.

If a question is complicated, try to break it down into small sections that are easy to understand.

Intelligent Guessing If you don't know the answer, eliminate those answers that you know or suspect are wrong. Pay attention to distracters, such as *always, never, all, none,* or *every*. Qualifiers make it easy to find an exception that makes a choice incorrect. Mark answers you aren't sure of and go back to them at the end of the test.

Chances are that you will leave your answers alone, but you may notice something that will make you change your mind—a qualifier that affects meaning or a remembered fact that will enable you to answer the question without guessing.

Watch the Clock Keep track of how much time is left and how you are progressing. Wear a watch or bring a small clock with you to the test room.

Some students are so concerned about time that they rush through the exam and have time left over. The best approach, however, is to take your time. Stay until the end so that you can check your answers.

KEYS TO SUCCESS!

- Study, review, and practice
- Keep a positive, confident attitude
- Follow all directions on the examination
- Do your best

Good luck!

Some of the study and test-taking tips were adapted from *Keys to Effective Learning*, 2nd edition, by Carol Carter, Joyce Bishop, and Sarah Lyman Kravits.

The following are the exams to qualify a massage therapist as nationally certified or licensed in participating states.

- National Licensing Examination for Therapeutic Massage and Bodywork (NCETMB)
- National Certification Examination for Therapeutic Massage (NCETM)
- Massage and Bodywork Licensing Examination (MBLEx)

	NCETMB License	NCETM License	MBLEx License
Question Content	Human anatomy, massage techniques, craniosacral, shiatsu—eastern medicine	Human anatomy, massage techniques (no eastern medicine)	Human anatomy, massage techniques, history, craniosacral, shiatsu—eastern medicine
Exam Fee	$185	$185	$195
Number of Questions	125 multiple choice	125 multiple choice	125 multiple choice
Test Time	2 h	2 h	2 h 30 min
Qualifications for the Exam	Graduate of an NCB-approved program with school code	Graduate of an NCB-approved program with school code	Verify education and training in the content subject areas
Application Time	3 weeks	3 weeks	3 weeks
Passing Grade	pass/fail	pass/fail	630
Contact Information	800-296-0664 www.ncbtmb.com	800-296-0664 www.ncbtmb.com	866-962-3926 www.fsmtb.org/mblex

Reviewers of the Fifth Edition

Lorena Haynes, BSEd, LMT
Westside Tech
Winter Garden, Florida

Karen M. Hobson, LMT, CMT, NCTM
Virginia College
Richmond, Virginia

Holly Huzar, LMT
Center for Natural Wellness School of Massage Therapy
Albany, New York

Tara McManaway, LMT
College of Southern Maryland
La Plata, Maryland

Lisa Mertz, PhD, LMT
Queensbororugh Community College
Bayside, New York

Karen A. Jackson, NCTMB, LMT
St. Louis College of Health Careers
St Louis, Missouri

Erika Monge MTP, LMT
Dade Medical College
Hialeah, Florida

Kenneth J. Nelan, RM/T, STL, MA, NCBTMB
Sacred Wandering Continuing Education
Tucson, Arizona

Jennifer O'Connell, LMT
Abaton Center of Healing Arts
Albuquerque, New Mexico

Kevin Pierce, MBA, NCBTMB
Anthem Education Group
Orlando, Florida

Margie Schaeffer
Synergy Massage
Blue Ridge Summit, Pennsylvania

Jean Wible, RN, BSN, NCTMB, LMT, HTCP
The Community College of Baltimore County
Baltimore, Maryland

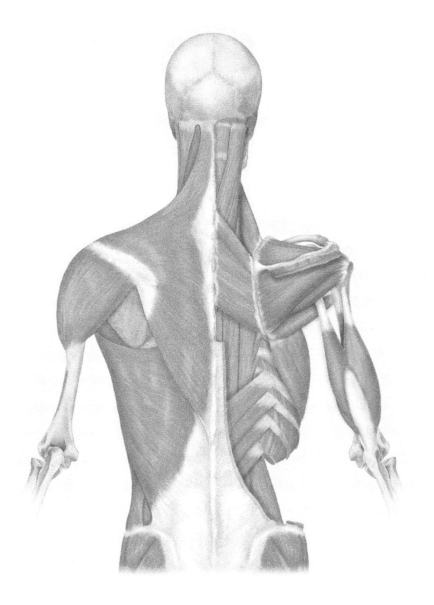

PART

1

Anatomy, Physiology, and Kinesiology

Part 1 contains medical terms, how the body is organized, Anatomy and Physiology, general and detail of each system, and 300 related questions, which is 25% MBLEx–35% NCTMB of the national exam content.

Medical Terminology

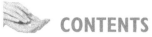

CONTENTS

DEFINITIONS	
Prefix	At the beginning of the word to alter or modify meaning
Word Root	Word or word element from which other words are formed
Suffix	At the end of a word to alter or modify meaning

GENERAL PREFIXES	
Prefix	**Meaning**
a, an-	without, lack of
ad-	toward
anti, contra-	against
auto-	self
bi-	two
brachy-	short
brady-	slow
cac-, mal-	bad
cardio-	heart
circum-	around
dia-	through
dys-	bad, difficult
epi-	on, up, against, high
eu-	good, normal
hemi-	half
hetero-	different
homeo-	similar, same
hydro-	water

Prefix	Meaning
hyper-	above, excessive
hypo-	below, deficient
infra-	below, underneath
intra-	within, inside, during
macro-	large, great
meta-	between
micro-	small
multi-	many
myo-	muscle
oligo-	scanty, little, few
osteo-	bone
pan-	all
pre-	before
pseudo-	false
supra-	above
sym-, syn-	together
tachy-	rapid
trans-	across
ultra-	beyond

GENERAL SUFFIXES

Suffix	Meaning	Suffix	Meaning
-algia	pain	-pathy	disease
-blast	immature or germ cell	-plasia	formation, to produce
-cyte	cell	-philia	attraction
-derma	skin	-physis	growth
-emia	blood condition	-plasty	surgical repair
-globin	protein	-pnea	breathing
-ist	one who specializes	-poiesis	formation
-itis	inflammation	-therapy	treatment
-logy	study of	-thorax	chest
-oma	tumor	-trophy	nourishment, development
-osis	abnormal condition	-uria	urine condition

COMBINING FORMS

Combining Form	Meaning	Combining Form	Meaning
acr/o	extremities	oste/o	bone
agglutin/o	clumping	path/o	disease
alveol/o	alveolus; air sac	pharmac/o	drug
anter/o	front	phleb/o	vein
arteri/o	artery	pneum/o	lung, air
articul/o	joint	pod/o	foot
blast/o	primitive cell	poster/o	back
bronchi/o	bronchiole	prosth/o	addition
bucc/o	cheek	proxim/o	near to
carcin/o	cancer	pulmon/o	lung
cardi/o	heart	ren/o	kidney
carp/o	wrist	seb/o	oil
caud/o	tail	somat/o	body
cervic/o	neck, cervix	stern/o	sternum
chondr/o	cartilage	super/o	above
coron/o	heart	synov/o	synovial membrane
cost/o	rib	tars/o	ankle
crani/o	skull	tend/o	tendon
cry/o	cold	therm/o	heat
cyt/o	cell	thorac/o	chest
dermat/o	skin	tox/o	poison
neur/o	nerve	varic/o	varicose veins
onc/o	tumor	vertebr/o	vertebra

MEDICAL TERMS

Term	Definition
abscess	A localized collection of pus, which may occur in any part of the body
active range of motion (AROM)	Patient performs own joint movement
acute	Sudden, sharp, severe; referring to a disease that has a sudden onset, severe symptoms, and a short course
adhesion	The process of being stuck together
afferent	Carrying impulses toward a center
allergy	Hypersensitive to a substance or medication
ambulatory	The condition of being able to walk, not confined to bed
antidote	A substance given to counteract a poison and its effects
anoxia	Lack of oxygen
antiseptic	Pertaining to an agent that works to kill bacteria at wound
aseptic	Without decay; sterile, free from all living microorganisms
atrophy	Lack or loss of normal development; muscle atrophy
autonomy	The condition of being self-governed; to function independently
axillary	Pertaining to the armpit
benign	Not cancerous
biopsy	Surgical removal of a small piece of tissue for microscopic examination; used to determine a diagnosis of cancer of other disease process in the body
cachexia	A condition of general ill health, malnutrition, and wasting
carcinogen	Substance that produces cancer
centigrade	Having 100 steps or degrees, like the Celsius temperature scale where boiling point is at 100°C and freezing point at 0°C
centrifuge	A device used in a laboratory to separate solids from liquids
chronic	Pertaining to time; a disease that continues over a long time, showing little change in symptoms or course
cryotherapy	Using cold for therapy
diagnosis	Determination of the cause and nature of a disease
disinfectant	A chemical substance that destroys bacteria
efferent	Carrying impulses away from a center
etiology	The study of the cause(s) of disease
excision	The process of cutting out; surgical removal
febrile	Pertaining to fever
gait	Manner of walking

(continued)

MEDICAL TERMS (continued)	
Term	**Definition**
homeostasis	Steady state of balance within the body
incision	The process of cutting into
kilogram	Unit of weight in the metric system; 1000 g (roughly equal to 2.2 pounds)
laser	Use of controlled beam of light as heat
liter	A unit of volume in the metric system, equal to 33.8 fluid ounces or 1.0567 quarts
malaise	A bad feeling; a condition of discomfort, uneasiness; often felt by a patient with a chronic disease
malformation	The process of being badly shaped, deformed
metastasis	Pertaining to the spreading process of cancer from one area of the body to another
microgram	A unit of weight in the metric system; 0.001 mg
microorganism	Small living organism that is not visible to the naked eye
milligram	A unit of weight in the metric system; 0.001 g
milliliter	A unit of volume in the metric system; 0.001 L
necrosis	A condition of death of tissue
neopathy	A new disease
oncology	Dealing with tumors
pallor	Paleness, a lack of color
pathology	Study of disease
prognosis	A condition of foreknowledge; the prediction of the course of a disease and the recovery rate
prophylactic	Pertaining to preventing or protecting against disease
pyrogenic	Pertaining to the production of heat or fever
spasm	Involuntary muscle contraction
syndrome	A combination of signs and symptoms occurring together that characterize a specific disease
toxicity	Extent of being poisonous
triage	The sorting and classifying of injuries to determine priority of need and treatment
visceral	Pertaining to internal organs
x-ray	High energy wave to produce an image on photo film

2 Organization of Body, Definitions, and Cytology

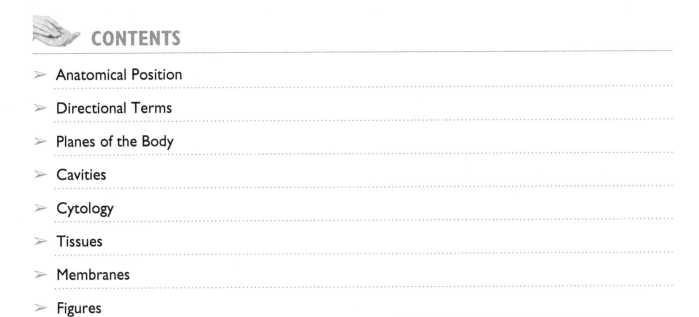 CONTENTS

ORGANIZATION OF BODY, DEFINITIONS, AND CYTOLOGY	
Anatomical Position	Body standing erect, face forward, palms forward
Directional Terms	***Anterior/Ventral***—Toward *front* of body
	Coronal/Frontal—Lengthwise plane dividing body into anterior and posterior
	Distal—*Away* from trunk or point of origin
	Inferior/Caudal—Toward sacrum; in lower position
	Lateral—Toward *side* of body, away from midline of body
	Medial—Toward *midline* of body
	Posterior/Dorsal—Toward *back* of body
	Proximal—Toward the *trunk*
	Superior/Cranial—Toward the *head* of body
Planes of the Body	***Coronal/Frontal***—Divides body into anterior and posterior halves
	Transverse—Divides body into superior and inferior
	Midsagittal—Divides body into left and right halves
	Sagittal—Divides body into left and right sections
Cavities	***Dorsal (posterior)***—Cranial (brain) and vertebral (spinal cord) cavities
	Ventral (anterior)—Thoracic above diaphragm (heart and lungs)
	Abdominopelvic—below (digestive, excretory, reproductive organs)
Cytology	***Cell membrane***—A phospholipid bilayer that is selectively permeable to wastes, gases, and salts
	Cytoplasm—Semifluid substance that contains organelles of specific function
	Mitochondria—"Powerhouse of cell" produces cell energy ATP by the aerobic respiration of O_2 + glucose
	Nucleus—Contains the genetic material dioxyribonucleic acid (DNA) in the 23 pairs of chromosomes, 22 pair autosomes, sex chromosome XX female, XY male
	Ribosomes—Assembles proteins along the rough ER
	Golgi apparatus—Transports, packages, and stores proteins and lipids to plasma membrane for secretion
	Cilia—Extension of cell membrane to aid in movement, mucus, fluids
	Endoplasmic reticulum (ER)—Tubules that collect proteins manufactured on ribosomes for use in or out of cell, rough ER and smooth ER, no ribosomes

	Lysosomes—Digest foreign material within cell by digestive enzymes
	Mitosis—Cell division into two identical cells
	Meiosis—Produces egg and sperm cells
	Transport and Movement:
	Diffusion—Movement of a substance from higher to lower concentration
	Osmosis—Diffusion of water through semipermeable membrane
	Active transport—Energy required transport in or out of cell
	Phagocytosis—Solids ingulfed by cell membrane
	Pinocytosis—Fluids engulfed by cell membrane
Tissues	Made up of cells that are similar in structure and function: epithelial, connective, muscle, nervous
	Epithelial tissue—Tissues that line and cover body surfaces and cavities and undergo rapid mitosis to replace and repair old or injured epithelial cells, types include squamous, cuboidal
	Connective tissue—Tissue that binds and holds other tissue:
	Adipose—Fat
	Reticular—Loose
	Tendon—Connects muscle to bone
	Ligament—Connects bone to bone
	Fascia—Lining of muscle, vessels, nerves
	Bone—Hard structure osteocytes and salts
	Cartilage—Elastic connective tissue, i.e., ears, nose, joints
	Blood—Liquid, blood cells, and plasma
	Muscle tissue—Tissue responsible for movement:
	Skeletal—Voluntary; attached to bone for body movement
	Smooth—Involuntary; contraction of blood vessels, intestines, diaphragm, and uterus
	Cardiac—Involuntary; contraction of heart to pump blood
	Nervous tissue—Controls all body functions by nerve impulses consisting of nerve cells and myelin sheath
Membranes	***Mucous***—Secrete mucus, line cavities of respiratory and digestive systems to protect and lubricate
	Serous—Secrete serous fluid, a lubricant that covers internal organs in thoracic, abdominal, and pelvic cavities
	Synovial—Membranes inside of joints; secrete synovial fluid, which is a lubricant for mobility of joints
	Fascial—Fibrous connective tissue that connects skin to muscles and underlying structures

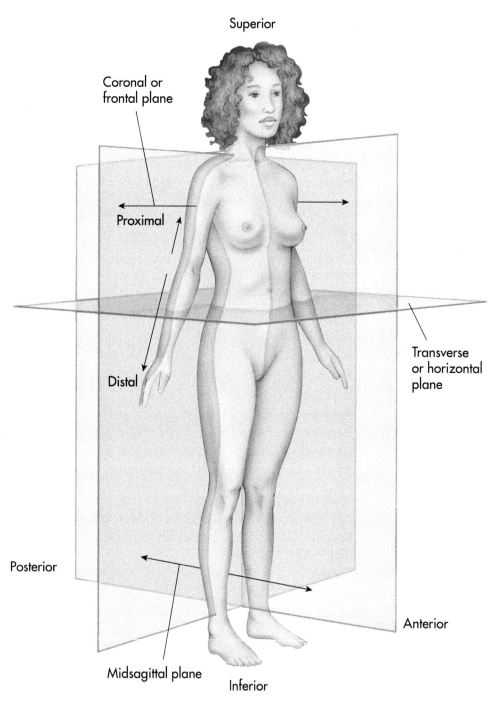

FIGURE 2-1
Body Planes.

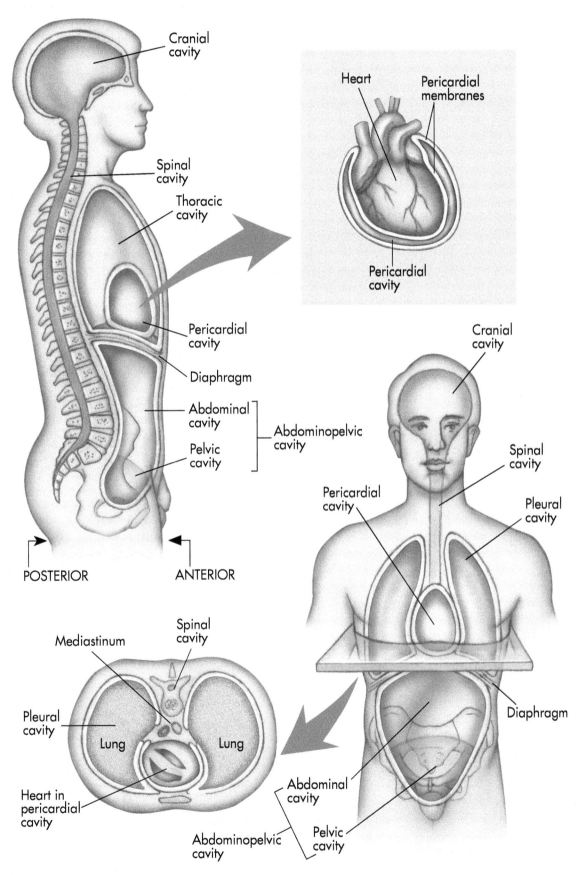

FIGURE 2-2
Body Cavities.

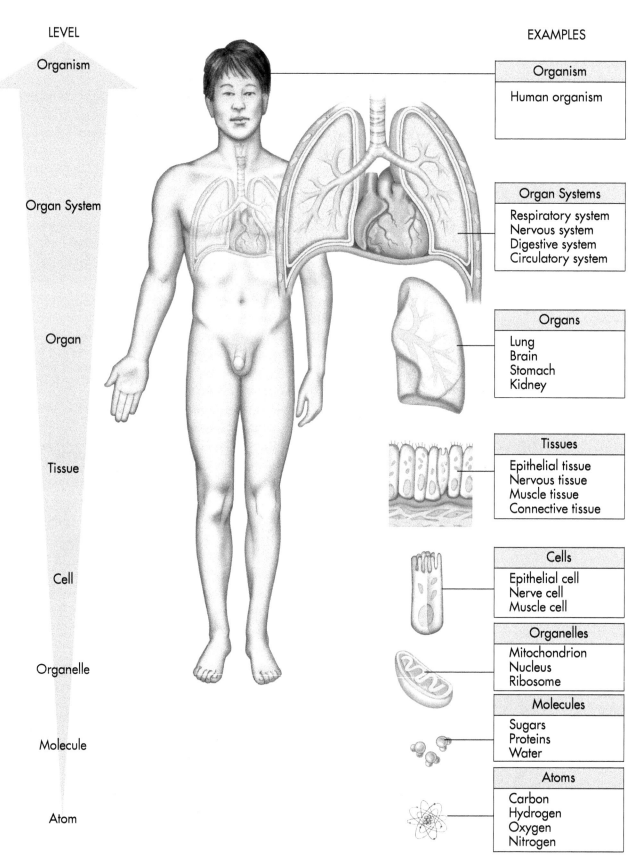

FIGURE 2-3
Levels of Organization.

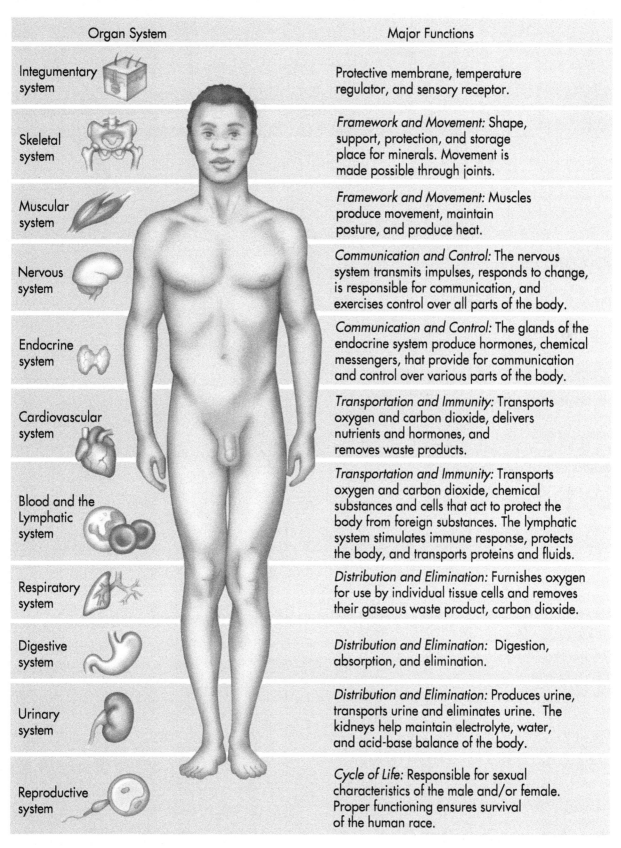

Organ System	Major Functions
Integumentary system	Protective membrane, temperature regulator, and sensory receptor.
Skeletal system	*Framework and Movement:* Shape, support, protection, and storage place for minerals. Movement is made possible through joints.
Muscular system	*Framework and Movement:* Muscles produce movement, maintain posture, and produce heat.
Nervous system	*Communication and Control:* The nervous system transmits impulses, responds to change, is responsible for communication, and exercises control over all parts of the body.
Endocrine system	*Communication and Control:* The glands of the endocrine system produce hormones, chemical messengers, that provide for communication and control over various parts of the body.
Cardiovascular system	*Transportation and Immunity:* Transports oxygen and carbon dioxide, delivers nutrients and hormones, and removes waste products.
Blood and the Lymphatic system	*Transportation and Immunity:* Transports oxygen and carbon dioxide, chemical substances and cells that act to protect the body from foreign substances. The lymphatic system stimulates immune response, protects the body, and transports proteins and fluids.
Respiratory system	*Distribution and Elimination:* Furnishes oxygen for use by individual tissue cells and removes their gaseous waste product, carbon dioxide.
Digestive system	*Distribution and Elimination:* Digestion, absorption, and elimination.
Urinary system	*Distribution and Elimination:* Produces urine, transports urine and eliminates urine. The kidneys help maintain electrolyte, water, and acid-base balance of the body.
Reproductive system	*Cycle of Life:* Responsible for sexual characteristics of the male and/or female. Proper functioning ensures survival of the human race.

FIGURE 2-4
Organ Systems and Function.

3 Integumentary System

 CONTENTS

INTEGUMENTARY SYSTEM	
Skin	An organ that: • Protects internal structures • Regulates body temperature • Sense of touch • Excretes salt, water, oils • Synthesizes vitamin D
Epidermis	Superficial layer that contains: ***Stratum corneum***—Cells that shed, outermost layer ***Stratum lucidum***—Cells located on hands and feet ***Stratum granulosum***—Produces keratin for waterproofing ***Stratum germinativum***—Divides cells
Dermis	Below epidermis; contains connective tissue, glands, blood vessels, nerve endings, muscle, hair follicles ***Arrector pili***—Muscle at hair root, produces "goosebumps" ***Blood vessels***—Regulate body temperature, fill with blood to heat skin, and transport blood to hair follicle ***Nerve ending***—Sensory receptor for pressure, temperature, and pain ***Cells***—Fibroblasts produce fibrin for clotting, macrophage for immune system ***Hair follicle***—Contains shaft, root, and bulb ***Glands***—Sebaceous oil glands connect to hair follicle; sudoriferous sweat glands located especially in palms and soles called eccrine glands
Subcutaneous Hypodermis	• Superficial fascia • Composed of adipose tissue
Nails	• Appendage to integument • Hardened layer of the stratum corneum found at ends of fingers and toes
Benefits of Massage to Skin	• Improves circulation • Stimulates sweat and oil glands • Stimulates sensation of touch (especially for infants and elders)

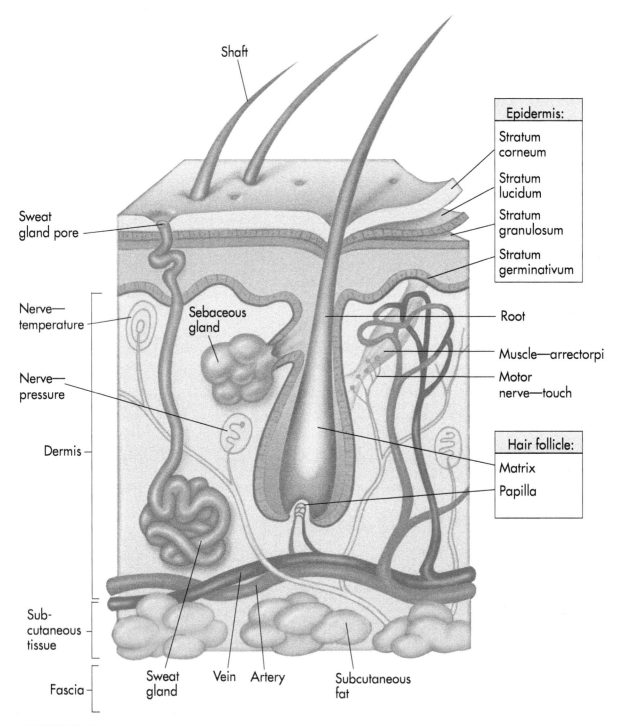

FIGURE 3-1
The Integument and Appendages.

4   Skeletal System

CONTENTS

SKELETAL SYSTEM	
Function	• **Support, protection, body framework** • **Red blood cell production** • **Calcium storage** • **Levers for muscles**
Cells	*Osteocytes*—Cells that maintain bone and produce collagen *Osteoblasts*—Cells that form bone *Osteoclasts*—Cells that break down bone
Bone Anatomy	*Diaphysis*—Shaft of long bone *Epiphysis*—End of long bone *Articular cartilage*—Surface of epiphysis for cushioning *Periosteum*—Covers bone where ligaments and tendons attach *Medullary canal*—Bone marrow canal *Spongy bone*—Porous bone containing red marrow *Compact bone*—Bone cells embedded in collagen calcified material
Bone Types, Shapes	Long, short, flat, irregular, sesamoid

Skeletal Divisions	*Axial*
	
	    Skull 22 bones
	
	    Hyoid Supports tongue
	
	    Ribs 12 pairs, 7 true, 3 false, 2 floating
	
	    Sternum Manubrium, body, xiphoid process
	
	    Vertebrae 7 cervical, #1 atlas, #2 axis, C1–C7
	
	                    12 thoracic, T1–T12
	
	                    5 lumbar, L1–L5
	
	                    1 sacral, (S1–S5)
	
	                    4 coccyx
	
	Appendicular—Pectoral girdle, clavicle, scapula with articulation at the acromioclavicular and sternoclavicular
	
	Upper limb—Humerus, radius, ulnar, carpals, metacarpals, phalanges
	
	Pelvic girdle—Ilium, ischium, pubis, and coxal bones
	
	Lower limbs—Femur, fibula, tibia, patella, tarsals, metatarsals, phalanges

Bony Landmarks	**Head**
	Zygomatic bone
	Mastoid process
	Shoulder
	Clavicle
	Sternal notch
	Sternum
	Chest
	Xiphoid process
	Ribs
	Arms
	Lateral epicondyle of humerus
	Medial epicondyle of humerus
	Head of radius
	Olecranon process of ulna
	Posterior border of ulna
	Styloid process of ulna
	Styloid process of radius
	Metacarpal heads
	Pisiform
	Back
	Spine of scapula
	Acromion process of scapula
	Vertebral border of scapula
	Inferior angle of scapula
	Axillary border of scapula
	Pelvic Girdle
	Iliac crest
	Sacrum
	Coccyx
	Ischial tuberosity
	Anterior superior iliac spine
	Posterior superior iliac spine
	Pubic symphysis

(*continued*)

SKELETAL SYSTEM *(continued)*	
	Leg
	Greater trochanter of femur
	Medial epicondyle of femur
	Lateral epicondyle of femur
	Patella
	Head of fibula
	Tuberosity of tibia
	Anterior shaft of tibia
	Medial malleolus of tibia
	Lateral malleolus of fibula
	Calcaneus of tarsal
Terminology	***Depressions and openings***—Hollow or depressed areas
	Foramen—Rounded hole in bone
	Fossa—Shallow depression in bone
	Groove—Furrow in bone
	Sinus—Cavity in bone
	Meatus—Canal in bone
	Processes—Bumps found on the surfaces of bones
	Tubercle—Small, round bump
	Tuberosity—Large, rough bump
	Spine—A sharp bump
	Condyle—Rounded bump
	Crest—Ridge
	Epicondyle—A bump above a condyle
Ligaments and Joint Structure and Function	• Ligaments are dense fibrous connective tissue high in elastin holding bone to bone
	• Ligaments maintain joint space
	• Joints contain synovial membrane secreting fluid for lubrication
	• Joints have a hard or soft end feel at limit of range of motion (ROM)
Joint Classification	**Synarthrotic** (fibrous)—Immovable joints found at epiphyseal plates and sutures
	Amphiarthrotic (cartilaginous)—Slightly movable joints found at pubic symphysis and intervertebral discs
	Diarthrotic (synovial)—Freely movable joints that possess a joint cavity of ligaments, synovial membrane, and fluid

Diarthrotic Joints	*Hinge joint*—Movement in one direction (elbow, knee)
	Gliding joint—Side-to-side movement (spine)
	Saddle joint—Movement in two planes (thumb carpometacarpal)
	Ball-and-socket joints—Movement of round convex surface in socket, in all planes (hip and shoulder)
	Pivot joint—Rotation (atlas on axis)
	Ellipsoidal joint—Convex on concave articulation, movement in two planes (base of phalanges)
Benefits of Massage on the Skeletal System	• Improve ROM of joints • Improve flexibility of joints through stretching ligaments • Improve curvature of spine by relaxing muscles

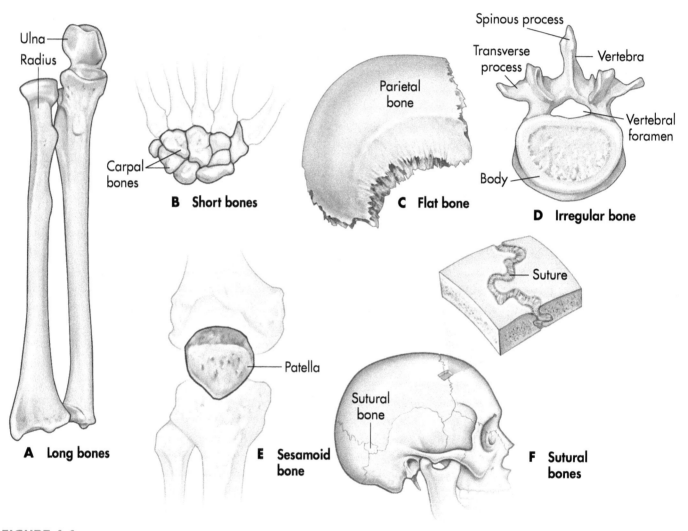

FIGURE 4-1

Classification of Bones by Shape.

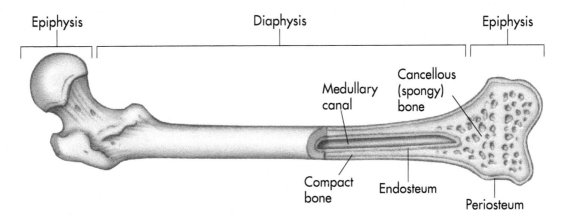

FIGURE 4-2
Typical Bone Structure.

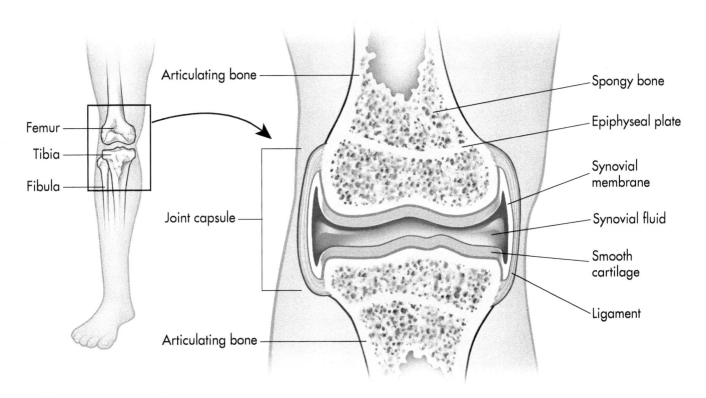

FIGURE 4-3
Typical Joint.

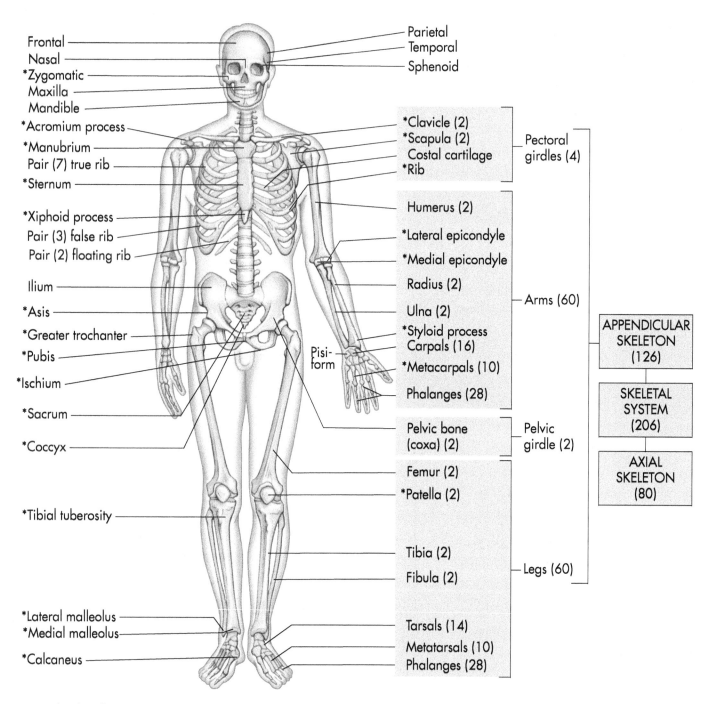

Frontal
Nasal
*Zygomatic
Maxilla
Mandible
*Acromium process
*Manubrium
Pair (7) true rib
*Sternum
*Xiphoid process
Pair (3) false rib
Pair (2) floating rib
Ilium
*Asis
*Greater trochanter
*Pubis
*Ischium
*Sacrum
*Coccyx
*Tibial tuberosity
*Lateral malleolus
*Medial malleolus
*Calcaneus

Parietal
Temporal
Sphenoid

*Clavicle (2)
*Scapula (2)
Costal cartilage
*Rib

Pectoral
girdles (4)

Humerus (2)
*Lateral epicondyle
*Medial epicondyle
Radius (2)
Ulna (2)
*Styloid process
Carpals (16)
*Metacarpals (10)
Phalanges (28)

Arms (60)

Pisi-
form

Pelvic bone
(coxa) (2)

Pelvic
girdle (2)

Femur (2)
*Patella (2)

Tibia (2)
Fibula (2)

Legs (60)

Tarsals (14)
Metatarsals (10)
Phalanges (28)

APPENDICULAR
SKELETON
(126)

SKELETAL
SYSTEM
(206)

AXIAL
SKELETON
(80)

*Bony landmarks

FIGURE 4-4
Principle Bones.

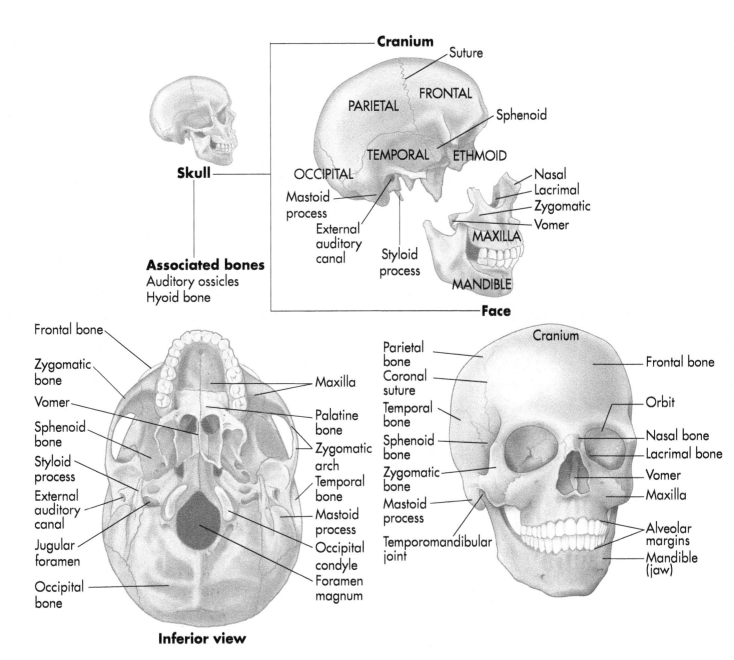

FIGURE 4-5
Bones of the Skull.

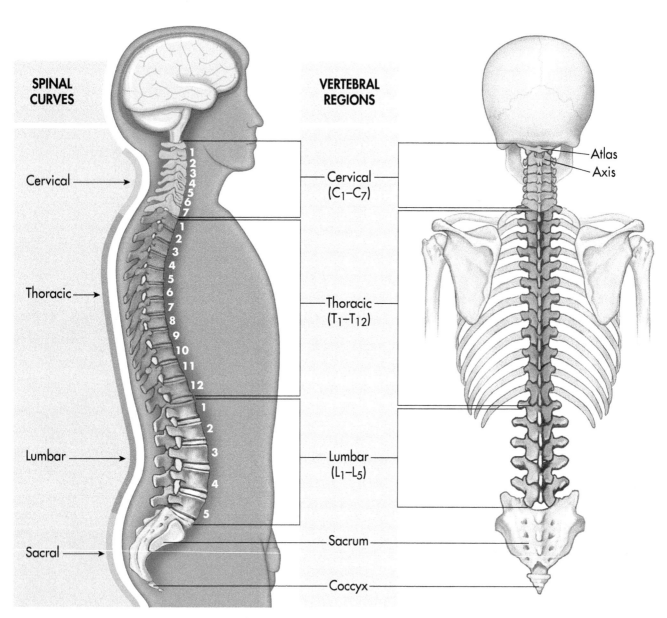

FIGURE 4-6
Vertebral Regions.

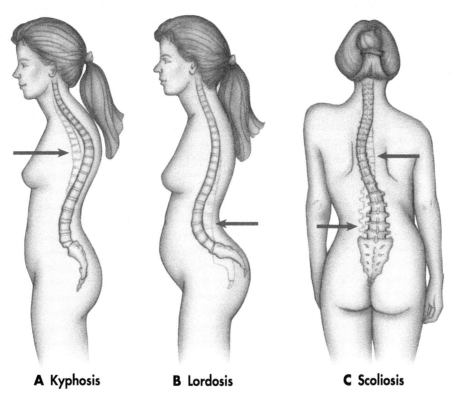

A Kyphosis   **B** Lordosis   **C** Scoliosis

FIGURE 4-7
Abnormal Curvature of the Spine.

CONTENTS

MUSCULAR SYSTEM	
Function	• **Body movement** • **Posture and support** • **Heat generation**
Muscle Anatomy	*Motor unit*—Contractile unit made up of sarcomeres and a neuron that innervates it *Actin protein*—Thin filaments of motor unit *Myosin protein*—Thick filaments of motor unit with heads for movement *Sarcolemma*—Membrane around muscle *Epimycium*—Muscle fibers connective tissue neuromuscular junction where nerve synapse meets muscle fibril
Muscle Attachments	*Tendon*—Dense, fibrous connective that connects muscle to bone, high concentration of collagen *Origin*—Attachment to more stationary bone of action *Insertion*—Attachment to more movable bone of action *Aponeurosis*—Sheet of connective tissue *Superficial connective tissue*—Areola below the skin attached to muscle
Characteristics of Muscle	• Ability to stretch (extensibility) • Return to resting position (elasticity) • Transmission of stimuli (conductivity) • Response to stimuli (excitability) • Ability to shorten (contractibility)
Muscle Types	*Skeletal*—Attach to bone for movement, voluntary (over 600 muscles) *Smooth*—Blood vessels, stomach, intestine, bladder, involuntary *Cardiac*—Heart, involuntary
Muscle Movement	*Agonist*—The primary muscle of the contraction *Synergist*—The muscle that helps the primary *Antagonist*—The muscle that works against the primary muscle *All-or-none law*—The entire muscle fiber contraction, no partial

(*continued*)

MUSCULAR SYSTEM (*continued*)	
Contraction of Skeletal Muscle	A motor unit consists of muscle fibers (cells) innervated by a branch from an axon
	Impulses received by brain/spinal cord → stimulate motor unit → release acetylcholine → stimulates muscle fiber to release calcium → causes actin and myocin to bind in presence of Adenosine Triphosphate (ATP) → contraction
Action Potential	Motor unit responds to nerve stimulation at neuromuscular junction during *latent period;* followed by release of neurotransmitter and Na^+ ions entering, resulting in muscle contracting, *contracting period;* and ending in muscle relaxation and breakdown of neurotransmitter acetylcholine, *relaxation period*
Benefits of Massage on the Muscular System	• Relaxes muscle • Improves muscle tone and elasticity • Improves rehabilitation of muscle injury and function • Relieves muscle spasms, pain, and soreness • Releases metabolic waste • Stimulates circulation • Improves athletic performance • Relieves trigger point activity

KINESIOLOGY MUSCLE MOVEMENT	
Types of Muscle Contractions	***Muscle twitch***—Single muscle contraction in motor unit
	Isometric—Contraction without changing length (push against wall)
	Isotonic—Contraction with change of length (concentric; brings origin/insertion of muscle together against pressure)
	Spasm—Involuntary contraction
	Tetanus—Sustained contraction
	Contracture—Inability of muscle to relax after contraction
	Treppe—Repeated stimulation

Joint Movements	***Abduction***—Moving body part away from midline ***Adduction***—Moving body part toward midline ***Circumduction***—Rotation of extremity from shoulder to hand ***Flexion***—Bending movement, decreasing angle ***Extension***—Straightening movement, increasing angle ***Lateral flexion***—Side bending, ear to shoulder ***Plantar flexion***—Pointing foot to floor ***Dorsiflexion***—Pointing toes to ceiling ***Pronation***—Palms turned down ***Supination***—Palms turned up ***Inversion***—Soles of feet face each other ***Eversion***—Soles of feet face laterally ***Protraction***—Moving shoulder forward ***Retraction***—Moving shoulder backward ***Elevation***—Lifting shoulder upward ***Depression***—Moving shoulder downward
Muscles that Move the Head	***Flexors***—Bring the chin to the chest; antagonists to the extensors Sternocleidomastoid Scalenes ***Extensors***—Bring the head backward; antagonists to the flexors Splenius capitis Splenius cervicis ***Rotation of head***—To same side Splenius capitis Sternocleidomastoid Scalenes (unilaterally) ***Lateral flexion***—Bring ear toward shoulder; unilateral Sternocleidomastoid Scalenes Splenius capitis ***Mandible protraction*** Masseter ***Mandible retraction*** Temporalis

(*continued*)

KINESIOLOGY MUSCLE MOVEMENT (*continued*)	
Muscles that Move the Scapula	**Upward rotators**—Raise humerus; antagonists to downward rotators Upper trapezius Lower trapezius Serratus anterior **Downward rotators**—Drop humerus; antagonists to upward rotators Levator scapulae Rhomboids Pectoralis minor **Abductors**—Move scapulas together Serratus anterior Pectoralis minor **Elevators**—Raise shoulders; antagonists to depressors Upper trapezius Levator scapulae **Depressors**—Drop shoulders; antagonists to elevators Pectoralis minor Trapezius, lower portion **Protractors**—Roll shoulders forward; antagonists to elevators Serratus anterior Pectoralis minor **Retractors**—Roll shoulders back; antagonists to protractors Middle trapezius Rhomboids
Muscles that Move the Humerus	**Flexors**—Raise the arm overhead; antagonists to extensors Anterior deltoid Pectoralis major Coracobrachialis Biceps (short head) **Extensors**—Straighten the arm; antagonists to flexors Latissimus dorsi Teres major Posterior deltoid Infraspinatus Teres minor Triceps Pectoralis major **Adductors**—Bring the arm toward the body; antagonists to abductors Pectoralis major Coracobrachialis Latissimus dorsi Teres major

	Rotator Cuff
	  S—Supraspinatus
	  I—Infraspinatus
	  T—Teres minor
	  S—Subscapularis
	
	Abductors—Move arm away from the body; antagonists to adductors
	  Supraspinatus
	  Middle deltoid
	
	Internal (medial) rotators—Roll the head of the humerus forward; antagonists to external rotators
	  Anterior deltoid
	  Pectoralis major
	  Subscapularis
	  Teres major
	  Latissimus dorsi
	
	External (lateral) rotators—Roll the head of the humerus back; antagonists to internal rotators
	  Infraspinatus
	  Teres minor
	  Posterior deltoid

Muscles that Move the Elbow	***Flexors***—Bring forearm toward upper arm; antagonists to extensors
	  Brachialis
	  Biceps
	  Brachioradialis
	  Pronator teres
	
	Extensors—Straighten elbow; antagonists to flexors
	  Triceps
	  Anconeus

Muscles that Move the Forearm	***Supinators***—Turn palms up; antagonists to pronators
	  Biceps
	  Supinator
	
	Pronators—Turn palms down; antagonists to supinators
	  Pronator teres
	  Pronator quadratus

Muscles that Move the Wrist	***Flexors***—Move fingers toward palm; antagonists to extensors
	  Flexor carpi radialis
	  Flexor carpi ulnaris
	  Palmaris longus
	
	Extensors—Move fingers away from palm; antagonists to flexors
	  Extensor carpi radialis longus
	  Extensor carpi radialis brevis
	  Extensor carpi ulnaris

(*continued*)

KINESIOLOGY MUSCLE MOVEMENT (*continued*)	

	Adductors—Move hand toward the body; antagonists to abductors
	     Extensors carpi ulnaris
	     Flexor carpi ulnaris
	
	 Abductors—Move hand away from the body; antagonists to adductors
	     Flexor carpi radialis
	     Extensor carpi radialis longus

Muscles that Move the Fingers	**Flexors**—Move fingers toward palm; antagonists to extensors
	     Flexor digitorum superficialis/profundus
	     Flexor pollicis longus (flexes thumb)
	
	 Extensors—Straighten the hand; antagonists to flexors
	     Extensor digitorum
	     Extensor digiti minimi
	     Extensor pollicis longus/brevis

Muscles that Move the Ribs	**Elevators**—Raise the ribs during inspiration; antagonists to depressors
	     External intercostals
	     Scalenes (forced inspiration)
	     Sternocleidomastoid (SCM)
	     Pectoralis minor (accessory respiratory muscle)
	     Quadratus lumborum
	
	 Depressors—Lower the ribs during expiration; antagonists to elevators
	     Internal intercostals
	     Rectus abdominus
	     Quadratus lumborum

Muscles that Move the Trunk	**Flexors**—Make the body bend forward; antagonists to extensors
	     Rectus abdominis
	     External oblique
	     Internal oblique
	
	 Extensors—Make the trunk stay upright; antagonists to flexors
	     Erector spinae (transversospinalis)
	
	 Rotation of trunk—To opposite side
	     External oblique
	     Transversospinalis
	     Internal oblique
	
	 Lateral flexion—Side bending
	     External oblique (unilaterally)
	     Internal oblique (unilaterally)
	     Quadratus lumborum

Muscles that Move the Femur	**Hip flexors**—Bring the femur upward; antagonists to extensors
	     Iliopsoas (psoas)
	     Pectineus
	     Tensor fasciae latae
	     Adductors (brevis, longus, magnus)

	Rectus femoris
	Sartorius
	Hip extensors—Bring the femur back to neutral; antagonists to flexors
	Gluteus maximus
	Hamstrings (semimembranosus, semitendenosus, biceps femoris)
	Abductors—Lift leg away from the midline; antagonists to adductors
	Gluteus medius
	Gluteus minimus
	Tensor fasciae latae
	Sartorius
	Adductors—Bring leg toward the midline; antagonists to abductors
	Adductors (brevis, longus, magnus)
	Gracilis
	Pectineus
	External (lateral) rotators—Antagonists to internal rotators
	Piriformis
	Gluteus maximus
	Iliopsoas
	Sartorius
	Internal (medial) rotators—Antagonists to external rotators
	Gluteus medius
	Gluteus minimus
	Tensor fasciae latae
	Pectineus
	Adductors (brevis, longus, magnus)
Muscles that Move the Knee	***Flexors***—Bend the knee; antagonists to extensors
	Hamstrings (semimembranosus, semitendenosus, biceps femoris)
	Sartorius
	Gracilis
	Gastrocnemius
	Plantaris
	Popliteus
	Extensors—Straighten the knee; antagonists to flexors
	Quadriceps (rectus femoris, vastus lateralis, medius and intermedialis)
	Tensor fascia latae
Muscles that Move the Ankle	***Dorsiflexors***—Bring toes toward the leg; antagonists to plantarflexors
	Tibialis anterior
	Extensor digitorum longus
	Extensor hallucis longus
	Peroneus

(*continued*)

KINESIOLOGY MUSCLE MOVEMENT (continued)	
	Plantarflexors—Toes away from the leg; antagonists to dorsiflexors
	Soleus
	Gastrocnemius
	Plantaris
	Peroneus longus and brevis
	Tibialis posterior
	Flexor hallucis longus
	Flexor digitorum longus
	Invertors—Antagonists to evertors
	Tibialis anterior
	Tibialis posterior
	Evertors—Antagonists to invertors
	Peroneus longus
	Peroneus brevis
	Peroneus tertius
Muscles that Move the Toes	***Flexors***—Point the toes toward the floor; antagonists to extensors
	Flexor digitorum longus
	Flexor hallucis
	Extensors—Bring the toes toward the body; antagonists to flexors
	Extensor digitorum longus
	Extensor hallucis longus

ORIGIN AND INSERTION OF SELECTED MUSCLES				
	Muscle	**Origin**	**Insertion**	**Action**
Face, Head, and Neck	Frontalis	Orbicularis oculi	Epicranial aponeurosis	Raise eyebrow
	Orbicularis oculi	Bones medial to eye	Eyelid	Close eyes
	Orbicularis oris	Oral fascia	Lips	Close lips
	Buccinator	Maxilla and mandible	Mouth	Cheek movement
	Zygomaticus	Zygomatic bone	Corner of mouth	Elevates corner of mouth
	Masseter	Zygomatic arch	Ramus of mandible	Elevates mandible
	Temporalis	Temporal fossa	Coronoid process	Elevates and retracts mandible
	Platysma	Fascia	Mandible	Depresses lower jaw
	Sternocleido-mastoid	Manubrium	Mastoid process	Neck flexion

	Scalenes (anterior middle posterior)	Transverse process of C-vertebrae	1st and 2nd rib	Raise ribs 1 and 2, neck flexion
Chest and Trunk	Pectoralis major	Clavicle, sternum, ribs 1–6	Bicipital groove of humerus	Rotation of humerus, adduction
	Pectoralis minor	Ribs 3–5	Coracoid process	Rotation, depression of scapula
	Serratus anterior	Ribs 1–8	Vertebral border scapula	Up rotation/protraction
	Subscapularis SITS	Surface of scapula	Tubercle of humerus	Medial rotation humerus, adduction
	Rectus abdominis	Pubic spine	Costal cartilages for ribs 5, 6, and 7	Trunk (spine) flexion
	External oblique	Lower eight ribs 5–12	Abdominal aponeurosis and anterior iliac crest	*Bilaterally:* Trunk flexion *Unilaterally:* Lateral flexion, trunk rotation
	Internal oblique	Inguinal ligament and anterior iliac crest	Costal cartilages of the last four ribs (9–12) and abdominal aponeurosis	*Bilaterally:* Trunk flexion *Unilaterally:* Lateral flexion, trunk rotation
	Transverse abdominis	Inguinal ligament, iliac crest	Abdominal aponeurosis	Compresses abdominal contents
Back	Levator Scapulae	C_1–C_4 spine process	Vertebral border of scapula from superior angle to root of spine	Elevation, downward rotation
	Trapezius Upper	Occipital bone	Lateral clavicle and acromion	Elevation upward rotation scapula
	Middle	C_7–T_5 spinous process	Spine of scapula	Retraction of scapula
	Lower	T_5–T_{12}	Root of spine of scapula	Depression, upward rotation scapula
	Rhomboids; major, minor	Spinous process T_2–T_5, C_7–T_1	Vertebral border of scapula	Retract, rotate scapula downward
	Supraspinatus SITS	Supraspinous fossa of scapula	Greater tubercle humerus	Abduction of humerus
	Infraspinatus SITS	Infraspinous fossa of scapula	Greater tubercle humerus	Lateral rotation humerus
	Teres Minor SITS	Axillary border of scapula	Greater tubercle humerus	Medial rotation humerus
	Teres Major	Lateral border of the scapula	Biceptal groove humerus	Extension, adduction, medial rotation

(continued)

ORIGIN AND INSERTION OF SELECTED MUSCLES (continued)

	Muscle	Origin	Insertion	Action
	Quadratus lumborum	Posterior iliac crest	12th rib and transverse processes of the lumbar vertebrae	Lateral flexion, hip elevation
	Latissimus Dorsi	T_7–iliac crest, lower ribs	Bicipital groove humerus	Extension, adduction, medial rotation
Shoulders and Arms	**Deltoid** *Anterior:* *Middle:* *Posterior:*	 Lateral third of clavicle Lateral acromion process Scapular spine	Tuberosity of humerus	Flexion, adduction, abduction, extension, rotation
	Biceps brachii	Short Head: Coracoid process of scapula Long Head: Supraglenoid Tubercle of scapula	Tuberosity of radius Bicipital aponeurosis	Flexion of elbow Supination of forearm
	Brachialis	Lower shaft of humerus	Ulnar tuberosity	Elbow flexion
	Brachioradialis	Lateral ridge of humerus	Styloid process of radius	Elbow flexion
	Triceps brachii *Long head:* *Lateral head:* *Medial head:*	 Tuberosity of scapula Posterior humerus above spiral groove Posterior humerus below spiral groove	Olecranon process of ulna	Elbow extension
	Pronator	Medial epicondyle of humerus	Shaft of radius	Pronation of forearm
	Supinator	Lateral aspect of elbow	Anterior proximal radius	Supination of forearm
	Extensor carpi radialis	Supracondylar ridge Lateral epicondyle of humerus	Base of 2nd metacarpal	Wrist extension, abduction
	Extensor carpi ulnaris	Lateral epicondyle of humerus	Lateral base 5th metacarpal	Wrist extension, abduction

	Flexor carpi radialis	Medial epicondyle humerus	Base of 2nd and 3rd metacarpals	Wrist flexion, abduction
	Flexor carpi ulnaris	Medial epicondyle humerus, ulna olecranon	Humeral head, pisiform, base of 5th metacarpal	Wrist flexion, abduction
Hip and Thigh	Gluteus maximus	Posterior ilium and sacrum	Gluteal tuberosity of femur and iliotibial tract	Hip extension, external rotation
	Gluteus medius	Lateral surface of the ilium	Greater trochanter of femur	Hip abduction, internal rotation
	Gluteus minimus	Lateral surface of the lower ilium	Greater trochanter of femur	Hip abduction, internal rotation
	Piriformis	Anterior sacrum	Greater trochanter of femur	Lateral rotation of femur at hip
	Tensor fascia latae	Anterior one third of the iliac crest	Tibia via the iliotibial tract	Hip abduction, flexion, internal rotation, and knee extension
	Iliopsoas			
	Psoas major:	Bodies of the lumbar vertebrae T12–L5	ASIS, lesser trochanter of the femur	Hip flexion, external rotation, abduction
	Iliacus:	Inner surface of illium (iliac fossa)	Lesser trochanter of the femur	Flexion of femur external rotation, abduction
	Sartorius	Anterior superior iliac spine	Upper medial shaft of the tibia	Flexion, abduction, lateral rotation of femur at hip Flexion, medial rotation of knee
	Gracilis	Inferior ramus of anterior pubis	Medial proximal shaft of the tibia	Hip adduction, flexion and medial rotation of knee
	Quadriceps	Body of pubis and inferior ramus of pubis	Tibial tuberosity via the patellar tendon	
	Rectus femoris:	Anterior inferior iliac spine	Patella	Assists hip flexion, knee extension
	Vastus lateralis:	Linea aspera on posterior femur	Patella	Knee extension
	Vastus medialis:	Linea aspera on posterior femur	Patella	Knee extension
	Vastus intermedialis:	Anterior and lateral femoral shaft	Patella	Knee extension
	Pectineus	Anterior pubis	Between the lesser trochanter and the linea aspera of posterior femur	Hip flexion, hip adduction, and internal rotation

(*continued*)

ORIGIN AND INSERTION OF SELECTED MUSCLES (continued)

	Muscle	Origin	Insertion	Action
	Adductor longus	Anterior pubis	Linea aspera on posterior femur	Hip adduction, hip flexion, and internal rotation
	Adductor brevis	Anterior pubis	Linea aspera on posterior femur	Hip adduction, hip flexion, and internal rotation
	Adductor magnus	Anterior (adductor) head: Inferior ramus of pubis Posterior (hamstring) head: Ischial tuberosity and ramus of ischium	Anterior head: Linea aspera of femur Posterior head: Adductor tubercle of femur	Anterior head: Assists flexion and medial rotation of femur at hip Posterior head: Assists extension and lateral rotation of femur at hip
	Hamstrings *Biceps femoris:*	Long head: Ischial tuberosity Short head: Linea aspera	Head of the fibula	Long head: Extension of hip Both heads: Flexion of knee lateral rotation of flexed knee
	Semitendinosus:	Ischial tuberosity	Posterior medial tibial condyle	Hip extension, flexion of knee, medial rotation of knee
	Semimembranosus:	Ischial tuberosity	Anterior proximal tibial shaft	Hip extension, flexion of knee, medial rotation of knee
Lower Leg	Gastrocnemius	Medial and lateral epicondyles of the femur	Calcaneus via the tendo Achilles	Assists knee flexion, ankle plantarflexion
	Soleus	Posterior tibia and fibula	Calcaneus via the tendo Achilles	Ankle plantarflexion
	Popliteus	Lateral condyle of the femur	Posterior proximal tibial shaft	Knee flexion
	Tibialis anterior	Anterolateral shaft of tibia	Base of 1st metatarsal and 1st cuneiform bones	Ankle dorsiflexion, ankle, inversion of foot
	Extensor hallucis longus	Anterior shaft of fibula and interosseous membrane	Base of 1st distal phalanx of the great toe	Great toe extension, assists in ankle dorsiflexion
	Peroneus longus	Head and lateral shaft of fibula (upper 2/3)	Base of 1st metatarsal	Eversion of foot, assists plantar flexion of ankle
	Peroneus brevis	Lateral shaft of fibula (lower 2/3)	Base of 5th metatarsal	Eversion of foot, assists plantar flexion of ankle
	Flexor hallucis longus	Posterior shaft of fibula	Distal phalanx of great toe	Great toe flexion, assists in ankle planterflexion

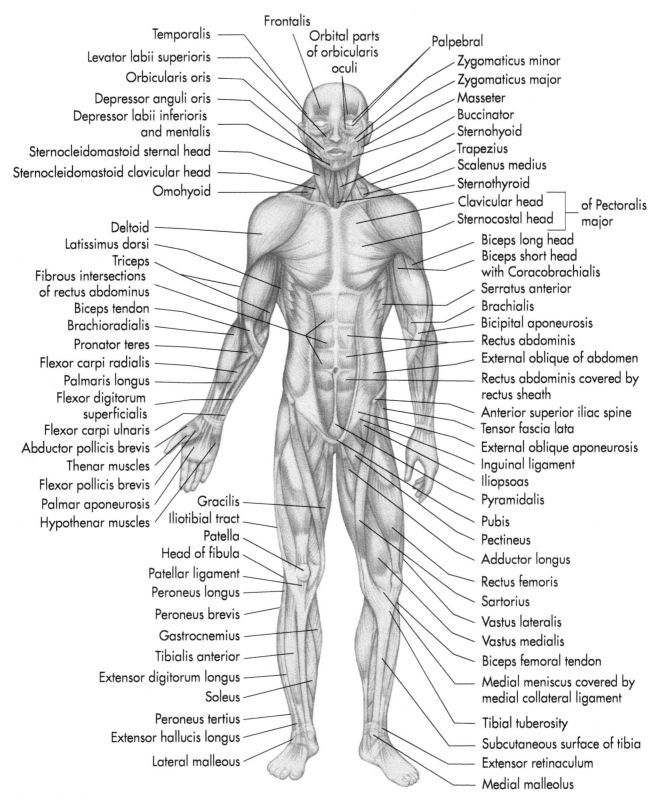

Temporalis
Levator labii superioris
Orbicularis oris
Depressor anguli oris
Depressor labii inferioris
and mentalis
Sternocleidomastoid sternal head
Sternocleidomastoid clavicular head
Omohyoid

Frontalis
Orbital parts
of orbicularis
oculi

Palpebral
Zygomaticus minor
Zygomaticus major
Masseter
Buccinator
Sternohyoid
Trapezius
Scalenus medius
Sternothyroid
Clavicular head
Sternocostal head
of Pectoralis major

Deltoid
Latissimus dorsi
Triceps
Fibrous intersections
of rectus abdominus
Biceps tendon
Brachioradialis
Pronator teres
Flexor carpi radialis
Palmaris longus
Flexor digitorum
superficialis
Flexor carpi ulnaris
Abductor pollicis brevis
Thenar muscles
Flexor pollicis brevis
Palmar aponeurosis
Hypothenar muscles

Biceps long head
Biceps short head
with Coracobrachialis
Serratus anterior
Brachialis
Bicipital aponeurosis
Rectus abdominis
External oblique of abdomen
Rectus abdominis covered by
rectus sheath
Anterior superior iliac spine
Tensor fascia lata
External oblique aponeurosis
Inguinal ligament
Iliopsoas
Pyramidalis
Pubis
Pectineus
Adductor longus

Gracilis
Iliotibial tract
Patella
Head of fibula
Patellar ligament
Peroneus longus
Peroneus brevis
Gastrocnemius
Tibialis anterior
Extensor digitorum longus
Soleus
Peroneus tertius
Extensor hallucis longus
Lateral malleous

Rectus femoris
Sartorius
Vastus lateralis
Vastus medialis
Biceps femoral tendon
Medial meniscus covered by
medial collateral ligament
Tibial tuberosity
Subcutaneous surface of tibia
Extensor retinaculum
Medial malleolus

FIGURE 5-1
Major Anterior Muscles and Related Structures.

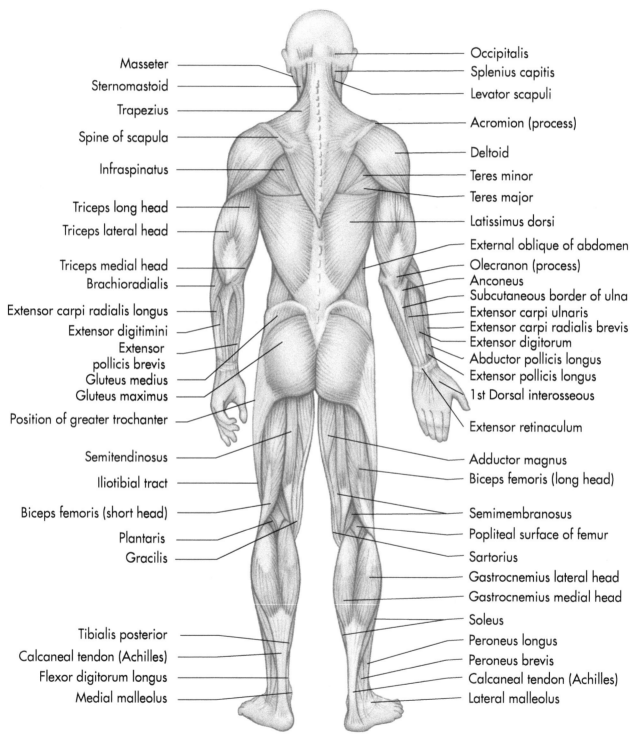

FIGURE 5-2

Major Posterior Muscles and Related Structures.

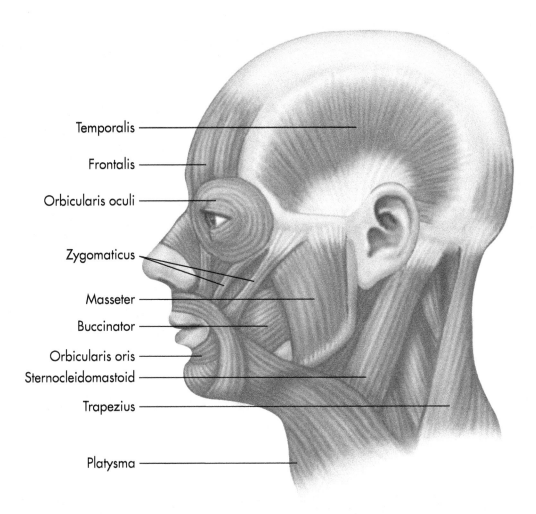

FIGURE 5-3
Skeletal Facial Muscles.

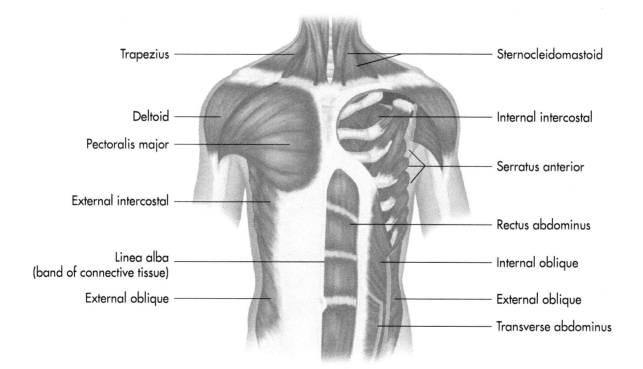

Anterior

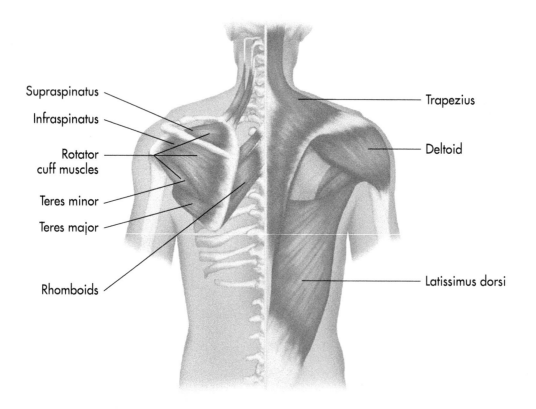

Posterior

FIGURE 5-4
Skeletal Muscles of the Anterior and Posterior Trunk.

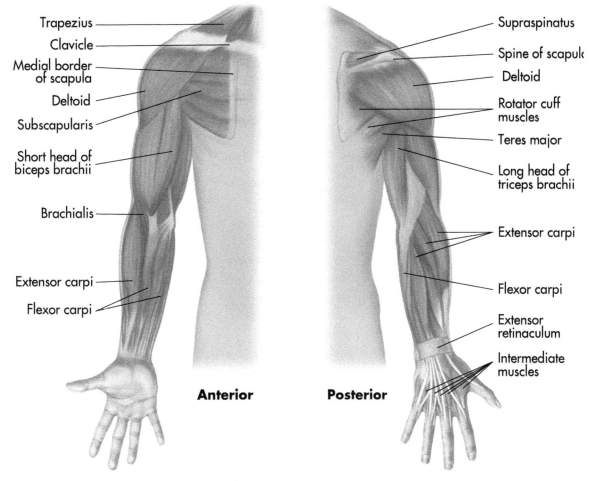

Trapezius

Clavicle

Medial border
of scapula

Deltoid

Subscapularis

Short head of
biceps brachii

Brachialis

Extensor carpi

Flexor carpi

Anterior

Supraspinatus

Spine of scapula

Deltoid

Rotator cuff
muscles

Teres major

Long head of
triceps brachii

Extensor carpi

Flexor carpi

Extensor
retinaculum

Intermediate
muscles

Posterior

FIGURE 5-5
Skeletal Muscles of the Shoulder, Arm, and Hand.

Muscles of the posterior left hip and thigh

Muscles of the anterior left hip and thigh

Muscles of the lateral left leg

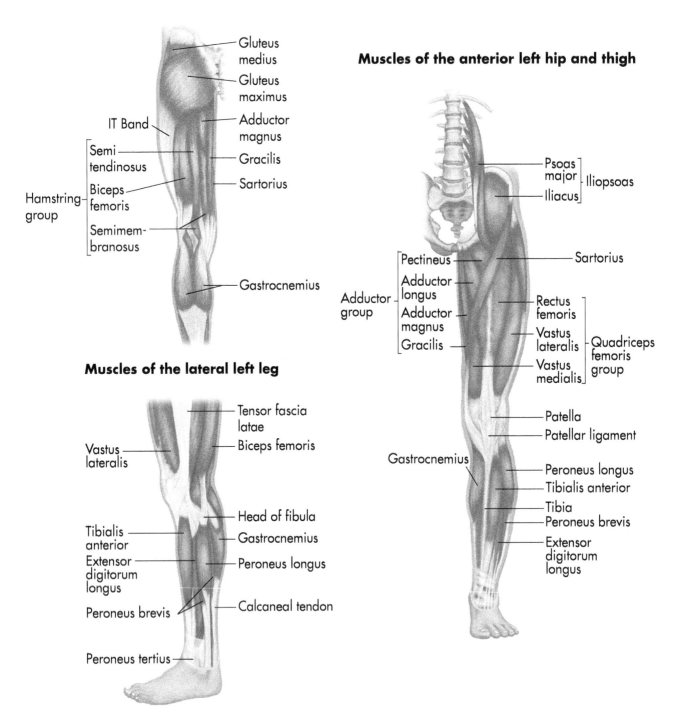

FIGURE 5-6
Skeletal Muscles of the Hip and Leg.

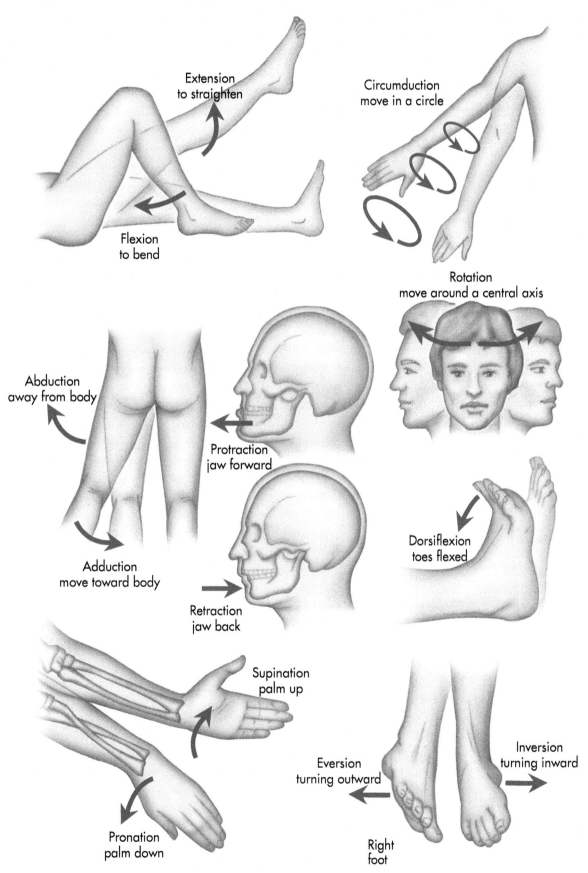

FIGURE 5-7
Body Movement.

6 Cardiovascular System

CONTENTS

CARDIOVASCULAR SYSTEM	
Function	• **To circulate blood around body to cells and various organs**
	• **Pumped by the heart to allow for exchange of gases, nutrients, and wastes between blood and body cells**
	• **Helps regulate temperature**
	• **Helps regulate acid/base balance**
Anatomy	*Heart*—A four-chambered cardiac muscle pump separating oxygen-rich blood on left and oxygen-poor blood on right by an atria ventricular septum
	• *Right atrium (RA)*—Receives oxygen-poor blood from vena cava
	• *Right ventricle (RV)*—Pumps oxygen-poor blood through pulmonary arteries to lungs for oxygen
	• *Left atrium (LA)*—Receives oxygen-rich blood from pulmonary veins
	• *Left ventricle (LV)*—Pumps oxygen-rich blood into aorta and all arterial branches
	• *Valves*—Tricuspid on right, bicuspid on left, both between atria and ventricles; sounds are the closing of valves
	• *Myocardium*—Heart tissue is striated and involuntary
	• *Coronary vessels*—Supply heart tissue with blood
	• *Purkinje fibers*—Stimulate contraction of myocardium
	• *AV and SA node (pacemaker)*—Cells in right atrium initiate contraction, pulse to ventricles
	Blood vessels—The vessels that carry oxygen-rich blood away from the heart and oxygen-poor blood to the heart
	• *Arteries*—Thick, smooth muscles that carry oxygen-rich blood away from heart except pulmonary artery branch into arterioles
	• *Arterioles*—Smaller blood vessels branching from arteries
	• *Veins*—Thin, superficial smooth muscles that carry blood toward heart and have valves and branch into venules
	• *Venules*—Smaller blood vessels branching from veins
	• *Capillaries*—Microscopic blood vessels permeable to gases by diffusion
	Blood—Liquid connective tissue composed of plasma and red and white blood cells
	• *Plasma*—90% water, 10% nutrients, gases, electrolytes, and hormones

(*continued*)

CARDIOVASCULAR SYSTEM (*continued*)	
	• *Cells*—Red blood cell (erythrocyte), formed in bone marrow, carries oxygen on hemoglobin, life span of 120 days; white blood cells (leukocytes, neutrophils, lymphocytes, basophils, cosinophils), formed in bone marrow and lymph nodes, body's defense mechanism forming antibodies against foreign antigens (bacteria, virus, toxins) • *Typing*—genetic antigen on RBC–A, B, AB (universal receiver), O (universal donor) • *Clotting*—Involves platelets (WBC) and prothrombin protein, which converts to the protein fibrin clot
Types of Circulation	*Systemic*—Blood to all parts of body from left ventricle to right atrium *Pulmonary*—Blood flow to lungs and back through pulmonary veins *Coronary*—Blood flow to coronary arteries around heart *Hepatic portal*—Veins from digestion, spleen, and pancreas to hepatic portal vein of liver and drained into vena cava *Cerebral*—Blood flow to the brain
Physiology	*ECG*—Graph of the contraction (systole 'R' wave) and relaxation (diastole 'T' wave) of the heart muscle; PQRST wave *Pulse*—Heart rate, or number of beats per minute *Blood pressure*—Systolic pressure, heart contraction over diastolic pressure, heart relaxation at rest; 120/80 mmHg normal average *CPR*—Cardiopulmonary resuscitation; emergency procedure to artificially return heartbeat and breathing after cardiac arrest by manually compressing chest and forcing air into lungs.
Pathway of Blood Through Heart	*From Body*—vena cava → RA → tricuspid valve → RV → pulmonic valve → pulmonary arteries → lungs *From Lungs*—pulmonary vein → LA → bicuspid valve → LV → aortic semilunar valve → aorta → body
Benefits of Massage on the Cardiovascular System	• Improves and increases arterial circulation • Assists venous and lymphatic circulation • Aids in lowering blood pressure • Improves flow of interstitial fluid

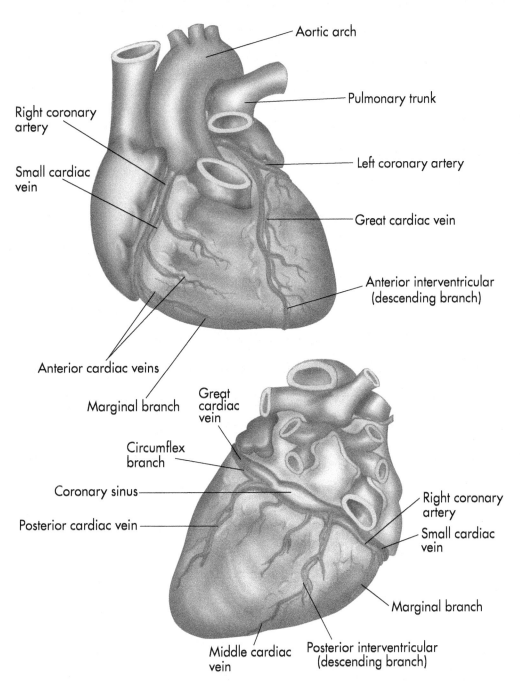

FIGURE 6-1

Anatomy of the Heart.

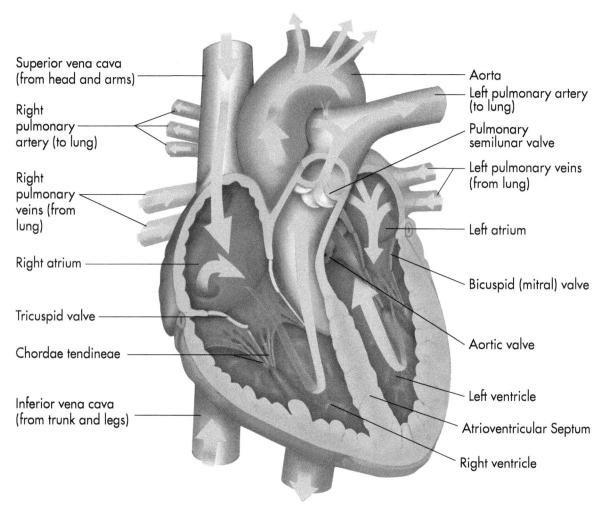

Superior vena cava
(from head and arms)

Right
pulmonary
artery (to lung)

Right
pulmonary
veins (from
lung)

Right atrium

Tricuspid valve

Chordae tendineae

Inferior vena cava
(from trunk and legs)

Aorta

Left pulmonary artery
(to lung)

Pulmonary
semilunar valve

Left pulmonary veins
(from lung)

Left atrium

Bicuspid (mitral) valve

Aortic valve

Left ventricle

Atrioventricular Septum

Right ventricle

FIGURE 6-2

Internal Anatomy and Blood Flow through the Heart.

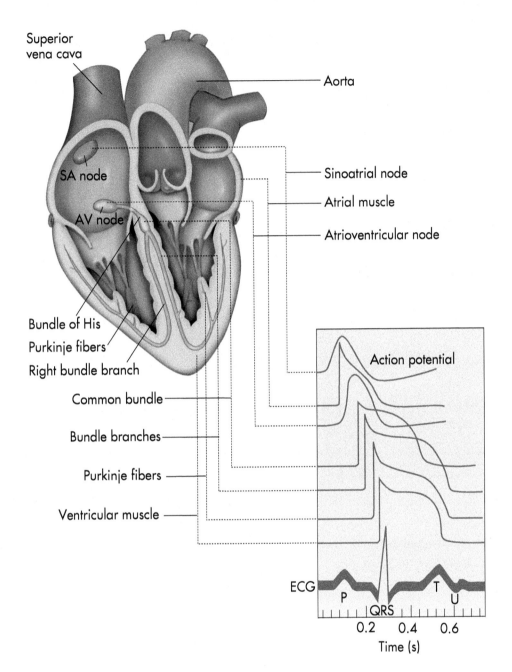

FIGURE 6-3

Electrocardiogram Activities.

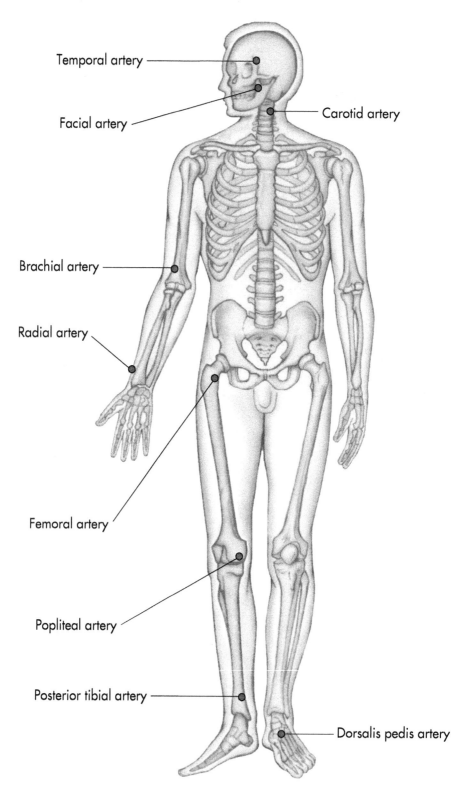

Temporal artery

Facial artery

Carotid artery

Brachial artery

Radial artery

Femoral artery

Popliteal artery

Posterior tibial artery

Dorsalis pedis artery

FIGURE 6-4

The Pulse Points.

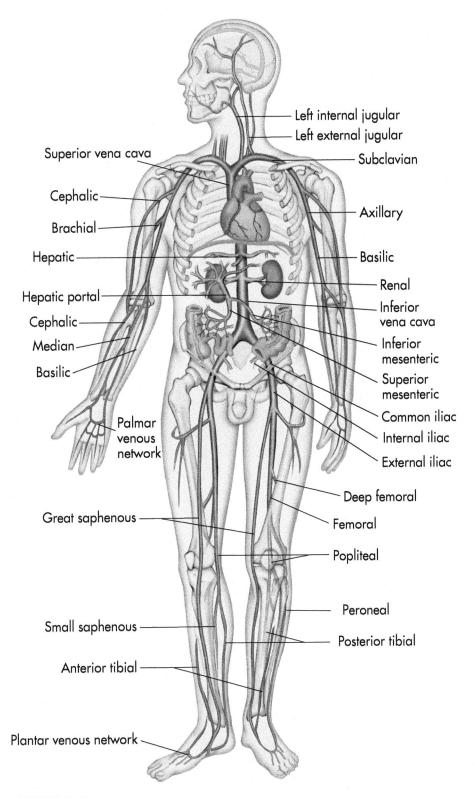

FIGURE 6-5

The Venous System.

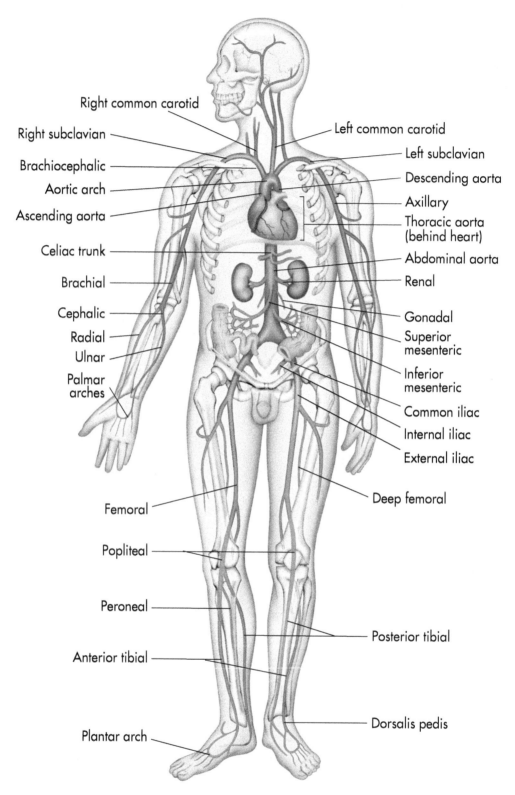

FIGURE 6-6
The Arterial System.

Lymphatic System

CONTENTS

LYMPHATIC SYSTEM	
Function	**Immunity and transport of antibodies (proteins that attack invading body organisms) and antigens (any substance that provokes an immune response)**
Cells	***Antibodies*** (immunoglobulins)—Attach to specific antigens ***T lymphocytes*** (T cells)—Special white blood cells that identify an antigen as foreign ***B cells***—Lymphocytes that differentiate into plasma cells to produce antibodies

Anatomy	***Lymph***—Fluid similar to plasma that travels in lymphatic vessels
	
	Lymphatic vessels—Microscopic capillaries composed of epithelial cells
	
	Right lymphatic duct—Drains right quadrant of body into right subclavian vein
	
	Thoracic duct—Drains left quadrants and lower body into left subclavian vein
	
	Lacteals—Lymph vessels in villi of intestine to absorb lymph and fat
	
	Lymphatic organs
	
	  Lymph nodes—Produce lymphocytes; arranged in clusters in areas of the axillaries, parotid, cervical, inguinal, mesenteric, popliteal, lumbar
	
	  Spleen—Left side of body under ribs 11 and 12
	
	  Tonsils—Three pair in pharynx: adenoids, palatine, lingual
	
	  Thymus—Mediastinum above heart
	
	  Red bone marrow—Located in long bones

Types of Immunity	***Nonspecific Immunity***—Defenses that are present from birth and work to prevent any foreign substance from entering the body. This includes physical barriers, phagocytes, immunologic surveillance from "Natural Killer" lymphocytes, chemicals such as cytokines, complement system, histamine, etc., the inflammatory process and fever.
	
	Specific immunity—An immune response directed toward a specific agent such as bacteria, fungi, toxins, viruses, etc., that the body recognizes as foreign. These are called antigens. T cells and B cells are the lymphocytes that mediate specific responses. There are two types of Specific Immunity:
	
	  Innate Immunity—Immunity that is genetically predetermined. For example, certain viruses or bacteria that infect animals cannot infect humans.
	
	  Acquired Immunity—Immunity that results from an immune system response to an antigen exposure. There are four different types of Acquired Immunity:
	
	    • ***Passive immunity naturally acquired***—Antibodies formed by the mother are given to the child in the womb and by breast milk. This is temporary immunity.

	• **_Passive immunity induced_**—Antibodies already formed by another or in a lab are injected into the individual. This is temporary immunity.
	• **_Active immunity naturally acquired_**—The individual in response to exposure to the specific antigen forms Antibodies.
	• **_Active immunity induced_**—Antibodies are formed by the individual in response to being deliberately exposed to modified or dead antigens in a vaccine.
Lymph Function	• Lymph fluid (water, electrolytes, lymphocytes) travels through lymphatic vessels containing valves to lymph nodes where lymph filtration and phagocyte activity takes place
	• Lymph vessels carry lymph fluid through the body until it reaches the junction of the jugular and superior vena cava where it is returned to the cardiovascular system/blood
Benefits of Massage on the Lymphatic System	• Increases and improves free flow of lymph
	• Moves lymphatic waste for elimination
	• Promotes good circulation of lymph to act as detoxification

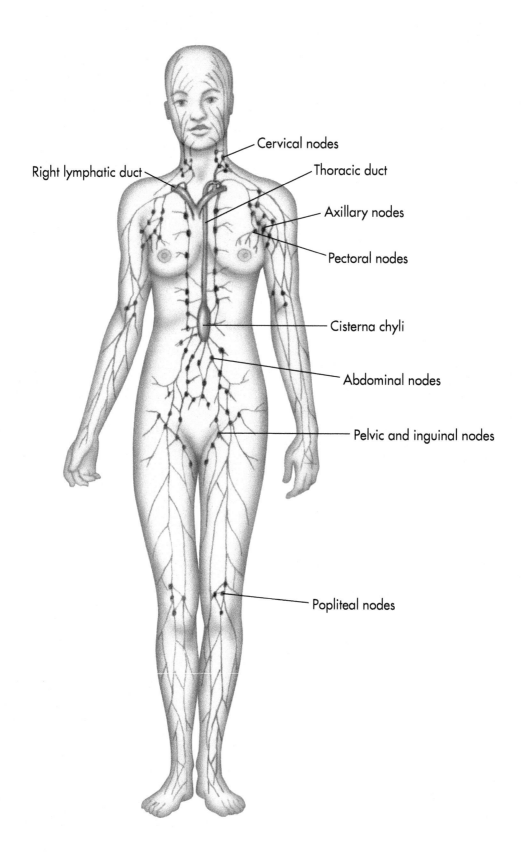

FIGURE 7-1
The Lymphatic System.

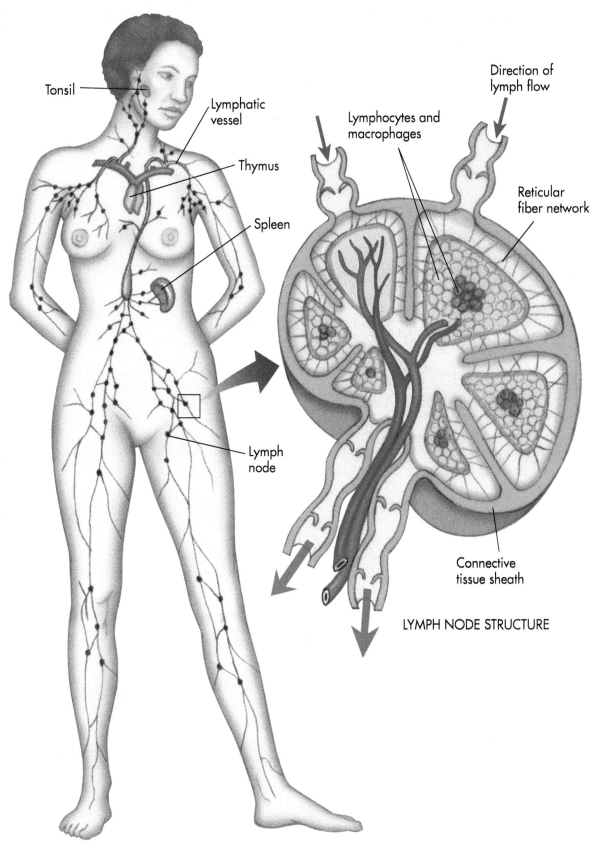

Tonsil

Lymphatic vessel

Thymus

Spleen

Lymph node

Direction of lymph flow

Lymphocytes and macrophages

Reticular fiber network

Connective tissue sheath

LYMPH NODE STRUCTURE

FIGURE 7-2
The Lymph Nodes and Organs.

CHAPTER 8

Respiratory System

 CONTENTS

RESPIRATORY SYSTEM	
Function	**Distribute air and exchange gas** • *External respiration*—Exchange of CO_2 and O_2 in lungs • *Internal respiration*—Exchange of gas between cells and capillaries • *Cellular respiration*—Use of O_2 to produce Adenosine Triphosphate (ATP) in mitochondria
Anatomy of the Respiratory Tract	*Nose*—Leads to the nasal cavity, lined with mucous membranes that moisten and filter air continuously with the sinus cavities *Pharynx*—Throat; common passage for air and food *Larynx*—Passageway for air at top of trachea, composed of vocal cords, muscle, and cartilage *Trachea*—Windpipe that extends into left and right bronchi with C-shaped cartilage to maintain structure *Bronchi*—Carry air into smaller branches of bronchioles *Alveoli*—Microscopic air sacs at distal ends of bronchioles that function to allow gas exchange between air and blood *Lungs*—Right, three lobes; left, two lobes separated by mediastinum and enclosed by diaphragm; each lobe contains blood vessels from heart, supporting tissue, and alveoli
Muscles of Respiration	Muscles of inhalation: Diaphragm, scalenes, SCM, and external intercostals Muscles of exhalation: External obliques, internal obliques, transverse abdominus, and internal intercostals
Blood Vessels	Pulmonary arteries and veins
Physiology of Breathing	*Inspiration*—Diaphragm contracts (moves down) to increase space, air moves in nasal cavity to reach alveoli for gas exchange (O_2 for CO_2) *Expiration*—Diaphragm relaxes (moves up) and moves air up and out nasal cavity *Tidal volume*—One inspiration and expiration air, 0.5L *Vital capacity*—Deep inspiration and maximum expiration, 4.8L *Respiratory rate*—At rest = 16 to 20 breaths per minute, increasing with exercise, low oxygen, smoking, disease
Benefits of Massage on the Respiratory System	• Aids in relaxation with deep breaths • Tapotement to dorsal thoracic for respiratory congestion • Slows respiratory rate

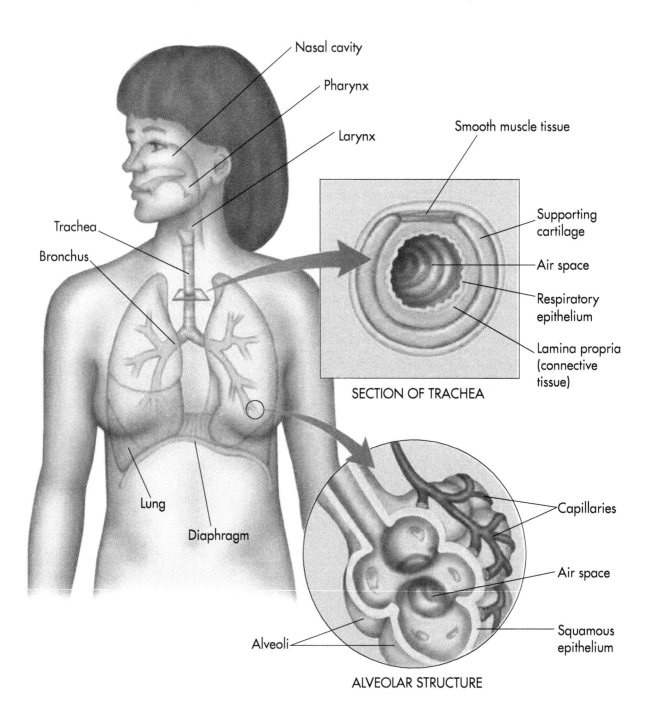

FIGURE 8-1
The Respiratory System.

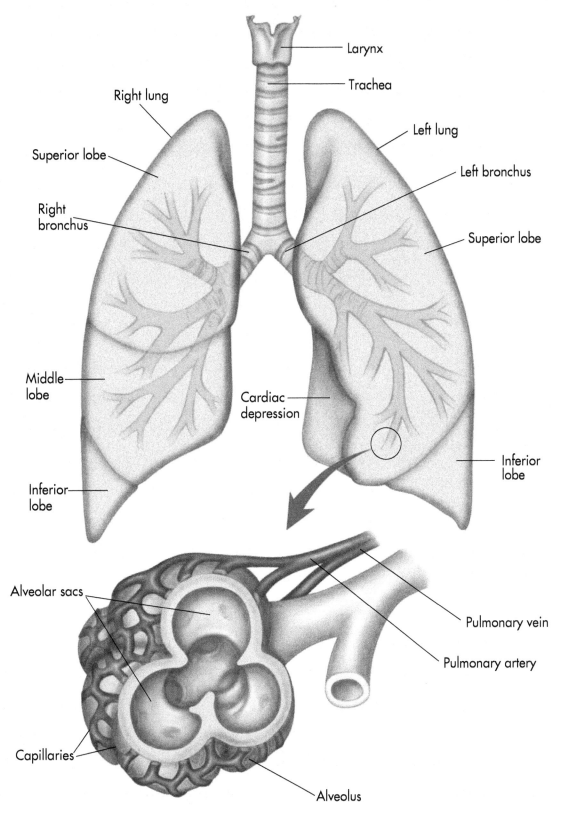

Larynx

Trachea

Right lung

Left lung

Superior lobe

Left bronchus

Right
bronchus

Superior lobe

Middle
lobe

Cardiac
depression

Inferior
lobe

Inferior
lobe

Alveolar sacs

Pulmonary vein

Pulmonary artery

Capillaries

Alveolus

FIGURE 8-2
The Lungs and Alveolus.

9 Nervous System

CONTENTS

NERVOUS SYSTEM	
Function	• **To interact with the external and internal environment through the stimuli of touch, sound, sight, taste, and speech** • **The body receives stimuli and responds voluntarily or automatically**
Nervous Tissue	*Neuron*—Nerve cell that conducts action potential and carries impulses • Axon—Takes information away from cell body • Dendrite—Sends information from cell to cell *Nerve bundle*—Nerve fibers (axon or dendrites) that extend from CNS to tissue *Synaptic vesicles*—Contain neurotransmitters at axon terminal for release *Myelin sheath*—Made of neuroglial cells
Anatomy of the CNS, PNS	*Central nervous system* (CNS)—Composed of brain and spinal cord *Peripheral nervous system* (PNS)—Composed of spinal nerves and cranial nerves • The PNS is composed of two systems: **Somatic nervous system**—Nerves that control skeletal muscle contraction; relay information to CNS regarding pain temperature touch and pressure from skin via somatic sensory nerves **Autonomic nervous system** (ANS)—Nerves that control smooth and cardiac muscle, glands • The ANS has two divisions: **Sympathetic**—Prepares body for stress; called "fight or flight" system, speeds up **Parasympatic**—Prepares the body for rest; called "rest and digest" system, slows down
Central Nervous System	*Meninges*—Three layers of tissue: • Dura mater—Thickest external layer • Arachnoid membrane—Web-like layer, space for cerebrospinal fluid that cushions brain • Pia mater—Thin and innermost layer supporting blood vessels that give elasticity and support to the spinal cord itself *Brain* • Cerebrum—80% of total brain mass, left and right hemispheres and subdivided into lobes, gyri, and sulci; contains sensory and motor pathways of frontal, parietal, and temporal lobes—"the seat of intelligence"—**gray matter cells** • Cerebellum—Second largest portion for coordination, balance, and equilibrium—**white matter** • Midbrain—Visual and auditory reflexes • Pons—Connects spinal cord and brain center for respiration control, white matter • Medulla oblongata—Cardiac control, vasomotor, respiratory center, white matter

(continued)

NERVOUS SYSTEM (*continued*)	
	• Thalmus—Controls pain perception, relays impulses from skin to cerebrum • Hypothalamus—Links nervous and endocrine system, acts as endocrine organ controlling the autonomic nervous system ***Spinal cord***—Descends from foramen magnum to about L4, **gray and white matter**

Peripheral Nervous System (all parts except brain and spinal cord)	***Cranial nerves***—12 pairs arise from underside of brain, (S) are sensory, (M) motor, (MS) are mixed (sensory & motor), include;
	
	1. (S) olfactory—smell
	
	2. (M) optic—sight
	
	3. (M) oculomotor—eye muscles
	
	4. (MS) trochlear—eye muscles
	
	5. (M) trigeminal—jaw muscles
	
	6. (MS) abducens—eye muscles
	
	7. (M) facial—muscles of face
	
	8. (S) auditory—hearing
	
	9. (MS) glossopharyngeal—taste
	
	10. (MS) vagus smooth muscle—organs
	
	11. (MS) spinoaccessory—head, neck muscles
	
	12. (M) hypoglossal—tongue muscle
	
	Spinal nerves mixed (sensory & motor)
	
	31 pairs of spinal nerves include:
	    Cervical—8 pairs
	    Thoracic—12 pairs
	    Lumbar—5 pairs
	    Sacral—5 pairs
	    Coccygeal—1 pair

Somatic Nervous System Sensory Receptor Nerves	***Proprioceptors***—Detect position and rate of movement • ***Muscle spindle cells***—Belly of muscle; lengthen, stretch, and control how fast a muscle is moving • ***Golgi tendon organs***—In tendon; monitor stretching ***Nociceptors***—Pain receptors ***Thermoreceptors***—Temperature receptors ***Photoreceptors***—Light receptors ***Visceroreceptors***—Internal organ receptors
Dermatomes	***Dermatomes***—Cutaneous/skin distribution of spinal nerve sensation including: • Cervical segments C1–C8 • Thoracic segments T1–T12 • Lumbar segments L1–L5

	• Sacral segments S1–S5 • Coccygeal segment Can be affected by massage techniques that stimulate the skin
Nerve Impulse Transmissions	**Synapse**—The space between a dendrite and axon terminal **Action potential**—Na⁺ enters and electrical current causes contraction of muscle **Neurotransmitters**—Hormones or chemical messengers contained at the synaptic vesicle and released to stimulate or inhibit action potential, e.g., acetylcholine, cholinesterase **Neuromuscular junction**—Where axon terminal meets sarcolemma of muscle fibers
Plexus	**A network of interconnecting nerves:** **Cervical plexus**—Nerve roots C1–C4, sensory and motor innervation for skin and muscles of head, neck, shoulders **Brachial plexus**—Nerve roots C5–T1, sensory and motor innervation to upper extremity and neck, gives rise to radial, (forearm, shoulder, wrist, fingers) axillary, (lateral deltoid) median, (elbow wrist, fingers, thumb) ulnar, (4th and 5th fingers) and musculocutaneous nerves of shoulder, arm, and hand muscles (biceps, bracial forearm) **Lumbosacral plexus**—Arises from nerve roots L1–S4 and provides sensory and motor innervation for lower extremities; gives rise to obturator, (medial thigh and adductors) femoral, (anterior and lateral thigh, quadriceps, sartorius, ilipsoas, pectineus) and sciatic nerve **Sciatic nerve**—L4–S3 (sensory-posterior thigh; motor-hamstrings) divides into tibial and peroneal nerves of calf and foot, tibial (sensory-posterior calf; motor-flexors) Peroneal (sensory-anterior calf; motor-extensors and peroneal muscles)

Neuroendocrine	Massage *increases* blood levels of hormones serotonin, dopamine, endorphins, and oxytocin
	
	Massage *reduces* hormone cortisol and regulates epinephrine and norepinephrine
	
	Massage is beneficial to:
	
	    A depressed, lonely person
	
	    A child with Attention Deficit Hyperactivity Disorder (ADHD)
	
	    A person suffering a chronic condition
	
	    A person with HIV
	
	    An infant
	
	    A person after surgery
	
	    Anyone who wants to feel better and give rise to higher thought

Benefits of Massage on the Nervous System	• Relaxation or calming effect • Stimulates parasympathetic–endorphin release • Can interrupt pain cycle • Increases body awareness through touch • Reflex effects to organs, pain receptors, and muscle and joints

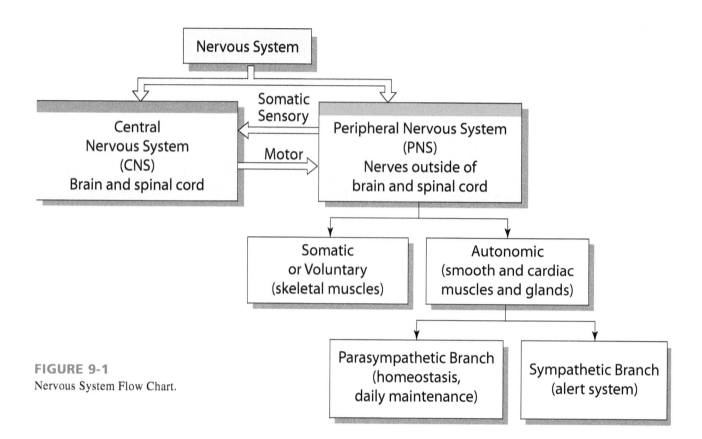

FIGURE 9-1
Nervous System Flow Chart.

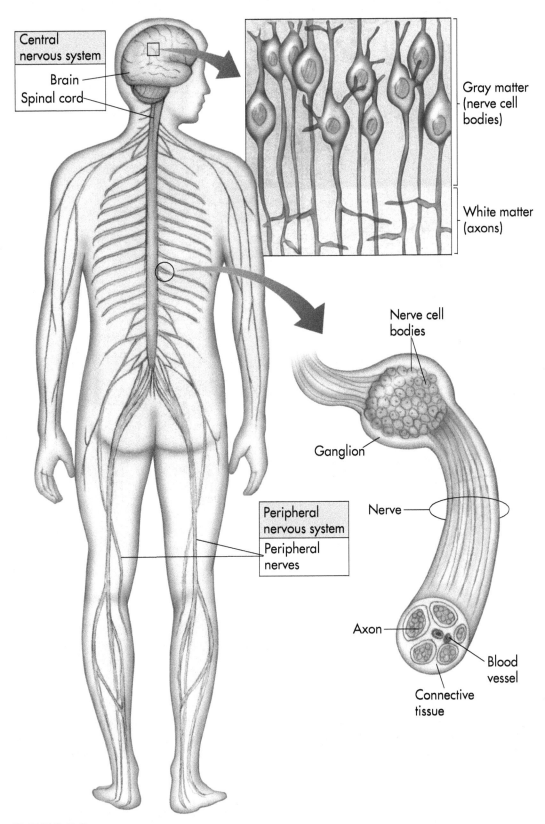

Central nervous system
- Brain
- Spinal cord

Gray matter (nerve cell bodies)

White matter (axons)

Nerve cell bodies

Ganglion

Nerve

Peripheral nervous system
- Peripheral nerves

Axon

Blood vessel

Connective tissue

FIGURE 9-2
The Central and Peripheral Nervous System.

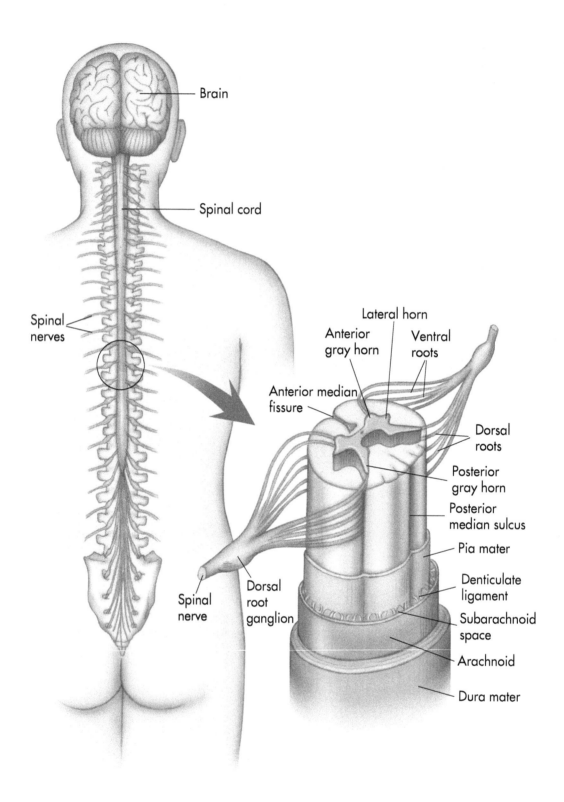

FIGURE 9-3

The Central Nervous System.

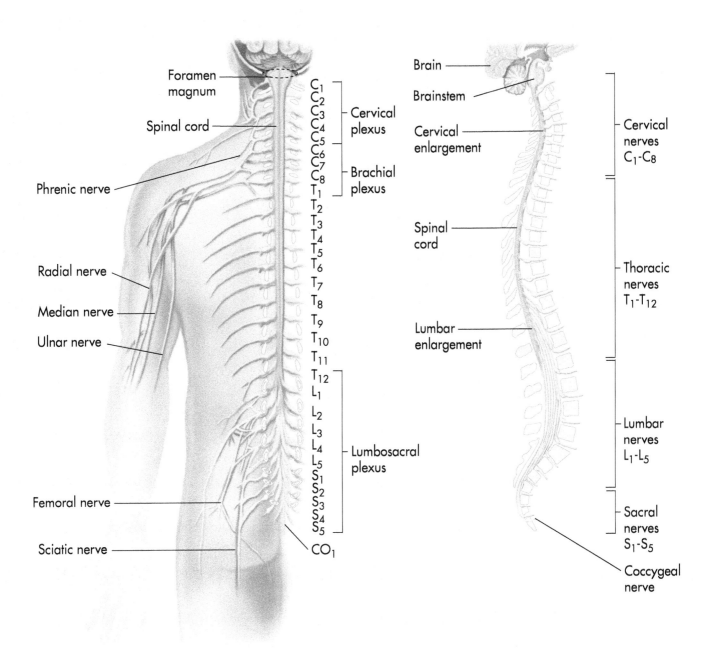

FIGURE 9-4

The 31 Pairs of Spinal Nerves.

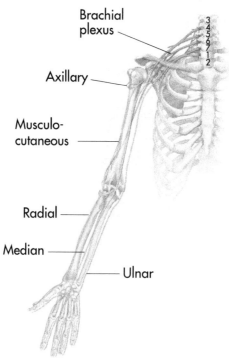

A. Brachial plexus

Brachial plexus

Axillary

Musculo-
cutaneous

Radial

Median

Ulnar

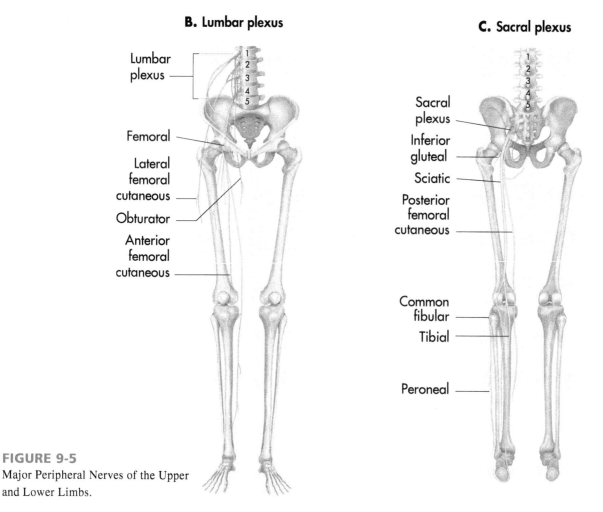

B. Lumbar plexus

Lumbar plexus

Femoral

Lateral femoral cutaneous

Obturator

Anterior femoral cutaneous

C. Sacral plexus

Sacral plexus

Inferior gluteal

Sciatic

Posterior femoral cutaneous

Common fibular

Tibial

Peroneal

FIGURE 9-5

Major Peripheral Nerves of the Upper and Lower Limbs.

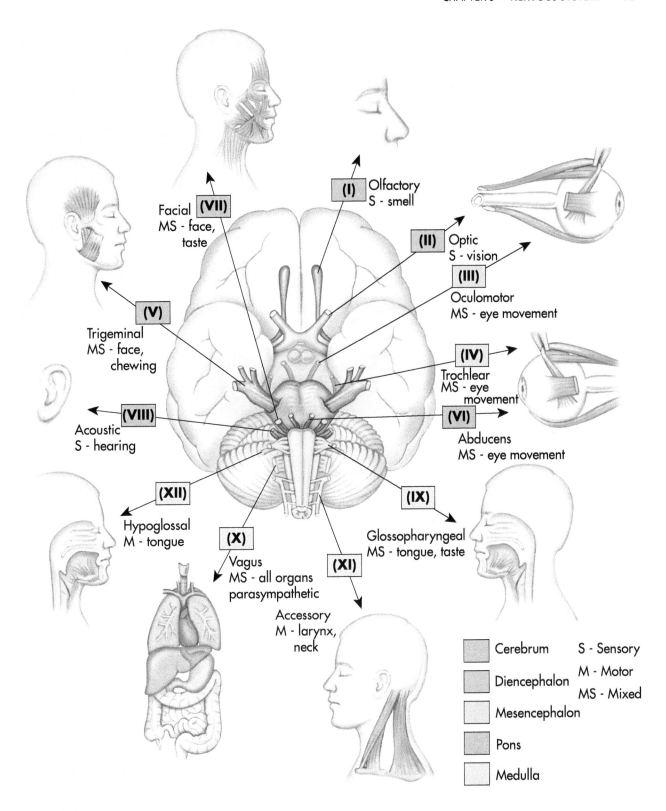

(I) Olfactory
S - smell

(II) Optic
S - vision

(III)
Oculomotor
MS - eye movement

Facial **(VII)**
MS - face,
taste

(V)
Trigeminal
MS - face,
chewing

(IV)
Trochlear
MS - eye
movement

(VIII)
Acoustic
S - hearing

(VI)
Abducens
MS - eye movement

(XII)
Hypoglossal
M - tongue

(X)
Vagus
MS - all organs
parasympathetic

(XI)
Accessory
M - larynx,
neck

(IX)
Glossopharyngeal
MS - tongue, taste

Cerebrum   S - Sensory

Diencephalon   M - Motor

Mesencephalon   MS - Mixed

Pons

Medulla

FIGURE 9-6

The Cranial Nerves: Function, Type, and Their Origins in the Brain.

CHAPTER

10 Urinary System

 CONTENTS

URINARY SYSTEM	
Function	**The urinary system regulates blood pressure, electrolyte balance, and eliminates excess water and toxins (waste) through a process of filtration in the nephrons of the kidneys that creates urine for excretion**
Anatomy	***Kidneys*** • Located between last thoracic vertebrae and L3 • Composed of capsule, cortex, medulla, calyces, pervis • Functional unit is nephron made up of glomeruli, bowman's capsule, and tubules ***Bladder***—Stores urine until voided by urethra ***Ureter***—Smooth muscle tube collecting urine and bringing to bladder
Urine Formation	***Filtration, secretion, and reabsorption***—Process the wastes of urine including urea, uric acid, creatine, and ammonia in the microscopic nephrons ***Excess water, hormones, sugar, amino acids, and electrolytes***—also filtered out of the blood
Benefits of Massage on the Urinary System	• Aids elimination of excess fluid and toxins from body

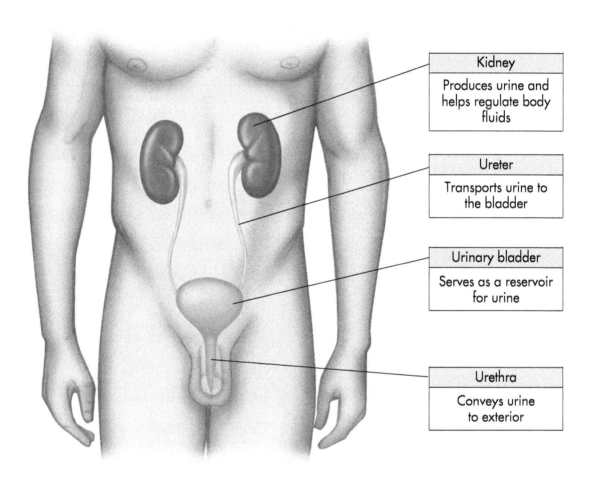

FIGURE 10-1
The Urinary System.

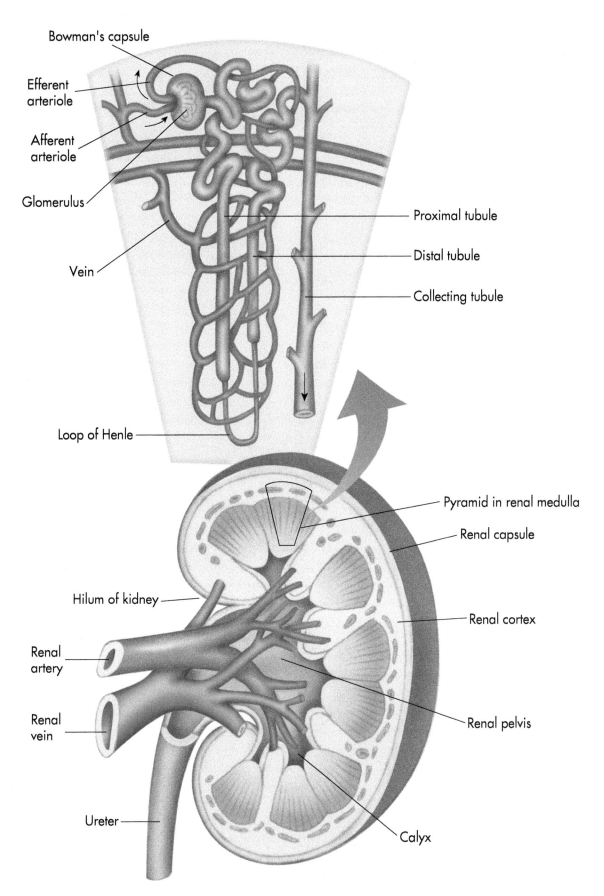

FIGURE 10-2
The Kidney and Nephron.

11 Digestive System

 CONTENTS

DIGESTIVE SYSTEM	
Function	• **Mechanical and chemical breaking down of food** • **Catabolic metabolism** • **Ingest food, carbohydrates, fats, and proteins** • **Secretion of enzymes, amylases, proteases, and lipases** • **Absorption of glucose, fatty acids, and amino acids by the gastrointestinal wall**
Organs of Digestion	*Mouth*—Teeth, salivary glands, tongue, pharynx *Stomach*—Esophagus *Small intestine*—Duodenum, jejunum, ilium, liver, gall bladder, pancreas *Large intestine*—Cecum, ascending, transverse, descending, sigmoid colon, rectum, anus
Mechanics of Digestion	*Mechanical digestion*—Converting large particles of food into small particles *Mastication lubrication*—Chewing in mouth, secretion of saliva *Peristalsis*—Muscular contraction that pushes food/bolus along alimentory canal *Villi*—Where absorption of end products takes place, glucose, amino acids, fatty acids *Rectum*—Stores solid waste *Anus*—Sphincter valve controls defecation
Anatomy of Digestive Tract Walls	*Serosa*—External epithelial membrane, peritoneum and mesentery *Muscularis*—Smooth muscle performs peristaltic action *Submucosa*—Contains blood vessels, nerves, and lymph vessels *Mucosa*—Mucous membrane *Villi*—Finger-like projections for absorption of nutrients *Lacteals*—Lymph vessels absorb fatty acids within villi
Accessory Organs	*Salivary glands*—Parotid, submandibular, and sublingual glands secrete lubricating saliva into mouth to break down carbohydrates *Liver*—Stores glycogen, synthesizes blood proteins, removes toxic substances, synthesizes urea, stores vitamins and minerals, manufactures bile to break down fats, destroys RBCs *Gallbladder*—Storage pouch for bile; connects to duodenum *Pancreas*—Below stomach, secretes alkaline pancreatic juice from acinar cells via pancreatic duct into duodenum to act on fats, carbohydrates, proteins, and nucleic acids *Veriform appendix*—Projects downward from cecum

(*continued*)

DIGESTIVE SYSTEM (continued)	
Chemical Digestion	*Mouth*—Saliva contains amylase enzyme ptyalin, which acts on starch
	Stomach—HCl and the protease pepsin act on protein
	Small intestine—Bile secreted emulsifies fats; pancreatic juice and intestinal juices act on lipids, carbohydrates, and peptides; absorption of end products, glucose, amino acids, and fatty acids by villi and lacteals
	Large intestine—Absorbs water and electrolytes, flora bacteria activity
Benefits of Massage on the Digestive System	• Improves digestive process through relaxation
	• Abdominal massage assists movement of food through descending, ascending, and transverse colon
	• Helps to regulate constipation

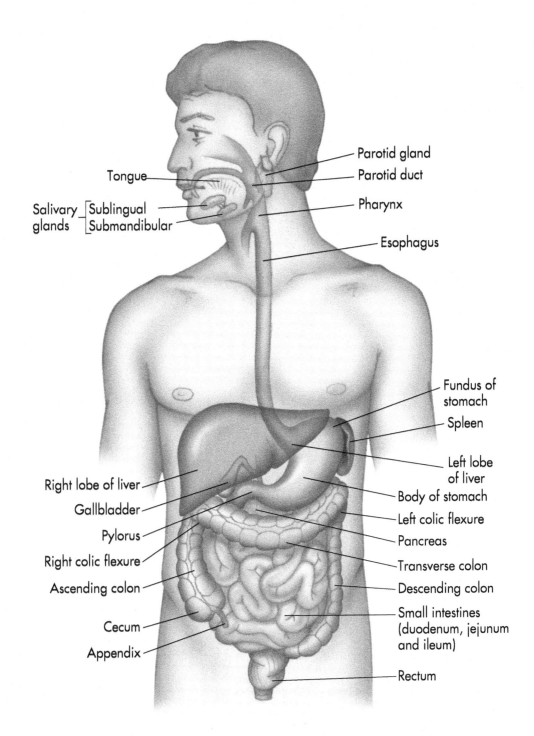

FIGURE 11-1
The Digestive System.

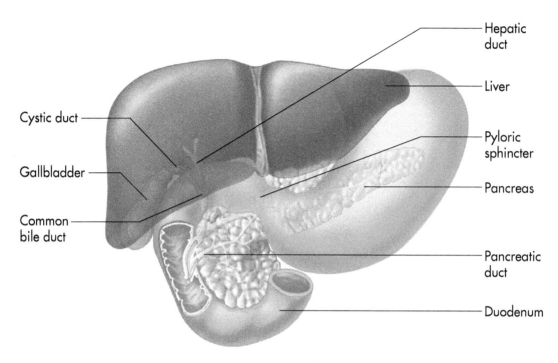

FIGURE 11-2
The Liver.

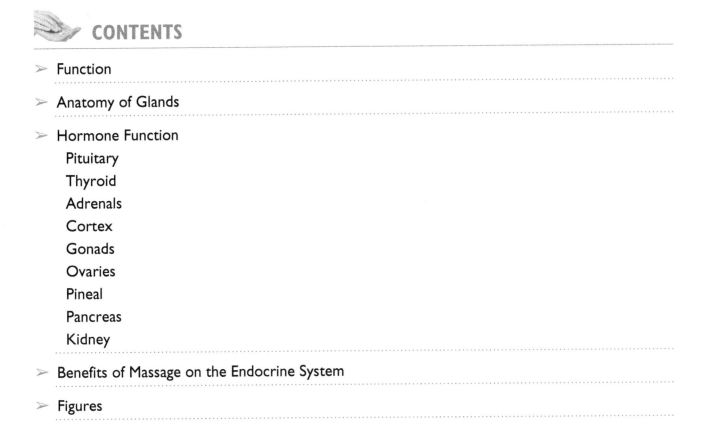

CONTENTS

ENDOCRINE SYSTEM	
Function	• **Consists of glandular organs to control and regulate metabolic processes** • **Maintains homeostasis** • **Secretes protein hormones directly into the blood**
Anatomy of Glands	*Hypothalamus*—Located in the center of the brain below the thalamus *Pituitary*—Anterior/posterior gland sits beneath thalmus and hypothalamus center of the brain *Thyroid*—Bowtie-shaped gland in neck below larynx *Parathyroids*—Four tiny glands embedded in posterior of thyroid *Pancreas*—Long gland inferior to stomach containing pancreatic islet cells *Adrenals*—Pyramid-shaped glands above the kidneys, divided into cortex and medulla *Pineal*—Small gland found in midbrain of brain stem *Kidneys*—Below adrenal gland *Ovaries*—In female lower pelvis left and right *Testes*—In male scrotum exterior to body

Hormone Function	*Hypothalamus*
	   TRH—Thyroid releasing hormone
	   GnRH—Gonadotropin releasing hormone
	   LHRH—Luteinizing hormone releasing hormone
	   PIH—Prolactin inhibiting hormone
	   PRH—Prolactin releasing hormone
	   GHRH, GHIH—Growth hormone inhibiting/releasing hormone
	   CRH—Corticotropic releasing hormone
	
	Pituitary
	Anterior:
	   • GH—Growth hormone
	   • TSH—Thyroid-stimulating hormone
	   • Prolactin—Milk production
	   • FSH—Follicle stimulating hormone
	   • ACTH—Adrenocortecotropic hormone; stimulates adrenal cortex
	   • LH—Leutinizing hormone egg release
	   • MSH—Melanocyte-stimulating hormone
	Posterior:
	   • ADH—Antidiuretic hormone; regulates excess water through kidneys
	   • Oxytocin—Regulates uterus and mammary glands; controls contractions during labor

	Thyroid (T4)
	Thyroxine—Increases metabolic rate
	Calcitonin—Decreases blood calcium
	Parathyroid (PTH)—Promotes calcium movement from bone to blood
	Adrenals and Medulla—Epinephrine increases heart rate, blood pressure and glucose, breathing; decreases digestion
	Cortex
	Cortisol—Response to stress, increases blood sugar levels
	Aldosterone—Kidneys conserve urine output, sodium uptake
	Testosterone—Male secondary sex traits
	Estrogen—Female sex traits
	Progesterone—Female sex traits
	Gonads—Testes; testosterone; regulate masculine changes
	Ovaries—Estrogen; regulate menstrual changes, sex drive, develop secondary sex traits
	Pineal—Melatonin; light response, circadian rhythms
	Pancreas
	Insulin—causes blood sugar level to fall, liver to produce glycogen
	Glucagons—blood sugar rise, glycogen to glucose
	Kidney—Erythropoietin; RBC stimulation
Benefits of Massage on the Endocrine System	• Massage changes hormone levels through interaction with the Autonomic Nervous Systems (ANS). For example, cortisol decreases with massage
	• Massage encourages release of endorphins (natural pain killers)
	• Increase oxytocin level
	• Decrease cortisol level

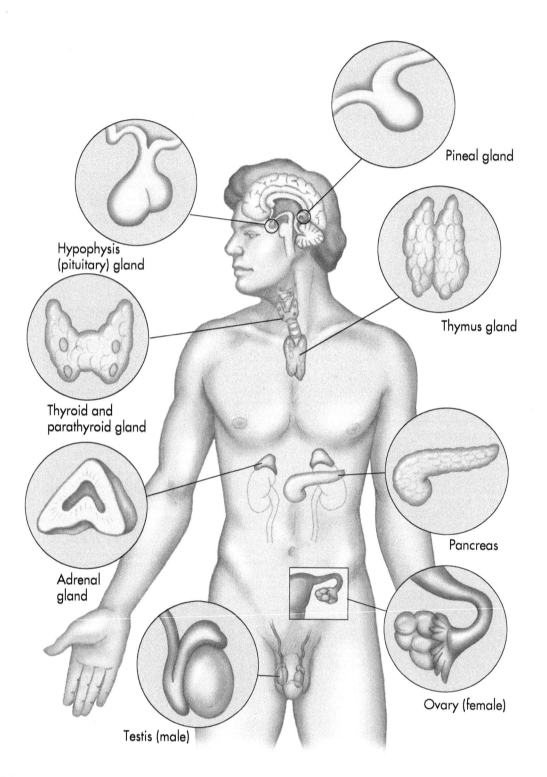

FIGURE 12-1
The Endocrine Glands.

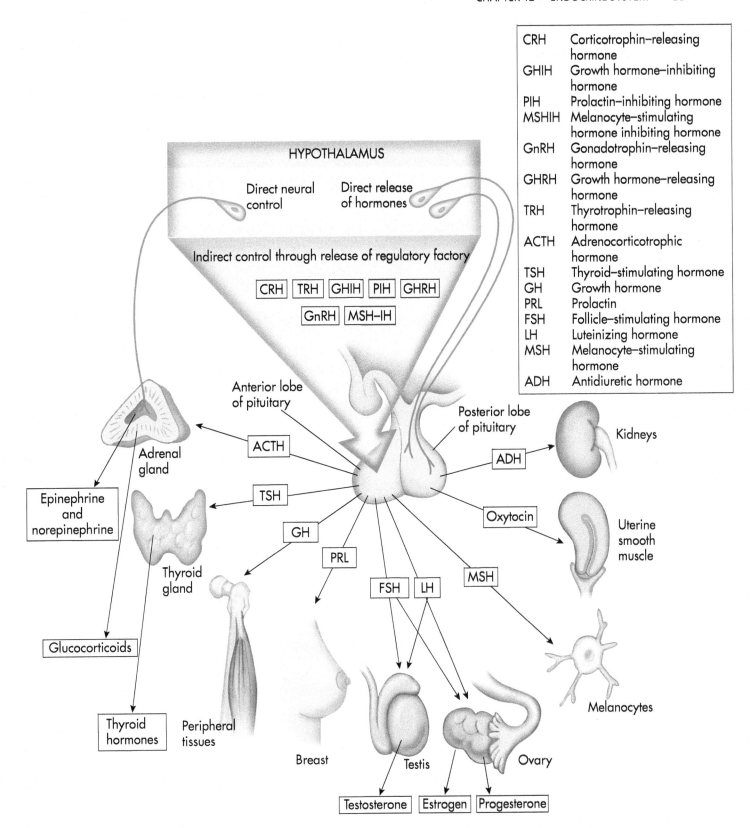

CRH	Corticotrophin–releasing hormone
GHIH	Growth hormone–inhibiting hormone
PIH	Prolactin–inhibiting hormone
MSHIH	Melanocyte–stimulating hormone inhibiting hormone
GnRH	Gonadotrophin–releasing hormone
GHRH	Growth hormone–releasing hormone
TRH	Thyrotrophin–releasing hormone
ACTH	Adrenocorticotrophic hormone
TSH	Thyroid–stimulating hormone
GH	Growth hormone
PRL	Prolactin
FSH	Follicle–stimulating hormone
LH	Luteinizing hormone
MSH	Melanocyte–stimulating hormone
ADH	Antidiuretic hormone

HYPOTHALAMUS

Direct neural control

Direct release of hormones

Indirect control through release of regulatory factory

CRH   TRH   GHIH   PIH   GHRH

GnRH   MSH–IH

Anterior lobe of pituitary

Posterior lobe of pituitary

Kidneys

ACTH

ADH

Adrenal gland

TSH

Oxytocin

Epinephrine and norepinephrine

GH

Uterine smooth muscle

PRL

Thyroid gland

FSH   LH

MSH

Glucocorticoids

Melanocytes

Thyroid hormones

Peripheral tissues

Breast

Testis

Ovary

Testosterone   Estrogen   Progesterone

FIGURE 12-2
The Pituitary Gland, Hormones, and Target Areas.

13 Reproductive System

 CONTENTS

REPRODUCTIVE SYSTEM	
Function	**To produce sex cells (gametes), eggs in female, sperm in male Fertilization with 23 pairs of chromosomes, half from each gamete**
Organs and Functions Male Female	*Penis*—External organ that contains urethra used to transport urine or deliver semen into female vagina during sexual intercourse *Scrotum*—External sac containing testes *Testes*—Reproductive glands located in scrotum that produce spermatozoa within the seminiferous tubules *Epididymus*—Site of sperm maturation and storage *Vas deferens*—Tubes conducting sperm from epididymus *Seminal vesicles*—Posterior to urinary bladder; produce and secrete semen; fluid, fructose, and prostaglandins with sperm *Prostate gland*—Small gland below bladder that contributes 25% fluid to semen for sperm motility *Urethra*—Long tube from bladder to tip of penis; transports semen and urine *Cowper's gland*—Secretes lubricant for urethra *Ovaries*—Female gonads that produce the ovum (egg) *Follicle*—Stores the immature eggs until ovulation *Fallopian tubes*—Oviducts propel egg from ovaries; fertilization occurs *Uterus*—Pear-shaped organ of smooth muscle holding embryo/fetus during pregnancy *Cervix*—Mouth of the uterus that protrudes down into the vagina *Vagina*—Part of birth canal; receives penis during intercourse *Vestibular glands*—Secrete mucus during sexual arousal *Mammary glands*—Found in breasts over the third to sixth ribs; secrete breast milk or lactate *Vulva*—Labia major and minor; two large and two small folds of tissue exterior and interior leading to vagina *Menses*—Onset of puberty; monthly sloughing off of the *endometrium,* the uterine lining, as blood; controlled by estrogen and progesterone hormones *Menopause*—Cessation of menstruation, reduced ovulation and hormone activity *Ovarian cycle*—Development of the immature follicle and ovum in ovary resulting with ovulation or rupture of the mature follicle
Benefits of Massage on the Reproductive System	Relaxation to body in general promoting an environment with less stress for conceiving

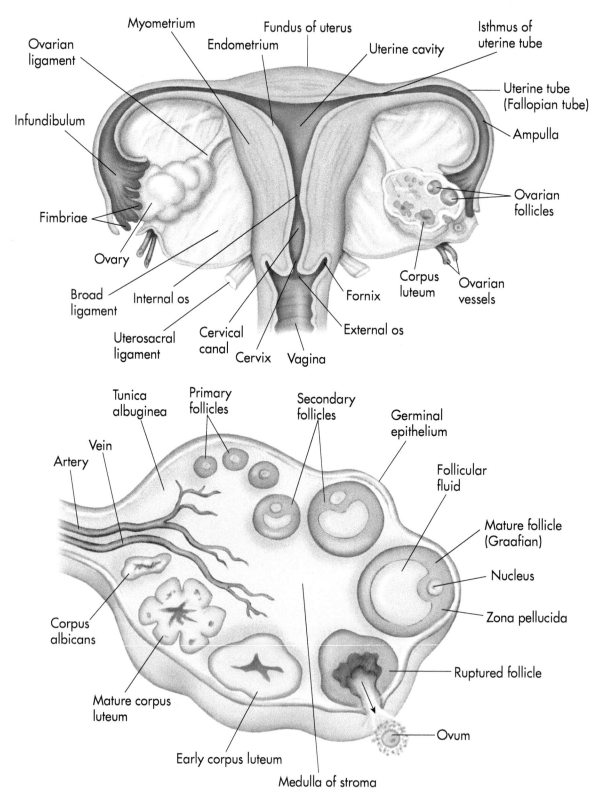

FIGURE 13-1
The Female Uterus and Ovary.

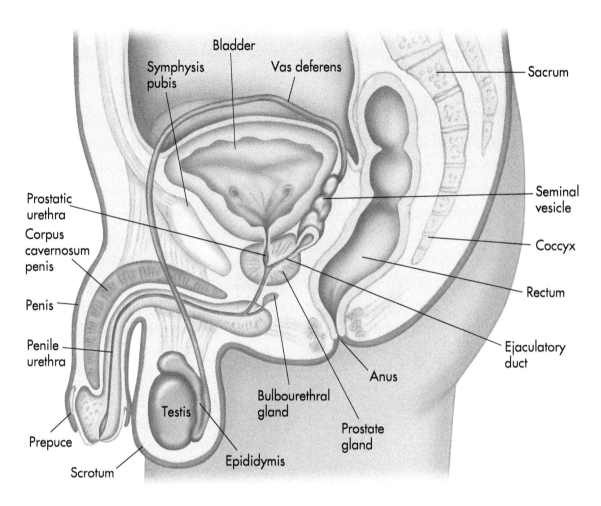

FIGURE 13-2
Male Reproductive System.

14

300 Questions with Answers and Rationales on Anatomy, Physiology, and Kinesiology

OBJECTIVES

Major areas of knowledge/content included in this chapter are based on the NCETMB, NCETM and MBLEx exam topics that cover general and detailed Anatomy, Physiology, and Kinesiology.

Exam Content Percentages:

NCETMB: 35%

NCETM: 33%

MBLEx: 25%

➤ Body Organization

➤ Medical Terminology

➤ Major Systems: Organs and Functions
Integumentary
Skeletal
Muscular
Nervous
Cardiovascular
Lymphatic
Respiratory
Digestive
Urinary
Reproductive

➤ Detailed Muscular Anatomy and Kinesiology

➤ Benefits of Massage

DIRECTIONS

Each of the questions or statements below is followed by four suggested answers or completions. Select **one answer** that is best in each case.

1. The tricuspid valve is found between the
   A. Right atrium and right ventricle
   B. Left ventricle and aorta
   C. Left ventricle and right ventricle
   D. Right atrium and left atrium

2. Which structure supports the body in the sitting position?
   A. Sacrum
   B. Coccyx
   C. Ischial tuberosity
   D. L5

3. Which statement is true about the Golgi tendon apparatus?
   A. Found in joint capsules
   B. Detects overall tension in tendon
   C. Originates in Purkinje fibers
   D. Activated by vagal reflex

4. Which muscles are major adductors?
   A. Pectoralis and deltoid
   B. Pectoralis and latissimus dorsi
   C. Deltoid and latissimus dorsi
   D. Biceps and deltoid

5. Which nerves supply the lower limbs?
   A. Dorsal primary rami
   B. Sciatic nerve
   C. Lumbosacral plexus
   D. Femoral nerve

6. There are _____ pairs of nerves arising from the spinal cord.
   A. 31
   B. 32
   C. 33
   D. 43

7. Which action does the sternocleidomastoid (SCM) not perform?
   A. Neck flexion
   B. Same side rotation
   C. Opposite side rotation
   D. Protraction of the head

8. The meninges include
   A. Spinal and cranial
   B. Cervical and abdominal
   C. Cervical and cranial
   D. Spinal and thoracic

9. The only joint in the upper body where the axial skeleton articulates with the appendicular skeleton is the
   A. Sternoclavicular
   B. Glenohumeral
   C. Sternoscapular
   D. Scapularclavicular

10. Which muscle adducts and medially rotates the femur at the hip?
    A. Gluteus medius
    B. Pectineus
    C. Quadratus femoris
    D. Tensor fascia latae

11. Which muscle is closest to the sciatic nerve?
    A. Gracilis
    B. Piriformis
    C. Gluteus medius
    D. Pectineus

12. Which is the most important element to combat infection?
    A. Red blood cells (RBCs)
    B. Platelets
    C. White blood cells (WBCs)
    D. Fibrinogen

13. Melatonin and serotonin are produced in the
    A. Pituitary gland
    B. Thyroid gland
    C. Sebaceous gland
    D. Pineal gland

14. The long tubules extending from the arachnoid and pia mater that act as one-way valves for the cerebrospinal fluid are the
    A. Erector pili
    B. Intake channels
    C. Arachnoid villi
    D. Pia mater

15. The movements at synovial joints may include flexion/extension, abduction/adduction, and
    A. Rotation
    B. Isolation
    C. Dynamics
    D. Pivot

16. The pericardial cavity is located within the
    A. Abdominopelvic cavity
    B. Cranial cavity
    C. Spinal cavity
    D. Thoracic cavity

17. A short, severe episode is referred to as
    A. Chronic
    B. Acute
    C. Terminal
    D. Minute

18. Which of the following factors contribute to muscle fatigue?
    A. Insufficient oxygen
    B. Depletion of glycogen
    C. Lactic acid buildup
    D. All of the above

19. A sudden involuntary contraction of a muscle is called a(an)
    A. Levator
    B. Proximal
    C. Isometric
    D. Spasm

20. Which type of lever is characterized as having the fulcrum between the effort and resistance? An example is the head resting on the vertebral column.
    A. 1st class
    B. 2nd class
    C. 3rd class
    D. 4th class

21. The prefix *ab* means
    A. Next to
    B. Away from
    C. Inner
    D. Soreness

22. Which facial muscle attaches into the mandible, angles of the mouth, and skin of the lower face?
    A. Buccinator
    B. Masseter
    C. Levator labii superioris
    D. Platysma

23. What is the spinal nerve contribution that composes the brachial plexus?
    A. C1–C4; T1
    B. C5–C8; T1
    C. C7–C8; T1
    D. T2–T12; L1

24. The prefix *macro* means
    A. Little
    B. Big
    C. Death
    D. Bacteria

25. Which of the following muscles are forearm flexors at the elbow joint?
    A. Biceps brachii, brachialis, triceps brachii
    B. Brachioradialis, anconeus, pronator quadratus
    C. Supinator, brachialis, biceps brachii
    D. Brachialis, brachioradialis, biceps brachii

26. What is the common origin for the scalenes?
    A. C2–C5
    B. C2–C7
    C. C1–T1
    D. C5–C7

27. Which of the following does not flex the wrist?
    A. Flexor carpi radialis
    B. Flexor carpi ulnaris
    C. Pronator quadratus
    D. Palmaris longus

28. Which of the following is not a hamstring muscle?
    A. Adductor magnus
    B. Biceps femoris

C. Semimembranosus

D. Semitendinosus

29. What muscle forms the outer layer of the lateral abdominal wall?

A. Rectus abdominis

B. Transversalis

C. Serratus anterior

D. External oblique

30. The primary flexor of the distal phalanges of the fingers is

A. Flexor carpi ulnaris

B. Pollices longus

C. Flexor digitorum profundus

D. Flexor carpi radialis

31. Inguinal nodes serve the purpose of draining lymph from the

A. Arm

B. Lower neck

C. Neck

D. Leg

32. The suffix *ism* means

A. Condition

B. Movement

C. Rate of exchange

D. Study of

33. The prefix *myo* means

A. Malignant

B. Muscle

C. Movement

D. Extensive

34. The membrane that surrounds the shaft of a long bone is the

A. Synovial membrane

B. Bursa

C. Periosteum

D. Peritoneum

35. With the elbow flexed, which muscle supinates the palm?

A. Pronator

B. Supinator

C. Quadrator

D. Brachialis

36. Muscle Energy Technique (MET) can be used to stretch the piriformis muscle in the supine position by

A. Rotating the knee laterally

B. Extending the knee to the chest

C. Adducting the knee over the opposite Anterior Superior Illiac Spine (ASIS)

D. Abducting the knee

37. Which is true of the adductor muscles along the medial femoral region of the hip?

A. Each has its origin on the pubic bone

B. Prevent hip flexion

C. Include the pectineus, and gracilis

D. Promote Abduction

38. Which of the following is true about terminal ganglia?

A. They are also known as collateral ganglia

B. They receive sympathetic preganglionic fibers

C. They lie close to the vertebral column and the large abdominal arteries

D. They are located at the end of an autonomic motor pathway

39. The prefix *nephro* means

A. Skin color

B. Bone

C. Kidney

D. Sleep

40. The function of lymph is to

A. Drain excess interstitial fluid

B. Transport lipids and red blood

C. Protect the body through immune response

D. A and C

41. Lymphocytes are also known as

A. B and C cells

B. L and C cells

C. B and T cells

D. D and C cells

42. Immunity acquired as the result of a vaccine is called

A. Passive naturally acquired immunity

B. Active naturally acquired immunity

C. Passive artificially acquired immunity

D. Active artificially acquired immunity

43. What muscle is the antagonist to the rhomboids?
    A. Latissimus dorsi
    B. Levator scapula
    C. Trapezius
    D. Serratus anterior

44. Which of the following moves an extremity away from the midline?
    A. Adductor
    B. Abductor
    C. Flexor
    D. Rotator

45. Which type of joint is found between the vertebrae?
    A. Ball and socket
    B. Gliding
    C. Condyloid
    D. Pivot

46. Which is a band of strong, fibrous tissue that connects the articular ends of bones and binds them together?
    A. Tendon
    B. Fascia
    C. Cancellous tissue
    D. Ligament

47. Which blood type is termed the "universal recipient"?
    A. O
    B. A
    C. B
    D. AB

48. An interosseous ligament of a syndesmosis area is located
    A. Near the articulation of a joint
    B. Between the radius and ulna to hold them together
    C. Around the patella bone
    D. Between the vertebrae

49. AIDS is the acronym for
    A. Active immunodeficiency syndrome
    B. Acquired immunodeficiency syndrome
    C. Antibody immunodeficiency syndrome
    D. Antigen immunodeficiency syndrome

50. The liver drains into the
    A. Hepatic portal vein
    B. Aorta
    C. Vena cava
    D. Pulmonary artery

51. The elbow is proximal to the hand and the hand is _____ to the elbow.
    A. Medial
    B. Anterior
    C. Distal
    D. Superior

52. Myelinated axon supported by neuroglia cells is
    A. White matter
    B. Gray matter
    C. Nucleus
    D. Ganglia

53. The _____ are the largest number of formed elements.
    A. Thrombocytes
    B. Leukocytes
    C. Erythrocytes
    D. Monocytes

54. The craniosacral system includes
    A. Nerves that control the parasympathetic division of the Autonomic Nervous System (ANS)
    B. Only the nerves that go to the head
    C. Nerves located in the thoracic area
    D. All periferial nerves

55. The plantar region is the most _____ of all the body regions.
    A. Distal
    B. Inferior
    C. Anterior
    D. Posterior

56. The radiocarpal joint is a(an)
    A. Hinge joint
    B. Ellipsoid joint
    C. Metacarpalphalangeal joint
    D. Pivot joint

57. Although the biceps brachii is the most visible flexor, another primary flexor muscle is the
    A. Brachialis
    B. Pronator quadratus
    C. Anconeus
    D. Triceps brachii

58. Where is the medial malleolus?
    A. Calcaneus
    B. Talus
    C. Fibula
    D. Tibia

59. The left coronary artery arises from the
    A. Ascending aorta
    B. Descending aorta
    C. Left atrium
    D. Left ventricle

60. Which part of a neuron carries impulses toward the cell body?
    A. Dendrite
    B. Axon
    C. Motor unit
    D. Schwann cell

61. The capitulum of the humerus articulates with the
    A. Radial tuberosity
    B. Head of the radius
    C. Olecranon of the ulna
    D. Coracoid

62. The median nerve is part of the
    A. Sacral plexus
    B. Sciatic nerve
    C. Brachial plexus
    D. Lumbar plexus

63. The joint that allows supination and pronation is the
    A. Radiocarpal joint
    B. Radioulnar joint
    C. Humeroradial joint
    D. Tibiofemoral joint

64. Which muscle does the axillary nerve innervate?
    A. Deltoid
    B. Brachial

65. C. Pectoralis major
    D. Bracioradialis

65. The wrist and fingers can be extended by the
    A. Extensor carpi radialis, longus, brevis, extensor digitorum, and ulnaris
    B. Brachioradialis
    C. Extensor carpi ulnaris and digitorum
    D. Extensor carpi radialis longus and brevis

66. Which is the most highly vascularized tissue?
    A. Muscle
    B. Ligament
    C. Nervous
    D. Tendon

67. Which is lower than normal adult body temperature?
    A. 37°C
    B. 98°F
    C. 98.6°F
    D. 39°C

68. The nervous system includes which two separate systems?
    A. CNS and PNF
    B. CVS and PNS
    C. CNS and PNS
    D. CIS and PNF

69. Which muscles abduct the scapula?
    A. Serratus anterior/pectoralis minor
    B. Rhomboids
    C. Latissimus dorsi
    D. Trapezius

70. Which is(are) not a part of the CNS?
    A. Cranial nerves
    B. Cerebellum
    C. White tracts
    D. Medulla oblongata

71. The external iliac artery supplies blood to
    A. The lower limbs
    B. All parts of the trunk
    C. The neck and back
    D. The pelvic organs

72. Which muscle plantar flexes and everts the foot?
    A. Tibialis anterior
    B. Gastrocnemius
    C. Plantaris
    D. Peroneus longus

73. The autonomic nervous system (ANS) is part of the
    A. Collating nervous system
    B. Enteric nervous system
    C. Peripheral nervous system
    D. Central nervous system

74. The normal resting pulse rate range is
    A. 70–80 beats per minute
    B. 80–90 beats per minute
    C. 120–130 beats per minute
    D. 130–140 beats per minute

75. Which muscle extends the femur?
    A. Soleus
    B. Gluteus minimus
    C. Gluteus maximus
    D. Peroneus

76. What is the normal systolic pressure?
    A. 80 mm/Hg
    B. 90 mm Hg
    C. 120 mm Hg
    D. 140 mm Hg

77. The diaphragm contracts on
    A. Inspiration
    B. Expiration
    C. Both
    D. Neither

78. Lymph is interstitial fluid consisting of
    A. Water, cell debris, gases, metabolic wastes, bacteria
    B. Water and gas
    C. Blood, lymphocytes, and bacteria
    D. Water alone

79. The nerve(s) that innervate the five flexor muscles of the forearm is(are) the
    A. Radial
    B. Median
    C. Median and ulnar
    D. Radial and ulnar

80. A medial collateral ligament
    A. Connects the femur to the tibia
    B. Connects the femur to the fibula
    C. Crosses the middle of the knee joint
    D. Attaches to the anterior cruciate ligament

81. Which muscle is not a part of the rotator cuff?
    A. Supraspinatus
    B. Infraspinatus
    C. Teres major
    D. Teres minor

82. The homeostatic responses of the body are regulated by which two systems?
    A. Digestive and urinary
    B. Reproductive and endocrine
    C. Endocrine and nervous
    D. Cardiovascular and respiratory

83. The most abundant inorganic substance in humans is
    A. Carbohydrate
    B. Lipid
    C. Oxygen
    D. Water

84. Which of the following is an acidic pH?
    A. 14
    B. 12
    C. 10
    D. 6

85. What type of synovial joint is the ankle?
    A. Pivot
    B. Gliding
    C. Hinge
    D. Ellipsoid

86. Neurotransmitters are
    A. Chemical messengers
    B. Short hairs that move the neurons
    C. Flagella
    D. Prokaryotes

87. The ball and socket joint associated with the pelvis is the
    A. Pubic symphysis
    B. Sacroiliac
    C. Iliofemoral
    D. Femoriliac

88. The space between two nerve cells is called the
    A. Borland gap
    B. Axolemma
    C. Renshaw opening
    D. Synapse

89. The outermost layer of epidermis is composed of
    A. Dermis epithelium
    B. Subcutaneous cuboidal epithelium
    C. Stratified columnar epithelium
    D. Stratified squamous epithelium

90. Which of the following is true about aging of the integumentary system starting with the late 40s?
    A. Collagen fibers increase
    B. Elasticity increases in elastic fibers
    C. Fibroblasts decrease in number
    D. Hair and nail growth tends to speed up

91. What is the salt that makes bone matrix hard?
    A. Calcium phosphate
    B. Potassium chloride
    C. Sodium chloride
    D. Calcium chloride

92. Which of the following processes forms a joint?
    A. Meatus
    B. Crest
    C. Tuberosity
    D. Condyle

93. Which of the following are paired cranial bones?
    A. Occipital and sphenoid
    B. Temporal and parietal
    C. Frontal and ethmoid
    D. Parietal and ethmoid

94. Which of the following is true with regard to the humerus?
    A. The olecranon fossa is an anterior depression that receives the ulna's olecranon process
    B. The medial and lateral epicondyles are rough projections on either side of the proximal end
    C. The radial fossa is a posterior depression that receives the head of the radius when the forearm is flexed
    D. Its trochlea articulates with the ulna

95. The prominence felt on the medial surface of the ankle is the
    A. Fibular notch
    B. Condyle
    C. Malleolus
    D. Tarsus

96. The largest and strongest tarsal bone is the
    A. Calcaneus
    B. Cuboid
    C. Lateral cuneiform
    D. Navicular

97. Which of the following joint classifications is described as freely movable?
    A. Amphiarthrosis
    B. Cartilaginous
    C. Diarthrosis
    D. Fibrous

98. The joint between the trapezium carpal bone and the thumb's metacarpal is which kind of joint?
    A. Ball-and-socket
    B. Ellipsoidal
    C. Gliding
    D. Saddle

99. Which subtype of diarthrosis joint is found in the knee, elbow, and ankle?
    A. Ball-and-socket
    B. Ellipsoidal
    C. Gliding
    D. Hinge

100. Which of the following is an intra-articular ligament of the knee?
    A. Anterior cruciate
    B. Arcuate popliteal
    C. Medial collateral
    D. Oblique popliteal

101. Which of the following is true concerning the microscopic anatomy of skeletal muscle?
    A. A sarcolemma is the muscle fiber's cytoplasm
    B. The skeletal muscle fiber is a long, cylindrical cell
    C. The sarcoplasma is the muscle fiber's plasma membrane
    D. Each skeletal muscle cell has several nuclei

102. Dopamine is
    A. A chemical neurotransmitter
    B. A hormone
    C. Both a neurotransmitter and a hormone
    D. Neither a neurotransmitter nor a hormone

103. The myelin sheath is a layer surrounding the neuron that
    A. Insulates
    B. Infiltrates
    C. Exfoliates
    D. Is gray matter

104. There are two main types of cells in the nervous tissue
    A. Neurons and Golgi cells
    B. Spine cells and neurons
    C. Protons and Schwann cells
    D. Neurons and axon cells

105. If a muscle is not used, the resulting condition is called
    A. Atrophy
    B. Myotrophy
    C. Hypertrophy
    D. Actintrophy

106. Which direction of muscle fiber is described as running parallel to the body's midline?
    A. Brevis
    B. Oblique
    C. Rectus abdominis
    D. Serratus

107. Which cheek muscle is a facial muscle?
    A. Buccinator
    B. Masseter
    C. Mentalis
    D. Platysma

108. At which vertebral level does the spinal cord end?
    A. 1st lumbar
    B. Between 1st and 2nd lumbar
    C. 5th lumbar
    D. 2nd sacral

109. Which of the following is not a functional component of a reflex arc?
    A. Brain
    B. Effector
    C. Motor neuron
    D. Receptor

110. Which reflex is essential to maintaining muscle tone and adjusts muscle performance during exercise?
    A. Crossed extensor
    B. Flexor
    C. Stretch
    D. Tendon

111. The deltoid muscle abducts the arm and is often used as a site of injection. Which nerve stimulates it?
    A. Axillary
    B. Median
    C. Musculocutaneous
    D. Radial

112. The sciatic nerve is actually two nerves. Which nerves compose the sciatic nerve?
    A. Common peroneal and pudendal
    B. Tibial and medial plantars
    C. Medial and lateral plantars
    D. Common peroneal and tibial

113. Which of the following are involved in the abduction of the arm?
    A. Deltoid and subscapularis
    B. Supraspinatus and infraspinatus
    C. Teres major and teres minor
    D. Supraspinatus and deltoid

114. Which of the following are involved in the adduction of the arm?
    A. Pectoralis major and latissimus dorsi
    B. Infraspinatus and teres major
    C. Teres minor
    D. Pectoralis major, teres major, teres minor, latissimus dorsi

115. Which of the following is not part of the erector spinae muscles?
    A. Iliocostalis
    B. Longissimus
    C. Spinalis
    D. Platysma

116. Which of the following muscles does not abduct the thigh?
    A. Gluteus maximus
    B. Gluteus medius
    C. Gluteus minimus
    D. Sartorius

117. Which of the following laterally rotates the thigh?
    A. Obturator externus
    B. Obturator internus
    C. Piriformis
    D. Obturator externus and piriformis

118. Which of the following is the longest muscle involved in crossing one's leg?
    A. Gastrocnemius
    B. Rectus femoris
    C. Sartorius
    D. Semimembranosus

119. Which of the following brain areas are thought to be associated with memory?
    A. Frontal lobe and temporal lobe association cortex
    B. Occipital lobe and parietal lobe association cortex
    C. Parts of the pons and medulla
    D. Both A and B

120. The major role for initiating and controlling precise, discrete muscular movements comes from the
    A. Center of the thalamus
    B. Bulk of the hypothalamus
    C. Area lateral to the septum
    D. Motor portions of the cerebral cortex

121. Which is a natural opiate produced by the brain to diminish pain?
    A. Endocrine
    B. Seratonin
    C. Endorphin
    D. Melatonin

122. Which part of the brain regulates the balance of sympathetic versus parasympathetic activity?
    A. Hypothalamus
    B. Medulla
    C. Pineal gland
    D. Pons

123. The sac that holds urine before it is expelled from the body is the
    A. Kidney
    B. Rectum
    C. Urinary bladder
    D. Nephron

124. Which is true of glucagon?
    A. Accelerates the formation of glycogen from glucose (glycogenesis)
    B. Promotes glucose formation from lactate and certain amino acids
    C. Lowers the blood glucose level
    D. Does all of the above functions

125. Which of the following is true about antidiuretic hormone (ADH)?
    A. During dehydration, ADH increases the rate of perspiration production
    B. Alcohol stimulates ADH secretion
    C. Pain, trauma, and anxiety suppress the secretion of ADH
    D. It is also called vasopressin

126. Blood pressure is lowest in
    A. Veins
    B. Capillaries
    C. Arteries
    D. Arterioles

127. Plasma constitutes what percentage of the blood?
    A. 20%
    B. 40%
    C. 55%
    D. 45%

128. Blood carries
    A. Carbon dioxide
    B. Metabolic waste
    C. Oxygen
    D. Gases, wastes, salts, and hormones

129. In the middle of the thoracic cavity is a space assigned to the heart called the
    A. Pleural space
    B. Pericardial space
    C. Mediastinum
    D. Sternal notch

130. A group of nerve cells that lie outside the CNS is called
    A. Gray matter
    B. White matter
    C. Ganglia
    D. Nucleus

131. The pulmonary circulation carries deoxygenated blood from the right ventricle to the air sacs of the lungs and returns oxygenated blood from the lungs to the
    A. Right atrium
    B. Left ventricle
    C. Left atrium
    D. Pulmonary valve

132. The 1st and largest branch of the arch of the aorta is the
    A. Subclavian
    B. Coronary
    C. Carotid
    D. Brachiocephalic

133. Within the brain, all veins drain into the
    A. Carotid artery
    B. Internal and external jugular veins
    C. Vertebral veins
    D. Cardiac veins

134. Lymph in the right leg would drain into the
    A. Right lymphatic duct
    B. Left thoracic duct
    C. Cisterna chyli
    D. Both B and C

135. In males, the tube that carries semen on its way out of the body is the
    A. Prostate
    B. Urethra
    C. Ureter
    D. Fallopian tube

136. The end product of glycolysis is pyruvic acid, and its fate depends on
    A. The body cellular need
    B. The availability of oxygen
    C. The transport in the bloodstream
    D. All of the above

137. The mineral that is found in the hemoglobin of blood and that carries oxygen to body cells is
    A. Phosphorus
    B. Calcium
    C. Magnesium
    D. Iron

138. Renal calculi are
    A. Tubes leaving the nephron
    B. Factors that cause a hardening of the kidneys
    C. Kidney stones
    D. Involved in urinary tract infections

139. An excessive amount of nitrogenous waste products in the blood is known as
    A. Nitrogena
    B. Toxemia
    C. Azotemia
    D. Enuresis

140. The primary method of water movement in and out of body compartments is
    A. Diffusion
    B. Osmosis
    C. Filtration
    D. Hydrolysis

141. Which of the following is true concerning cartilage?
    A. Except for that in the perichondrium, cartilage has no blood vessels or nerves
    B. The cells of mature cartilage are known as lacunae
    C. The resilience of cartilage is due to its collagen fiber
    D. There are three kinds of cartilage: hyaline, mosaic, and elastic

142. You have a headache so you rub your temple area immediately posterior to the zygomatic part of the orbit. You are rubbing the skin, connective tissue, and muscle over which bone?
    A. Frontal
    B. Parietal
    C. Sphenoid
    D. Temporal

143. Which of the following is true concerning the scapula?
    A. The end of the spine projects as the expanded process called the coracoid
    B. The coracoid articulates with the clavicle
    C. The glenoid fossa is where the scapula and humerus articulate
    D. The lateral border of the scapula is near the vertebral column

144. The average meal requires about _____ hours for complete absorption.
    A. 4
    B. 10
    C. 12
    D. None of the above

145. The principle of a negative feedback system is
    A. To regulate hormone levels in the blood
    B. The stimuli that triggers an endocrine gland
    C. Like a thermostat in a house
    D. All of the above

146. The pancreas is an endocrine gland that secretes _____ and _____ to maintain normal blood glucose levels.
    A. Insulin, parathormone
    B. Insulin, glucagon

C. Glucagon, pancreatic juice
D. Insulin, progesterone

147. A synaptic transmission of a nerve impulse is
    A. A one-way nerve conduction from the axon to dendrite
    B. A neurotransmitter chemical
    C. A two-way nerve conduction between two axons
    D. Controlled by the vagus nerve

148. An example of a neurotransmitter is
    A. Acetylcholine
    B. Dopamine
    C. Serotonin
    D. All of the above

149. A frequently used pulse point is the
    A. Jugular vein
    B. Carotid artery
    C. Popliteal artery
    D. Femoral artery

150. Which muscle tendons form the Achilles tendon?
    A. Soleus and tibialis
    B. Achilles and gastrocnemius
    C. Gastrocnemius and soleus
    D. Peroneus and soleus

151. _____ nerves regulate blood pressure.
    A. Parasympathetic
    B. Sympathetic
    C. Peripherial
    D. Cranial

152. Venous blood is found in which vessel?
    A. Pulmonary vein
    B. Pulmonary artery
    C. Aorta
    D. Arterioles

153. The kidneys are located
    A. In the gastrointestinal (GI) tract
    B. Below the 5th lumbar vertebra
    C. Below the 12th thoracic vertebra
    D. Above the liver

154. The acromion process is part of which bone?
     A. Humerus
     B. Thoracic vertebra
     C. Clavicle
     D. Scapula

155. Dorsiflexors of the ankle include
     A. Tibialis anterior, gastrocnemeius
     B. Extensor digitorum and Achilles tendon
     C. Peroneus longus, brevis
     D. Tibialis anterior, peroneus tertius

156. The deepest muscle at the back of the knee is
     A. Plantaris
     B. Popliteus
     C. Tibialis posterior
     D. Soleus

157. Medial and lateral condyles can be found on the
     A. Femur and tibia
     B. Pelvis
     C. Tibia and fibula
     D. Radius and ulna

158. The olecranon process is found on the
     A. Humerus
     B. Tibia
     C. Radius
     D. Ulna

159. The obturator innervates muscles in the lower body including the
     A. Quadraceps
     B. Hamstrings
     C. Rectus femoris
     D. Gracilus, adductors, obturator extermus

160. Endocrine glands
     A. Use ducts to transport their products to the site of action
     B. Include sebaceous and salivary glands
     C. Produce secretions that diffuse directly into the blood
     D. Both A and B

161. Chemicals that facilitate, arouse, or inhibit the transmission of nerve impulses across synapses are
     A. Hormones
     B. Histamines
     C. Steroids
     D. Neurotransmitters

162. The muscle that is responsible for the resisting or opposing action is called the
     A. Agonist or prime
     B. Synergist
     C. Antagonist
     D. Insertion

163. A sac-like membrane that contains synovial fluid and is provided around joints to prevent friction is the
     A. Suture
     B. Tendon
     C. Periosteum
     D. Bursa

164. The greatest range of motion (ROM) is from
     A. Pivot joints
     B. Hinge joints
     C. Ball-and-socket joints
     D. Saddle joints

165. The muscle causing the desired action is the
     A. Agonist or prime mover
     B. Retinaculum
     C. Antagonist
     D. Insertion

166. The three divisions of the small intestines start to finish are the
     A. Duodenum, ileum, and jejunum
     B. Ascending, transverse, and descending
     C. Jejunum, ileum, and duodenum
     D. Duodenum, jejunum, and ileum

167. The major type of muscle in the GI tract is the
     A. Cardiac
     B. Voluntary
     C. Skeletal
     D. Smooth

168. The mechanical and chemical process that occurs as food is converted into an absorbable state is called
     A. Ingestion
     B. Digestion
     C. Homeostasis
     D. Absorption

169. The main parts of the heart's conducting system is/are
   A. Sinoatrial (SA) node
   B. Septum
   C. Atrioventricular (AV) node
   D. Both A and C

170. Gas exchange between blood and the tissue is called
   A. Environmental respiration
   B. External respiration
   C. Internal respiration
   D. Diffusion of gas

171. The sounds created by a beating heart are due to the
   A. Contraction of the ventricles
   B. Closing of the heart valves
   C. Blood moving from one heart chamber to another
   D. Compression from the respiratory system

172. The main muscle of respiration is the
   A. Scalene
   B. SCM
   C. Diaphragm
   D. Rectus abdominus

173. The main venous portal system, which collects blood from the digestive organs and delivers this blood to the liver for processing, is called the portal system
   A. Digestive
   B. Intestinal
   C. Gastric
   D. Hepatic

174. During this phase of pulmonary ventilation, air moves out of the lungs during normal _____
   A. Inhalation
   B. Exhalation
   C. Pulmonary apnea
   D. Tissue respiration

175. Which of the following is *not* one of the functions of the cardiovascular system?
   A. Transportation and distribution of gases, nutrients, antibodies, and hormones
   B. Protection of the body through disease-fighting white blood cells

   C. Synthesis of vitamin A, D, and E
   D. Protection of the body through the clotting mechanism

176. Which of the following structures collect and filter lymph?
   A. Lymph nodes, arteries
   B. Spleen and gall bladder
   C. Liver
   D. Lymph nodes, spleen, tonsils

177. The functional contractile unit in muscle fibers composed of actin and myosin filaments is the
   A. Sarcomere
   B. Agonist
   C. Myofibril
   D. Penniform

178. In general, where do the flexors of the wrist originate?
   A. Lateral epicondyle of the humerus
   B. Greater tubercle of the humerus
   C. Medial epicondyle of the humerus
   D. Lesser tubercle of the humerus

179. Which muscle expands the thoracic cavity?
   A. Internal intercostals
   B. Diaphragm
   C. Multifidus
   D. Levator scapula

180. A synergist to the gluteus medius in abduction of the hip is the
   A. Gracilis
   B. Pectineus
   C. Tensor fascia latae
   D. Adductor magnus

181. Contraction of the iliopsoas will cause the pectineus to
   A. Lengthen
   B. Shorten
   C. Spasm
   D. Cramp

182. Engaging this muscle will bring the arm forward
   A. Latissimus dorsi
   B. Teres major
   C. Infraspinatus
   D. Coracobrachialis

183. This muscle is used when rising from a seated position:
    A. Gluteus maximus
    B. Gluteus medius
    C. Gluteus minimus
    D. Tensor fascia latae

184. External rotation of the humerus will cause the palm of the hand to
    A. Retract
    B. Protract
    C. Supinate
    D. Pronate

185. An antagonist to the biceps is the
    A. Triceps
    B. Brachialis
    C. Brachioradialis
    D. Supinator

186. This plane divides the body into equal right and left halves
    A. Midsagittal
    B. Coronal
    C. Sagittal
    D. Frontal

187. The body cavity that contains the thoracic and abdominopelvic regions is the
    A. Dorsal
    B. Ventral
    C. Vertebral
    D. Cranial

188. This muscle separates the thoracic and abdominopelvic regions
    A. Esophagus
    B. Rectus abdominis
    C. Diaphragm
    D. Serratus anterior

189. Which muscles are known as entrappers because they can entrap a nerve or nerve plexus?
    A. Brachioradialis, biceps, scalenes
    B. Scalenes, piriformis, pectoralis minor
    C. Biceps, piriformis, scalenes
    D. Pectoralis minor, biceps, brachioradialis

190. The action of the deltoid muscles working as a group is called
    A. Extension
    B. Adduction
    C. Abduction
    D. Flexion

191. In muscle contraction, the greatest amount of movement takes place at the
    A. Origin
    B. Insertion
    C. Belly
    D. Extensor

192. Which muscle stabilizes the scapula by preventing extreme elevation and protraction of the clavicle?
    A. Subscapularis
    B. Subclavius
    C. Supraspinatus
    D. Serratus anterior

193. Which abdominal muscle rotates the trunk to the same side?
    A. External oblique
    B. Internal oblique
    C. Rectus abdominis
    D. Transverse abdominis

194. The strongest elbow flexor is the
    A. Brachioradialis
    B. Biceps brachii
    C. Coracobrachialis
    D. Brachialis

195. The action of the triceps as a group is
    A. Extension of the humerus
    B. Extension of the elbow
    C. Flexion of the elbow
    D. Flexion of the humerus

196. Which is not an attachment of the SCM?
    A. Styloid process
    B. Mastoid process
    C. Medial clavicle
    D. Manubrium of the sternum

197. The muscle that does not attach to the humerus is the
    A. Pectoralis major
    B. Biceps brachii
    C. Subscapularis
    D. Brachialis

198. The longest muscle in the body is the
    A. Great saphenous
    B. Gracilis
    C. Sartorius
    D. Pectineus

199. When the humerus is rotated laterally, which muscle is stretched?
    A. Infraspinatus
    B. Teres minor
    C. Teres major
    D. Pectoralis minor

200. Which muscle has no attachments on the scapula?
    A. Pectoralis major
    B. Subscapularis
    C. Rhomboid
    D. Pectoralis minor

201. The functions of the erector spinae muscles are
    A. Unilateral flexion of the spine, extension of the hip bilaterally
    B. Bilateral flexion of the spine, flexion of the hip unilaterally
    C. Bilateral extension of the spine, lateral flexion of the spine
    D. Unilateral extension of the spine, bilateral flexion of the spine

202. Which muscles invert the foot?
    A. Peroneus longus and brevis
    B. Tibialis anterior and posterior
    C. Flexor and extensor digitorum longus
    D. Gastrocnemius and soleus

203. A muscular contraction in which the length of the muscle shortens is called
    A. Isometric
    B. Static
    C. Isotonic
    D. Eccentric

204. The aorta branches into which three trunks?
    A. Axillary, cranial, and femoral
    B. Brachiocephalic, thoracic, and abdominal
    C. Peroneal, cranial, and abdominal
    D. Brachiocephalic, femoral, and axillary

205. For muscular contraction to occur, which of the following molecules are needed?
    A. Actin, myosin
    B. Calcitonin, tropin
    C. Myosin, melanin
    D. Actin, tropin

206. A motor neuron sends information from
    A. CNS to muscles/glands
    B. Sensory receptors to CNS
    C. ANF to PNS
    D. PNS to ANF

207. Stimulation of the sympathetic nervous system will
    A. Increase heart rate
    B. Decrease heart rate
    C. Decrease tidal volume
    D. Increase insulin dependence

208. The passage of food throughout the intestinal tract is possible because of
    A. Mastication
    B. Fermentation
    C. Peristalsis
    D. Defibrillation

209. The pulmonary veins carry _____ blood from the lungs to the heart.
    A. Oxygenated
    B. Deoxygenated
    C. Carbon dioxide-rich
    D. Carbon monoxide-rich

210. Which of the following is not part of the axial skeleton?
    A. Hyoid
    B. Ribs
    C. Clavicle
    D. Vertebrae

211. Proprioceptors identify which of the following?
    A. Light changes in the environment and pupils
    B. Pain and directions of movement
    C. Receptors in muscles, joints, tendons respond to motion or movement of body
    D. Chemical changes

212. The direction of urine output is
    A. Bladder, ureters, urethra, kidneys
    B. Kidneys, urethra, ureters, bladder
    C. Urethra, ureters, kidneys, bladder
    D. Kidneys, ureters, bladder, urethra

213. The "master gland" of the endocrine system is the
    A. Thymus
    B. Pituitary
    C. Adrenal
    D. Thyroid

214. The nephron is the functional unit of the
    A. Cell
    B. Nervous system
    C. Circulatory system
    D. Kidney

215. After a muscular contraction, a muscle loses the ability to respond to stimulation. This is known as the _____ period.
    A. Latent
    B. Refractory
    C. Relaxation
    D. Contraction

216. The principal function of insulin is to
    A. Lower blood glucose levels
    B. Raise blood glucose levels
    C. Lower blood count
    D. Raise blood count

217. The part of the brain responsible for coordination and balance is called the
    A. Cerebellum
    B. Cerebrum
    C. Medulla
    D. Thalamus

218. The molecule that binds oxygen and carbon dioxide in erythrocytes is
    A. Antigen
    B. Thrombin
    C. Hemoglobin
    D. Globulin

219. The cells involved with the immune system are called
    A. Erythrocytes
    B. Leukocytes
    C. Thrombocytes
    D. Chondrocytes

220. A muscle contraction in which the muscle fiber length is constant is called
    A. Isotonic
    B. Isometric
    C. Concentric
    D. Eccentric

221. The ileocecal valve is located between the
    A. Stomach and small intestine
    B. Small intestine and large intestine
    C. Esophagus and stomach
    D. Gallbladder and liver

222. The Golgi tendon is responsible for detecting change in muscle
    A. Length
    B. Striation
    C. Composition
    D. Tension

223. Which of the following carries deoxygenated blood to the lungs?
    A. Pulmonary veins
    B. Pulmonary arteries
    C. Aorta
    D. Inferior vena cava

224. Which muscle(s) are involved in forced expiration?
    A. External intercostals
    B. SCM
    C. Internal intercostals
    D. Scalenes

225. Which nerve innervates the frontalis muscle?
    A. Vagus (X)
    B. Facial (VII)
    C. Trigeminal (V)
    D. Trochlear (IV)

226. What proprioceptor is involved while massaging a client and a muscle contraction releases?
     A. Spindle cells
     B. Golgi tendon
     C. Chemoreceptor
     D. Thermoreceptor

227. Irritability of a muscle is defined as the ability of a muscle to
     A. Return to its original shape after contraction
     B. Stretch
     C. Receive and react to stimuli
     D. Contract or shorten

228. An increase in the lumen of the vein is called
     A. Vasoconstriction
     B. Phlebitis
     C. Vasodilation
     D. Thrombosis

229. One complete cycle of inhalation and expiration is known as
     A. Cellular respiration
     B. Forced expiration
     C. Forced inspiration
     D. Tidal volume

230. The origin of the gluteus maximus is the
     A. Superior gluteal line
     B. Middle gluteal line
     C. Inferior gluteal line
     D. Linea aspera

231. Which muscle crosses two joints?
     A. Popliteus
     B. Brachialis
     C. Soleus
     D. Rectus femoris

232. The insertion of the triceps is the
     A. Lateral epicondyle of the humerus
     B. Medial epicondlyle of the humerus
     C. Olecranon process of the radius
     D. Olecranon process of the ulna

233. All of these muscle extend the humerus except
     A. Latissimus dorsi
     B. Biceps brachii
     C. Teres major
     D. Teres minor

234. The strongest lateral hip rotator is
     A. Iliopsoas
     B. Adductor magnus
     C. Piriformis
     D. Sartorius

235. Which muscles are located in the femoral region?
     A. Hamstrings
     B. Quadriceps
     C. Adductors
     D. Scalenes

236. Which tendons make up the Achilles tendon?
     A. Gastrocnemius and soleus
     B. Plantaris and semitendinosus
     C. Semitendinosus and soleus
     D. Biceps femoris and gastrocnemius

237. All of the following abduct the hip except
     A. Gluteus medius
     B. Sartorius
     C. Gracilis
     D. Tensor fascia latae

238. Which muscle would you be affecting when massaging lateral to the vastus lateralis?
     A. Pectineus
     B. Tensor fasciae late
     C. Vastus medialis
     D. Gracilis

239. Which muscle's action is elevation and downward rotation of the scapula?
     A. Levator scapula
     B. Trapezius
     C. Rhomboid
     D. Teres major

240. Which muscle stabilizes the humerus in the glenoid fossa and abducts the humerus?
     A. Teres major
     B. Trapezius
     C. Subscapularis
     D. Supraspinatus

241. The muscle that opposes the serratus anterior is the
     A. Teres major
     B. Infraspinatus
     C. Rhomboid major
     D. Levator scapula

242. The biceps femoris performs which two actions?
    A. Extension and medial rotation
    B. Flexion and medial rotation
    C. Extension and abduction
    D. Flexion and extension

243. Which muscle is shortened when a person is wearing high-heeled shoes?
    A. Tibialis anterior
    B. Peroneus tertius
    C. Popliteus
    D. Gastrocnemius

244. A client comes in for a massage, and the scapula is still abducted after the massage. Which muscle do you recommend that the client stretch?
    A. Pectoralis minor
    B. Rhomboids
    C. Subscapularis
    D. Latissimus dorsi

245. What do you call the bony prominence at the proximal end of the ulna?
    A. Medial epicondyle
    B. Lateral epicondyle
    C. Olecranon process
    D. Styloid process

246. When massaging the lateral head of the fibula, of which structure should you be careful?
    A. Popliteal endangerment site
    B. Peroneal nerve
    C. Tibial nerve
    D. Femoral nerve

247. With your client in the supine position, how do you expose the serratus anterior?
    A. Lateral rotation and adduction of the arm
    B. Medial rotation and adduction of the arm
    C. Horizontal abduction of the arm
    D. Horizontal adduction of the arm

248. Hypercontraction of the pectoralis minor causes rounded shoulders. Which muscle would be weak and overstretched?
    A. Pectoralis minor
    B. Rhomboid
    C. Subclavius
    D. Levator scapula

249. All of these muscles share a common attachment
    A. Biceps brachii, brachioradialis, coracobrachialis
    B. Coracobrachialis, brachioradialis, pectoralis minor
    C. Pectoralis minor, coracobrachialis, brachioradialis
    D. Biceps brachii, coracobrachialis, pectoralis minor

250. All of the following dorsiflex the ankle except the
    A. Tibialis anterior
    B. Extensor hallucis longus
    C. Peroneus longus
    D. Peroneus tertius

251. Which muscle is involved in shin splints?
    A. Soleus
    B. Tibialis anterior and posterior
    C. Poplitius
    D. Plantaris

252. The hamstring muscles from medial to lateral are
    A. Biceps femoris, semitendinosus, semimembranosus
    B. Semitendinosus, semimembranosus, biceps femoris
    C. Semimembranosus, semitendinosus, rectus femoris
    D. Semimembranosus, semitendinosus, biceps femoris

253. Where do you palpate the sciatic notch?
    A. Deep in the adductor region
    B. Deep in the gluteal region
    C. Deep in the femoral region
    D. Deep in the inguinal region

254. Which movement brings the arm closer to the midline?
    A. Abduction
    B. Adduction
    C. Circumduction
    D. Supination

255. We do not massage the SCM bilaterally because of the
    A. Femoral artery
    B. Common carotid artery

C. Peroneal artery
D. Tibial artery

256. The muscle(s) located in the posterior femoral region is/are the
   A. Quadriceps
   B. Hamstrings
   C. Latissimus dorsi
   D. Triceps brachii

257. The muscle of the rotator cuff responsible for medial rotation is
   A. Supraspinatus
   B. Infraspinatus
   C. Teres minor
   D. Subscapularis

258. This muscle initiates walking
   A. Gluteus medius
   B. Iliopsoas
   C. Semimembranosus
   D. Tibialis posterior

259. A bursa sac is usually located
   A. Inside of a joint
   B. Between the bone and a tendon
   C. Between muscle and tendon
   D. Between muscle and bone

260. What kind of joint allows movement in a single plane?
   A. Hinge joint
   B. Condyloid joint
   C. Ellipsoid joint
   D. Ball-and-socket joint

261. What movement is created when moving parallel to the sagittal plane and the angle at the joint increases?
   A. Abduction
   B. Extension
   C. Hyperextension
   D. Flexion

262. What movement is created when moving parallel to the coronal plane with the body part moving further from the midline?
   A. Flexion
   B. Abduction
   C. Adduction
   D. Extension

263. Medial rotation of the forearm is specifically termed
   A. Plantarflexion
   B. Dorsiflexion
   C. Supination
   D. Pronation

264. The term given to the action when the foot is pulled closer so the anterior angle decreases is
   A. Plantarflexion
   B. Dorsiflexion
   C. Supination
   D. Pronation

265. Which term refers to the movement of the feet where the soles of the feet are facing each other and the person's weight is on the lateral edges?
   A. Inversion
   B. Eversion
   C. Circumduction
   D. Pronation

266. What is the only saddle joint found in the body?
   A. Atlantoaxial
   B. Knee
   C. Hip
   D. Thumb

267. What is the bony landmark used to locate the distal end of the ulna?
   A. Medial epicondyle
   B. Lateral epicondyle
   C. Olecranon process
   D. Styloid process

268. What is the axis?
   A. 2nd cervical vertebrae
   B. 1st cervical vertebrae
   C. The joint between the skull and the 1st cervical vertebrae
   D. The joint between the radius and ulna

269. The joint between the skull and the 1st cervical vertebrae is called the
   A. Atlantoaxial joint
   B. Axioatlantal joint
   C. Atlantooccipital joint
   D. Intervertebral joint

270. What type of joint is the pubic symphysis?
    A. Gliding
    B. Synarthrodial
    C. Amphiarthrodial
    D. Diathrodial

271. Another name for the cartilage at the knee is the
    A. Collateral
    B. Cruciate
    C. Patella
    D. Meniscus

272. How many ribs are there in the body?
    A. 12
    B. 15
    C. 24
    D. 7

273. The shoulder joint is called the
    A. Humeroglenoid joint
    B. Humeroulnar joint
    C. Acromioclavicular joint
    D. Glenohumeral joint

274. What is the insertion for the SCM?
    A. Medial clavicle
    B. Mastoid process
    C. Superior sternum
    D. Inferior sternum

275. What muscle is the antagonist to the SCM?
    A. Anterior scalene
    B. Splenius cervicis
    C. Trapezius
    D. Splenius capitis

276. Which muscle can rotate the head?
    A. SCM
    B. Splenius capitis
    C. Trapezius
    D. Both A and B

277. What is the insertion of the brachioradialis?
    A. Styloid process of radius
    B. Lateral epicondyle of humerus
    C. Medial epicondyle of humerus
    D. Styloid process of ulna

278. What is the origin of the teres minor?
    A. Vertebral border of scapula
    B. Axillary border of scapula

C. Lesser tubercle
D. Greater tubercle

279. What muscle shares an attachment with the deltoids?
    A. Levator scapula
    B. Biceps brachialis
    C. Trapezius
    D. Supraspinatis

280. Which rotator cuff muscle (SITS) is positioned on the anterior on the scapula?
    A. Supraspinatis
    B. Infraspinatis
    C. Subscapularis
    D. Teres minor

281. What is the insertion for pectoralis major?
    A. Medial clavicle
    B. Medial bicepital groove
    C. Sternum
    D. Lateral bicepital groove

282. What name may be given to a muscle that acts on the thumb?
    A. Thallucis
    B. Longus
    C. Pollicis
    D. Brevis

283. Which erector spinae muscle is the most medial of the group?
    A. Spinalis
    B. Multifidous
    C. Longisimus
    D. Iliocostalis

284. What is the insertion site for the levator scapulae?
    A. Ribs 1–8
    B. Medial border of the scapula
    C. Superior angle of the scapula
    D. C1–C4

285. What is the action for the gluteus maximus?
    A. Flexion of hip, medial rotation
    B. Extension of hip, medial rotation
    C. Flexion of hip, medial rotation
    D. Extension of hip, lateral rotation

286. What action does piriformis play?
    A. Abducts and medially rotates
    B. Adducts and medially rotates
    C. Abducts and laterally rotates
    D. Adducts and laterally rotates

287. Which of the following muscles is not found in the anterior leg?
    A. Peroneus longus
    B. Tibialis anterior
    C. Extensor hallucis longus
    D. Extensor digitorum longus

288. Where is the origin of tennis elbow found?
    A. Medial epicondyle of humerus
    B. Styloid process of ulna
    C. Lateral epicondyle of humerus
    D. Styloid process of radius

289. A broad, flattened tendon-like sheet of connective tissue is called a
    A. Retinaculum
    B. Aponeurosis
    C. Slip
    D. Digitation

290. Which vessel takes the blood from the heart to the lungs?
    A. Pulmonary arteries
    B. Pulmonary veins
    C. Coronary arteries
    D. Coronary veins

291. The kidneys are positioned approximately between
    A. The 9th and 12th ribs
    B. The 12th rib and the 5th lumbar vertebra
    C. The 12th rib and 3rd lumbar vertebra
    D. The 8th and 12th ribs

292. What nerve branches into the tibial and common peroneal nerve?
    A. Superior gluteal
    B. Inferior gluteal
    C. Sciatic
    D. Femoral

293. The nerve that supplies the adductors of the thigh is the
    A. Femoral
    B. Superior gluteal
    C. Tibial
    D. Obturator

294. The parasympathetic nervous system causes the body to
    A. Increase heart rate
    B. Increase respiration
    C. Decrease adrenaline and heart rate
    D. Decrease excretory processes

295. What nerve innervates the quadriceps?
    A. Femoral
    B. Tibial
    C. Superior gluteal
    D. Obturator

296. How many pairs of cranial nerves are there?
    A. 35
    B. 31
    C. 12
    D. 11

297. The tibial nerve innervates which of the following muscles?
    A. Tibialis anterior
    B. Extensor hallucis longus
    C. Semitendonosis
    D. Tibialis posterior

298. What helps circulate or "pump" lymphatic fluid through out the body?
    A. Heart
    B. Lymph nodes
    C. Spleen
    D. Skeletal muscles

299. What is the name of the fascia that wraps the muscle bellies?
    A. Endomysium
    B. Perimysium
    C. Epimysium
    D. Sarcolemma

300. Where does the lymphatic system drain?
    A. Aorta
    B. Lymph nodes
    C. Subclavian vein
    D. Kidneys

ANSWERS AND RATIONALES

1. **A.** The blood flow from the right atrium to the right ventricle is through the tricuspid valve to keep the blood flowing in one direction.

2. **C.** The ischial tuberosity is the posterior portion of the ramus of the ischium, where the body weight is supported.

3. **B.** The Golgi tendon organ is a proprioceptor. Proprioceptors are multibranched sensory nerve endings in tendons that measure tension in the muscle.

4. **B.** Adductor muscles of the upper body that bring the arms toward the body include the pectoralis major and latissimus dorsi.

5. **C.** The lumbosacral plexus includes the spinal nerves from L1 to L5 that supply the lower limb.

6. **A.** There are 31 pairs of spinal nerves that arise from the spinal cord.

7. **B.** The SCM protracts the head, flexes the neck, and can do an opposite side rotation.

8. **A.** There are spinal and cranial meninges.

9. **A.** Sternoclavicular: The sternum of the rib cage of the axial skeleton articulates with the clavicle bone, which is part of the appendicular skeleton.

10. **B.** The pectineus, the uppermost medial thigh muscle attached to the pubis and femur, is for rotation and adduction.

11. **B.** The piriformis muscle is very close to the sciatic nerve as its origin is on the greater sciatic notch; it is innervated at L5 and S1 at the sacral plexus.

12. **C.** The WBCs fight any infection by engulfing and digesting bacteria and producing antibodies for protection from disease organisms.

13. **D.** The pineal gland produces the hormones melatonin and seratonin.

14. **C.** Long tubes are arachnoid villi.

15. **A.** The movement of bones occurring at a synovial joint is called ROM and includes flexion, adduction, and rotation.

16. **D.** The thoracic cavity contains the heart.

17. **B.** Acute is short and serious.

18. **D.** Many factors contribute to muscle fatigue, including a lactic acid buildup and depletion of oxygen, calcium, and glycogen.

19. **D.** A muscle spasm is a sudden involuntary contraction of the muscle when the nerve to the muscle is irritated.

20. **A.** The 1st-class lever is like a seesaw as the head is resting on the vertebrae. When the head is raised, the facial area is in resistance. The fulcrum is between the effort and resistance.

21. **B.** *Ab* means away from.

22. **D.** The platysma is the superficial muscle of the face that moves the lip downward and backward by inserting on the mandible.

23. **B.** The brachial plexus contributes spinal nerves through C5–C8 and T1 only.

24. **B.** *Macro* means big.

25. D. The flexors at the elbow joint include the brachialis, brachioradialis, and biceps brachii. All these muscles help to flex the forearm.

26. B. The origin for the scalene muscles is C2–C7.

27. C. The pronator quadratus is responsible for pronating the forearm and wrist.

28. A. The hamstring muscles of the posterior thigh include the biceps femoris, semimembranosus, and semitendinosus. The adductors do not flex.

29. D. Three muscles form the lateral abdominal wall, with the external oblique being the most superficial.

30. C. The distal phalanges are flexed by the flexor digitorum profundus.

31. D. The body has regional lymph nodes for drainage; the inguinal nodes drain the legs.

32. A. *Ism* means condition.

33. B. *Myo* means muscle.

34. C. Anatomically the structure of a bone has a membrane over the compact bone called the periosteum.

35. B. The supinator muscle is responsible for supination in the palm of the hand.

36. C. A short piriformis muscle will cause the affected side to be shortened and externally rotated. Adducting the knee across the opposite ASIS will stretch the muscle.

37. A. The five adductors of the hip all have their origin on the pubis to enhance hip flexion and pull the femur closer to the midline. They include the pectineus, adductor longus, adductor brevis, adductor magnus, and the gracilis.

38. D. Terminal ganglia are located at the end of an autonomic motor pathway.

39. C. *Nephro* is always related to the kidney.

40. D. Lymph drains, transports, and protects the body through immune response.

41. C. B and T cells are lymphocytes or WBCs.

42. D. A vaccine is artificially acquired immunity.

43. D. The serratus anterior muscle acts antagonistically to the rhomboids.

44. B. The abductor muscles move an appendage away from the body.

45. B. Between the vertebrae are gliding joints.

46. D. A ligament is the strong fibrous connective tissue that articulates bone to bone.

47. D. A person who is able to receive blood from any other blood type is AB—the universal recipient.

48. B. The broad surface of the radius bone is covered by a long fibrous connective tissue called the interosseous ligament, which holds the radius to the ulna and allows slight movement.

49. B. AIDS is the acronym for acquired immunodeficiency syndrome.

50. A. Blood returns to the heart through the hepatic portal system when digestion is completed.

51. C. Directional terminology is used in reference to a landmark that does not change. Two references make the statement correct: The elbow is proximal (closer to head) to the hand, and the hand is distal (farther from head) to the elbow.

52. **A.** The white matter is collectively the axons that are supported by the neuroglia cells.

53. **C.** There are approximately 5×10^6 mm^3 erythrocytes found in the blood, making them the largest number of formed elements.

54. **A.** The parasympathetic NS is part of the craniosacral system.

55. **B.** The foot is most inferior (below) to the head and not in back, in front, or away from the head as the body's point of reference.

56. **B.** The radius and proximal carpals form the radiocarpal joint (wrist). It is an ellipsoid joint that helps to pronate and supinate the forearm.

57. **A.** The brachialis is an important flexor of the arm, along with the biceps brachii.

58. **D.** The medial malleolus is found on the medial side of the tibia in the leg.

59. **A.** The ascending aorta gives rise to many arteries, including the left coronary artery of the heart.

60. **A.** The dendrite is the structure on the neuron that carries impulses toward the cell body.

61. **B.** The head of the radius articulates with the humerus at the capitulum.

62. **C.** The brachial plexus has many nerves that go into the shoulder and arm, including the median nerve.

63. **B.** Supination and pronation are a function of the radioulnar joint.

64. **A.** The axillary nerve is part of the brachial plexus that innervates the deltoid at the shoulder.

65. **A.** All the extensor muscles of the wrist and fingers create extension and are located between the brachioradialis and the shaft of the ulna.

66. **A.** Skeletal muscle is rich in blood for quick movement, which requires ATP and gas exchange.

67. **B.** Any body temperature below 98. 6°F or 37°C is lower than normal body temperature.

68. **C.** The central nervous system (CNS) and peripheral nervous system (PNS) together form the whole nervous system.

69. **A.** The pectoralis minor and serratus anterior control abduction of the scapula.

70. **A.** The 12 pairs of cranial nerves are motor or sensory and arise from the base of the brain apart from the CNS.

71. **A.** The iliac branches off the dorsal aorta to supply the legs.

72. **D.** The peroneus longus is responsible for the eversion of the foot and plantarflexion.

73. **C.** The peripheral nervous system contains the autonomic nervous system.

74. **A.** The adult normal pulse range is 60–100 beats per minute.

75. **C.** The gluteus maximus is an extender of the hip and femur.

76. **C.** Blood pressure is measured in systolic and diastolic measurements. A normal systolic pressure is 120 mm -Hg and diastolic 80 mm -Hg.

77. **A.** The diaphragm is a smooth muscle in breathing that contracts during inspiration (moves down).

78. **A.** Lymph fluid consists of water, cell debris, gases, metabolic waste, and bacteria.

79. C. The flexor carpi radialis and palmaris longus are innervated by the median and the ulnar nerve.

80. A. The medial collateral ligament is also called the tibial collateral ligament, which connects the femur to the tibia and to the medial meniscus.

81. C. The teres major is not part of the "SITS" muscles of the rotator cuff. It is located on the scapula and humerus for rotation and extension.

82. C. The nervous and endocrine systems respond to homeostatic responses.

83. D. Water is the most abundant inorganic molecule.

84. D. The pH of 6 is considered acidic, compared to water at a neutral pH of 7.

85. C. The ankle is a double hinge joint that is easily movable.

86. A. Chemical messages are neurotransmitters released by nerve endings.

87. C. The iliofemoral joint at the acetabulum.

88. D. The synapse is the space between two nerves.

89. D. The outermost layer of the skin is epidermis, composed of stratified squamous epithelium.

90. C. One of the aging factors is a decrease in fibroblasts.

91. A. The bone matrix is hard due to the salt of calcium phosphate.

92. D. Condyles are on the ends of long bones and form the joint.

93. B. The cranial bones in the skull contain two paired bones: the parietal and temporal.

94. D. The trochlea of the humerus articulates with the ulna.

95. C. The medial malleolus is the ankle bone projection on the medial side.

96. A. The tarsal bones include the calcaneus or heel for the Achilles tendon attachment.

97. C. The diarthrosis joints are classified as freely movable, which includes the ball and socket, hinge, and pivot.

98. D. The thumb is classified as a saddle joint for movement at the carpal and metacarpal articulation.

99. D. The single hinge of the knee and elbow and the double hinge of the wrist and ankle are types of diarthroses joints.

100. A. The knee contains many ligaments that are intra-articular and include the anterior cruciate ligament (ACL).

101. D. Skeletal muscles are the only types of muscle cells that are multinucleated.

102. C. Dopamine functions as a hormone and neurotransmitter.

103. A. Insulation protects the neuron.

104. A. Neurons and Golgi cells are found in nervous tissue.

105. A. Atrophy is a condition in which the muscle cannot be contracted or is very weakened and begins to waste away.

106. C. The abdominis muscle runs adjacent to the midline in a parallel direction.

107. **A.** The major cheek muscle is the buccinator.

108. **B.** The spinal cord in the adult ends between the 1st and 2nd lumbar vertebrae and is called the conus medullaris.

109. **A.** The reflex arc does not include the brain in the rapid adjustments to homeostatic balancing. Only the spinal cord integrates the reflex action.

110. **C.** The stretch reflex is important to maintaining and adjusting muscle tone through a monosynaptic reflex arc, one motor neuron and one sensory neuron.

111. **A.** The axillary nerve of the brachial plexus stimulates the deltoid muscle, which is used as an injection site.

112. **D.** The sciatic nerve of the sacral plexus is composed of the common peroneal and tibial nerves arising from L4 to S4.

113. **D.** The deltoid muscle of the shoulder and the supraspinatus accomplish the abduction of the humerus.

114. **D.** The adduction of the arm is accomplished by the pectoralis major, teres major, latissimus dorsi, and the coracobrachialis.

115. **D.** The erector spinae muscles are composed of three separate muscles: iliocostalis, longissimus, and spinalis. The platysma is found in the face.

116. **A.** The gluteus maximus extends and rotates the thigh laterally. It does not abduct the thigh.

117. **D.** The deep muscles, including the obturator externus, internus, and piriformis, accomplish lateral rotation of the thigh.

118. **C.** The sartorius muscle is the longest muscle found in the leg and laterally rotates when crossing over the knee.

119. **D.** The memory is associated with frontal, temporal, occipital, and parietal lobes, parts of the limbic system, and the diencephalon.

120. **D.** The cerebral cortex has areas for muscle movement that are action-specific for motor movements.

121. **C.** Endorphin is a natural pain killer.

122. **A.** The hypothalamus is the part of the brain that regulates the balance of sympathetic and parasympathetic activity.

123. **C.** Urine is stored in the urinary bladder before being expelled.

124. **B.** The hormone glucagon stimulates formation of glucose from lactate and amino acids.

125. **D.** Some hormones are known by alternate names, including vasopressin for ADH.

126. **A.** There is no blood pressure in the veins as compared to the arteries.

127. **C.** The liquid portion of the blood is plasma, which is 55% of the total volume.

128. **D.** The blood is the transport system for metabolic wastes, gases, nutrients, hormones, and salts.

129. **C.** The mediastinum is the medial part of the thoracic cavity containing the heart.

130. **C.** Ganglia are masses of neurons that extend along the outside of the spine and synapse with other neurons.

131. **C.** In blood flow, the lungs return oxygenated blood to the left side of the heart at the atrium.

132. **D.** The aorta artery branches with the major brachiocephalic after it leaves the heart.

133. **B.** The vena cava branches into the jugular vein, which drains the blood from the brain.

134. **D.** Drainage of lymph from the right leg enters the cisterna chyli and then the left thoracic duct.

135. **B.** The urethra carries semen in the male.

136. **D.** An aerobic process converts glucose into pyruvic acid, provided a blood supply and oxygen are available.

137. **D.** Iron is a mineral that is part of the hemoglobin in the RBC.

138. **C.** Kidney stones form in urinary system.

139. **C.** Azotemia are nitrogen wastes from the kidney.

140. **B.** The diffusion of water is called osmosis.

141. **A.** Cartilage is a connective tissue that has few or no blood vessels or nerves.

142. **C.** The sphenoid bone is the keystone of the cranial floor because it articulates with many bones and is a common area for a headache massage.

143. **C.** The glenoid fossa is where the scapula and humerus articulate.

144. **A.** In about a four-hour period, a meal has been completely digested.

145. **D.** The endocrine system functions as a negative feedback system by regulating the hormone levels in the blood. When the blood level reaches normal, the target organ is stimulated to stop secreting.

146. **B.** Insulin decreases blood glucose, and glucagon increases blood glucose levels. The alpha cells of the pancreas secrete both.

147. **A.** A synaptic transmission is one electrochemical method by which the nerve impulse from one axon bridges the synaptic gap (synaptic cleft) to the nerve dendrite of the next neuron.

148. **D.** There are 30 known neurotransmitters in the body that facilitate, arouse, or inhibit the transmission of nerve impulses between synapses. They include acetylcholine, serotonin, dopamine, epinephrine, histamine, and more.

149. **B.** The carotid artery is used frequently for pulse since it is easy to palpate on the neck area even if a person is dressed. There is no pulse in a vein.

150. **C.** The insertion of the soleus and gastrocnemius muscle is the Achilles tendon on the posterior surface of the calcaneus.

151. **B.** The sympathetic nervous system regulates the blood pressure to the arterioles. As the vessels become more remote from the heart, the pressure decreases.

152. **B.** The pulmonary artery carries carbon dioxide from the right ventricle to the lungs for gas exchange. It is the only artery that transports oxygen-poor blood away from the heart.

153. **C.** The kidneys are a pair of organs located bilaterally in the upper lumbar region below the 12th thoracic vertebrae.

154. **D.** The acromion process is found on the lateral end of the spine of the scapula, forms the top of the shoulder, and articulates with the clavicle with the acromioclavicular ligament.

155. **D.** The tibialis anterior, extensor digitorum, and peroneus longus perform the dorsiflexion of the ankle.

156. **B.** The popliteus muscle initiates knee flexion and is the deepest in the posterior of the knee.

157. **A.** The femur and the tibia each have a medial and lateral condyle, which serve for muscle attachment.

158. **D.** The olecranon process is at the elbow joint located on the proximal end of the ulna.

159. **D.** The obturator innervates the gracilis, adductors, and obturator externus of the thigh.

160. **C.** Endocrine glands secrete hormones directly into the blood stream; they are also called "ductless glands."

161. **D.** Neurotransmitters are the chemical cause of neural impulses that are facilitators across the synaptic cleft.

162. **C.** The antagonist or opposing muscle must resist, or yield to, the joint motion initiated by the agonist.

163. **D.** The bursae provide cushion and prevent rubbing of tendon during muscle contraction. They contain the synovial membrane that secretes synovial fluid for lubrication of joints.

164. **C.** The ball-and-socket joint, or sphenoid triaxial joint, has the greatest ROM as in the hip and shoulder.

165. **A.** The agonist or prime mover is the muscle most responsible for causing the desired joint action.

166. **D.** The small intestine has three divisions starting with the 10–12 inch duodenum, then the 6 foot jejunum, and 9 foot ileum.

167. **D.** The GI tract is made up of the involuntary smooth muscle that starts in the esophagus, stomach, and small intestine and ends with the large intestine.

168. **B.** Digestion occurs through chewing, peristalsis, chemical enzymes, and hydrolysis to prepare the food ingested for absorption.

169. **D.** The SA node, AV node, and atrioventricular bundle are all part of the conduction system of the heart; they are made up of modified cardiac cells.

170. **C.** Internal respiration or tissue respiration is the diffusion of oxygen from the blood capillaries to the tissue cells.

171. **B.** The sounds of a beating heart are due to the closing of the hearts valves: tricuspid and bicuspid, pulmonary and aortic.

172. **C.** The muscle of respiration is the diaphragm, a dome-shaped muscular partition that separates the thoracic cavity from the abdominal cavity.

173. **D.** The hepatic portal system collects blood from the digestive system to be processed before it enters systemic circulation.

174. **B.** During normal exhalation of pulmonary ventilation, the air is forced out of the lungs as the diaphragm relaxes.

175. **C.** The synthesis of vitamins A, D, and E is not a function of the cardiovascular system; it only produces clotting proteins and blood cells in the bone marrow.

176. **A.** The lymph flows into the afferent vessels and leaves through the efferent vessels of the lymph nodes.

177. **A.** The sarcomere is the microscopic contractile unit of the myofibril. It contains two predominant proteins called actin and myosin that move across according to the sliding filament theory of muscle contraction.

178. **C.** The flexors of the forearm have their origin on the medial epicondyle of the humerus and insert on the metacarpals.

179. **B.** The diaphragm is the breathing muscle that expands the thoracic cavity during inhalation.

180. C. The tensor fascia latae is a synergist to the gluteus medius.

181. B. The pectineus shortens when the iliopsoas contracts.

182. D. The coracobrachialis will bring the arm forward.

183. A. The gluteus maximus is used to stand up.

184. C. The palm supinates when the humerus rotates laterally.

185. A. The triceps is an antagonist to the biceps.

186. A. The midsagittal plane divides the body in half.

187. B. The thoracic and abdominopelvic cavities are in the ventral cavity.

188. C. The diaphragm divides the two body cavities.

189. B. Entrappers are scalenes, piriformis, and pectoralis minor.

190. C. The deltoid is an abductor.

191. B. Movement takes place at the insertion.

192. B. The subclavius stabilizes the scapula.

193. B. Internal oblique rotates to same side.

194. D. The brachialis is a strong flexor.

195. B. The triceps extends the elbow.

196. A. The styloid is not an attachment.

197. B. The biceps brachii attaches to the radius.

198. C. The sartorius is the longest muscle.

199. C. The teres major is stretched.

200. A. The pectoralis major inserts on the humerus.

201. C. The erector spinae muscle cause bilateral extension of the spine.

202. B. The tibialis inserts on medial side of foot.

203. C. Isotonic is when the muscle shortens.

204. B. The major trunks of the aorta are the thoracic, abdominal, and brachiocephalic.

205. A. Actin and myosin move along each other for muscle contraction.

206. A. CNS receives information from the motor neurons.

207. A. Fight or flight causes the heart rate to increase by the sympathic NS.

208. C. Peristalsis is muscle contraction.

209. A. Oxygenated blood from lungs is carried in the pulmonary veins.

210. C. The clavicle is part of the appendicular skeleton.

211. C. Proprioceptors identify movement of the body.

212. D. The output of urine is the kidneys, ureter, bladder, urethra.

213. B. The master endocrine gland is the pituitary.

214. D. There are 1 million nephrons in the kidney.

215. **B.** The refractory period is when a muscle loses ability to respond to stimulation.

216. **A.** Insulin lowers blood sugar levels.

217. **A.** Coordination in the brain is controlled by the cerebellum.

218. **C.** Hemoglobin binds the oxygen in the RBC.

219. **B.** Leukocytes or WBCs are involved in the immune system.

220. **B.** Isometric is a constant length, with increase in tension.

221. **B.** The cecum of large intestine is at the end of the small intestine.

222. **D.** The Golgi tendon organ detects tension, and the muscle spindle cells detect length.

223. **B.** The only arteries that carry oxygen-poor blood.

224. **C.** Forced expiration is done by the internal intercostals.

225. **B.** The facial nerve is part of the forehead.

226. **A.** Spindle cells release the muscle.

227. **C.** Stimuli can cause irritability of muscle.

228. **C.** Vasodilation is an increase in size of lumen.

229. **D.** A relaxed breath is tidal volume.

230. **A.** The superior gluteal line is the origin of the gluteus maximus.

231. **D.** The rectus femoris crosses the hip and knee.

232. **D.** The olecranon process of the ulna is the insertion of the triceps.

233. **B.** The biceps brachii does not extend the humerus.

234. **C.** The piriformis is the lateral hip rotator.

235. **C.** The adductors are located in the femoral region.

236. **A.** The Achilles tendon is the gastrocnemius and soleus.

237. **C.** The gracilis does not abduct the hip.

238. **B.** The tensor fascial latae is lateral to vastus lateralis.

239. **A.** The levator scapula elevates and rotates scapula downward.

240. **D.** The supraspinatus stabilizes the humerus.

241. **C.** The rhomboids oppose the serratus anterior.

242. **D.** Flexion and extension of hip and knee are actions of the biceps femoris.

243. **D.** High heels shorten the gastrocnemius.

244. **A.** The pectoralis minor will relieve the scapula.

245. **C.** The olecranon process at the end of ulna.

246. **B.** The peroneal nerve is lateral to the fibula.

247. **C.** The abduction of the arm exposes the serratus anterior.

248. **B.** The rhomboids stretch from rounded shoulders.

249. **D.** The corocoid process has three muscles attached to it.

250. **C.** The peroneus longus plantar flexes the ankle.

251. **B.** The tibialis anterior and posterior cause shin splints.

252. **D.** The semimembranosus, semitendinosus, and biceps femoris are all hamstring muscles.

253. **B.** The gluteal region at the bony landmark.

254. **B.** Adduction to the midline brings the arm close to the body.

255. **B.** The carotid artery is over the bilateral SCM.

256. **B.** The hamstrings are the posterior muscles.

257. **D.** The subscapularis rotates medially.

258. **B.** The iliopsoas initiates walking.

259. **B.** The bursa sac is only located between the bone and tendon.

260. **A.** Only the hinge joint moves in one direction.

261. **B.** When the angle of a joint increases, the movement is extension.

262. **B.** Abduction is the movement away from the midline.

263. **D.** To pronate is to rotate medially.

264. **B.** Dorsiflexion is pointing the toes toward the body.

265. **A.** When you put the soles of your feet together, the movement is inversion.

266. **D.** The thumb is the only location for a saddle joint.

267. **D.** The distal end of the ulna and radius is the styloid process.

268. **A.** The 1st cervical vertebrae is the atlas, and the 2nd is the axis.

269. **C.** The joint between the occipital bone and the atlas is the atlantooccipital.

270. **C.** The joint at the pubic symphysis is slightly movable.

271. **D.** The meniscus is a specialized cartilage at the knee joint.

272. **C.** There are 12 pairs of ribs for a total of 24.

273. **D.** The joint where the humerus articulates with the scapula is called the glenohumeral joint.

274. **B.** The SCM inserts on the mastoid process.

275. **D.** The SCM and splenius capitis are antagonistic and share an insertion.

276. **D.** The SCM and splenius capitis can both rotate the head.

277. **A.** The brachioradialis inserts on the styloid process of the radius.

278. **B.** The teres minor of the rotation has its origin on the axillary border of the scapula.

279. **C.** The deltoid shares an attachment with the trapezius.

280. **C.** The only anterior muscle of the SITS is the subscapularis.

281. **D.** The pectoralis major inserts on the lateral bicepital groove of the humerus.

282. C. The pollicis muscle is located in the thumb.

283. A. The spinalis erector spinae muscle is medial.

284. C. The levator scapula inserts on the superior angle of the scapula.

285. D. The gluteus maximus extends and laterally rotates the hip.

286. C. The piriformis muscle laterally rotates and abducts the hip.

287. A. The peroneus longus is a lateral muscle of the lower leg.

288. C. Tennis elbow pain originates on the lateral epicondyle of the humerus.

289. B. Sheets of connective tissue are called aponeurosis.

290. A. The only artery that carries oxygen-poor blood away from the heart is the pulmonary artery.

291. C. The kidneys are dorsal between the 12th rib and L3.

292. C. The sciatic nerve branches into the tibial and peronial nerves.

293. D. The obturator nerve supplies the adductor muscles.

294. C. A decrease in adrenaline and heart rate is an effect of the parasympathetic nervous system.

295. A. The quadricep muscles are innervated by the femoral nerve.

296. C. The brain has 12 pairs of cranial nerves.

297. D. The tibialis posterior is innervated by the tibial nerve.

298. D. The skeletal muscles help to move the lymph fluid through the body.

299. B. The perimysium is the fascia that surrounds the muscle bellies.

300. C. The lymph pumps into the subclavian vein.

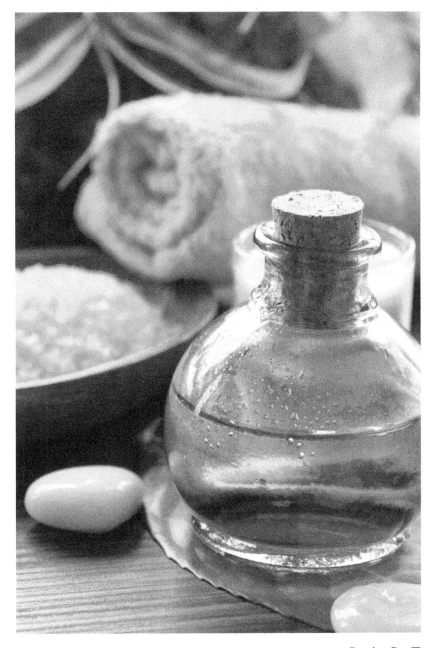

PART

2

Pathology and Pharmacology

Part 2 covers general Pathology, the common Pathology of
each system, basic types of medication. The 200 questions
make up 13% of the content in the NCETMB, NCETM and
MBLEx exams.

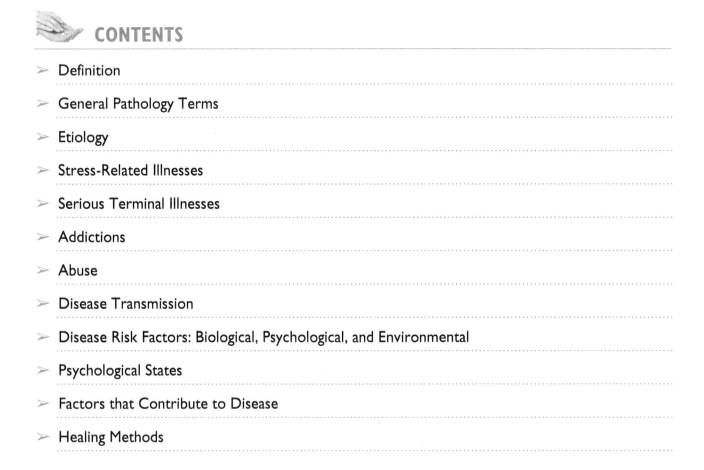

CONTENTS

GENERAL PATHOLOGY	
Definition	**The study of the structural and functional change caused by disease, which is the impairment of health condition or normal functioning of the body** **Types of disease: Genetic, congenital, metabolic, idiopathic**
General Pathology Terms	*Epidemiology*—The study of the occurrence, transmission, and distribution of a disease *Pandemic*—Worldwide disease outbreak *Diagnosis*—Identification of a specific disease or condition *Prognosis*—The expected outcome of a condition *Chronic*—Term used to describe a condition or disease that is long lasting and less intense *Acute*—Term used to describe a condition that is short term and more intense *Local*—Confined to specific part of body *Systemic*—Affecting the whole body or blood *Signs*—Observable abnormalities (fever, rash, bleeding) *Symptoms*—Nonobservable abnormalities that the patient complains of (aches, pains, fatigue) *Syndrome*—Group of signs and symptoms with a common cause
Etiology	The etiology of a disease indicates origin or cause of the disease: • *Trauma*—Physical, chemical, or radioactive damage to body • *Infection*—Invasion of a pathogenic microorganism • *Degeneration*—The breakdown of body tissue • *Autoimmunity*—Own immune system destroys its own tissue
Stress-Related Illnesses	Increased stress load or reduced ability to adapt, depleting energy and reserve capacity, can manifest itself as: • Cardiovascular problems • Hypertension • Digestive difficulties • Ulcers • Bowel syndromes • Sleep disorders • Endocrine dysfunction (adrenal, thyroid) • Pain and fatigue syndromes • post-traumatic stress disorder

(*continued*)

GENERAL PATHOLOGY (*continued*)	
Serious Terminal Illnesses	**Cancer**—Acute or chronic malignancies; massage is generally contraindicated, but research has shown that it can support the immune system if supervised by medical personnel
	HIV/AIDS—The human immunodeficiency virus caused by a retrovirus that attached the T-lymphocytes. Massage is indicated with standard Universal Precautions and can be relieving to the client in the terminal stage.
	Hepatitis—Infection of the liver caused by a virus that is transmitted through routes similar to HIV; vaccines are effective for A and B types. Massage is indicated for relaxation in clients without symptoms and contraindicated in acute stage of infection.
Addictions	• Addictions can take many forms: food, drugs, alcohol, tobacco, exercise, pain, sex, crisis, or loss
	• Behavioral changes are necessary through counseling or rehabilitation
	• Massage is beneficial to the addictive personality
Abuse	**Physical**—Forms of mistreatment to another person: Beating, rape, neglect, molestation, misuse, exploitation, crime
	Emotional—Verbal, criticism, or unrealistic expectations that affect the victim's self-worth
	Effects of abuse are in state-dependent memory that can be triggered by a place, smell, music, taste, or other stimulus that brings back the form of abuse in scattered or vague ways
	Massage can remind the body of abuse, but can also help resolve and integrate the experience
Disease Transmission	Pathogens are spread by:
	• Direct contact—body fluids and blood
	• Droplet—liquid
	• Airborne—inhale
	• Blood/body fluid—blood, saliva, urine, and feces
	• Ingestion—enter mouth
	• Vector transmission—virus, bacteria, parasite, fungi
	Agents of infection:
	Virus
	Bacteria
	Fungi
	Parasites
	Prions

Disease Risk Factors: Biological, Psychological, and Environmental	*Age*—Different age groups are more susceptible to certain diseases
	Gender—Some diseases are limited to male (prostate cancer) or female (breast and uterine cancer)
	Heredity and race—Diseases passed down genetically in families or ethnic groups; some groups are more prone to certain diseases
	Congenital—Some diseases are present from birth
	Sun—Exposure to excess sun causes skin cancer
	Nutrition—Improper diet or deficiency of vitamins or minerals
	Occupation—Some jobs cause certain diseases
	Obesity—Increases heart disease and diabetes, as well as other physical problems
	Pollution—Air, water, soil, chemical, and gas; all can affect health
	Smoking—Increases incidence of lung and other cancers
	Stress—Increases potential to contract many diseases
	Anxiety and depression—Increase nervous disorders, shingles, among others
Psychological States	*Depression*—Characterized by a decrease in vital functional activity and mood disturbances of emptiness, hopelessness, and melancholy with fatigue and pain syndromes; massage and bodywork help to relieve symptoms
	Anxiety—Uneasy feeling connected with sympathetic arousal, which massage helps to control
	Grief—A response to a loss of some kind and includes stimulation of the sympathetic autonomic nervous system to alarm, disbelief, anger, and guilt; massage and bodywork help to heal and calm
	Eating disorders—Involve mood disorders, physiologic response to food, and control issues
	• *Anorexia nervosa*—Starving disorder
	• *Bulimia*—Binge eating and purging by vomiting
Factors that Contribute to Disease	• Biological
	• Psychological
	• Environmental
	• Stress
	• Smoking
	• Obesity
	• Pollution
	• Genetic predisposition
Healing Methods	• Massage
	• Meditation
	• Yoga
	• Exercise

CHAPTER 16 Pathology of Systems

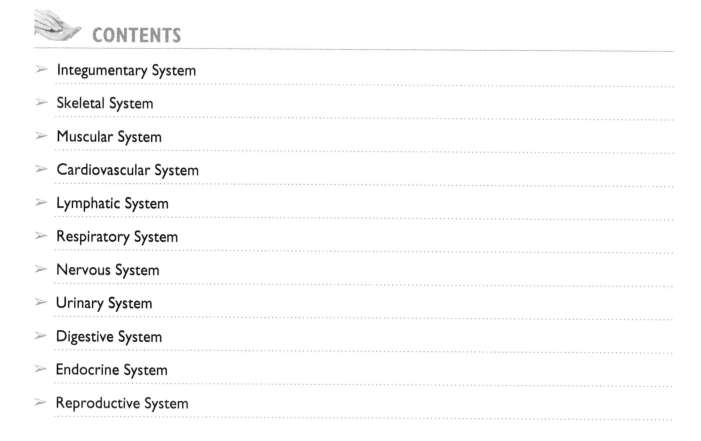

CONTENTS

PATHOLOGY OF SYSTEMS

Integumentary System	**Acne**—Disease of sebaceous glands characterized by inflamed lesions such as pustules
	Athlete's foot—Fungus found between toes
	Basal cell carcinoma—Skin cancer, usually due to sun overexposure

	Burns
	    1st degree: outer layer of skin
	    2nd degree: deeper, causing blisters
	    3rd degree: full depth of skin

	Callus—Thick area of keratin
	Cellulitis—Acute bacterial infection with swelling and redness
	Cold sore—Infected blister from herpes virus
	Contusion—Bruise, black and blue
	Corn—Keratinized horny layer of epidermis of foot
	Cyst—Benign fluid-filled sac
	Eczema—Inflammation of skin
	Fissure—Crack in skin, chapped lips
	Hives—Skin reaction to allergen or emotion; inflammatory
	Jaundice—Skin discoloration due to liver inflammation
	Melanoma—A malignant tumor arising from deep melanosomes of the skin
	Mole—A benign pigmented skin lesion
	Psoriasis—Chronic inflammatory squamous irritation
	Rosacea—Chronic skin inflammation
	Skin tag—Benign polyp-like growth of epidermis
	Wart—Epidermal protrusion caused by virus
Skeletal System	**Arthritis**—Inflammation of joints including rheumatoid (destructive disease of joints) and osteoarthritis (breakdown of cartilage at synovial joints) (contraindicated)
	Bursitis—Inflammation of the bursa with fluid buildup
	Bunion—Inflammation of bursa of the big toe

	Curvature of spine
	    • **Scoliosis**—Lateral curvature of spine
	    • **Kyphosis**—Thoracic curvation, "dowager's hump"
	    • **Lordosis**—Lumbar curvature, "swayback"

	Dislocation—Displacement of bone from normal location

(*continued*)

PATHOLOGY OF SYSTEMS (*continued*)	
	Fractures • **Closed**—simple • **Open**—skin broken • **Comminuted**—shattered • **Transverse**—across • **Greenstick**—break on one side only • **Colles**—wrist • **Spiral**—length of bone • **Pott's**—dislocation • **Compression**—vertebrae **Gout**—Uric acid buildup, usually presents as inflammation of big toe **Herniated disc**—Protrusion of intervertebral disc, which compresses on nerve root (contraindicated) **Osteomyelitis**—Inflammation of bone caused by bacteria (contraindicated) **Osteoporosis**—Loss of bone density **Spondylitis**—Unknown cause, degenerative joint disorder **Sprain**—Injury to ligaments from a few fibers to complete rupture **Subluxation**—Partial dislocation of bone at joint
Muscular System	**Adhesion**—Binding of fascial tissue **Atrophy**—With no activity and no use, muscle diminishes **Contracture**—Abnormal shortening of muscle, tendon, and fascia **Fibromyalgia**—Painful, tender spots in muscles, fatigue, numbness, and tingling in extremities **Flaccid**—No muscle tone **Hernia**—Tear in muscle wall **Lateral epicondylitis**—Inflammation of muscle to humerus, tennis elbow **Muscular dystrophy**—Muscle atrophy and degeneration **Myalgia**—Muscle pain **Myasthenia gravis**—Autoimmune, weakness of skeletal muscles due to lack of release of acetylcholine **Paralysis**—Loss of voluntary muscles to move **Shin splint**—Involves anterior tibialis and periosteum around tibia **Spasm (cramp)**—Involuntary contraction of skeletal muscle **Sprain** Ligament becomes stretched or injured 1st, 2nd, and 3rd degree severity

	Strain Tendon or muscle stretched or injured 1st, 2nd, and 3rd degree severity ***Tendinitis***—Inflammation of tendon attached to muscle ***Torticollis***—Wryneck caused by SCM muscle strain causing tilting of neck
Cardiovascular System	***Anemia***—A decrease in the oxygen-carrying capacity of blood (iron deficiency) ***Aneurism***—A bulge in the wall of the artery ***Angina pectoris***—Pain in the chest and arm caused by myocardial ischemia ***Arrhythmia***—Irregular heartbeat, can result in cardiac arrest ***Arteriosclerosis***—Thickening of the walls of the arteries ***Atherosclerosis***—Plaque buildup in arteries from cholesterol and lipids leading to decreased blood flow, caused by obesity, diabetes, and steroid use ***Cerebrovascular accident (CVA)***—Called stroke, loss of blood supply to brain caused by clot or hemorrhage ***Chronic obstructive pulmonary disease (COPD)***—Lungs lose capacity for inspiration and expiration ***Coronary artery disease (CAD)***—Blockage of coronary arteries causes low blood to heart ***Congestive heart failure***—Pulmonary or systemic edema, difficulty breathing ***Embolism***—Obstructing of blood vessel by clot or foreign substance ***Fibrillation***—Abnormal contraction of heart muscle-arrhythmia ***Hypertension***—High blood pressure: systolic 140 and above, diastolic 90 and above, caused by age, obesity, smoking, genetics, and stress ***Leukemia***—A cancer of the white blood cells (WBCs), overproduction of individual types of leukocytes ***Murmur***—Leaking heart valve, congenital ***Myocardial infarction (MI)***—Caused by a blockage of blood flow to the heart muscle that leads to death of the muscle cells and can be caused by worsening athero- and arteriosclerosis (CAD), thrombosis or embolism, spasm of coronary arteries or arrhythmias ***Phlebitis***—Inflammation of vein caused by obesity and inactivity ***Raynaud's disease***—Peripheral vasoconstriction, cause unknown ***Rheumatic heart disease***—Heart valve disease from rheumatic fever ***Spider veins***—Superficial dense network of veins, light massage only ***Thrombus***—Blood clot within a blood vessel ***Varicose veins***—A swelling of lower leg veins caused by pooling of blood due to incompetent valves in veins

(continued)

PATHOLOGY OF SYSTEMS (continued)	
Lymphatic System	***Allergy***—Hypersensitivity to a particular allergen, which causes bronchial or sinus congestion ***AIDS***—Autoimmune disease caused by HIV infection that destroys T cells in activating immune system ***Chronic fatigue syndrome***—Idiopathic, unexplained lethargy ***Hodgkin's disease***—Malignant lymphoma resulting in immunodeficiency ***Lupus***—Autoimmune, inflammatory disorder of connective tissue that causes pain, fatigue, and photosensitivity ***Lymph edema***—Swelling of extremities due to excessive lymph fluid ***Lymphoma***—Lymphatic tissue tumor ***Mononucleosis***—Swollen lymph nodes, fever, fatigue caused by Epstein-Barr virus
Respiratory System	***Asthma***—Narrowing of bronchial tubes, causing difficulty in breathing ***Apnea***—Temporary cessation of breathing ***Bronchitis***—Inflammation of bronchi ***Cystic fibrosis***—Genetic disorder resulting in thick mucus produced by respiratory tract ***Dyspnea***—Shortness of breath ***Emphysema***—Tissue deterioration in lung alveoli causing increased air retention ***Hiccup***—Spastic contraction of diaphragm ***Hyperventilation***—Abnormal deep, fast respiration; can result in fainting ***Influenza (flu)***—Acute viral infection of respiratory tract
Nervous System	***Alzheimer's disease***—Progressive death of nerve cells resulting in loss of memory ***Bell's palsy***—Neuritis of facial nerve causing paralysis ***Carpal tunnel syndrome***—Neuropathy of median nerve in wrist caused by compression of tendon flexor ***Encephalitis***—Inflammation of the brain, leading to nerve degeneration and brain damage ***Epilepsy***—Long-term disturbance of brain with seizures ***Meningitis***—Inflammation of meninges caused by bacteria or virus ***Migraine***—Vascular headache; caused by smoke, stress, oral contraceptives ***Multiple sclerosis***—Progressive demyelization of neurons in CNS ***Parkinson's disease***—Degenerative disorder affecting motor neurons; reduction of dopamine leads to tremors ***Sciatica***—Neuritis of sciatic nerve caused by tight surrounding muscles ***Stroke***—Cardiovascular accident (CVA) causing brain damage resulting from ischemia from blood vessel rupture (massage contraindicated)

Urinary System	Urine containing blood, WBCs, albumin, glucose, ketones
	Cystitis—Infection of urinary bladder
	Dialysis—Mechanical filtering of blood
	Enuresis—Incontinence
	Kidney stones—Calcium or uric acid
	Renal failure—Decline in renal function
	Urinary tract infection—Bacterial infection of urethra
Digestive System	*Acid reflux*—Abnormal return of stomach contents
	Cirrhosis—Scar tissue in liver with chronic inflammation
	Colitis—Inflammation of colon
	Crohn's disease—Chronic inflammation of GI tract
	Eating disorders—Anorexia and bulimia nervosa, characterized by lack of eating or self-induced purging
	Gallstones—Stones formed from bile that get caught in bile duct
	Hemorrhoids—Dilated blood vessels around anus
	Hepatitis A, B, C—Viral diseases transmitted through contaminated food, water, or bodily fluids
	Hiatal hernia—Stomach protrudes through diaphragm
	Irritable bowel syndrome—Recurrent abdominal cramps, diarrhea, or constipation caused by stress
	Peptic ulcer—Ulcer in esophagus, stomach, or small intestine caused by penetration of gastric juice into mucous membrane
Endocrine System	*Addison's disease*—Hyposecretion of glucocorticoids from the adrenal glands results in low blood pressure and energy
	Cretinism—Thyroid disorder causing stunted growth
	Cushing's disease—Excessive production of cortisol from adrenal cortex results in deposits of fat all over body
	Diabetes mellitus Type I—Deficiency in insulin due to autoimmune; insulin-dependent Type II—Adult onset over 40 due to overweight, poor diet, aging, insulin medication, or injection
	Giantism—A pituitary disorder causing excessive growth
	Goiter—Thyroid disorder in which gland becomes enlarged
	Hyperglycemia—Blood sugar is abnormally high, characteristic of diabetes
	Hypoglycemia—A deficiency in blood sugar caused by too little blood glucose

(continued)

PATHOLOGY OF SYSTEMS *(continued)*	
Reproductive System	***Amenorrhea***—Discontinuation of menstrual cycle
	Breast cancer—Uncontrolled growth of breast tissue
	Fibroid—A nonmalignant tumor in the uterus
	Candidiasis—A fungal infection, caused by *Candida,* affecting the vagina
	Endometriosis—Abnormal growth of tissue in lining of uterus causing infertility
	Genital herpes—Sexually transmitted disease caused by herpes virus
	Gonorrhea—Sexually transmitted disease caused by bacteria, with pus and painful urination
	Infertility—Inability to sexually reproduce
	Mastectomy—Removal of breast and lymph tissue
	Prostate cancer—Cancer of prostate gland in male; more prevalent in age 50 and over, indicated by elevated prostate-specific antigen (PSA)
	Syphilis—Sexually transmitted disease caused by *Spirochete* bacteria

17 Basic Pharmacology

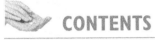 **CONTENTS**

BASIC PHARMACOLOGY	
Medication	Massage therapist should consult a *Physicians' Desk Reference* or similar drug reference book to identify any drug that might have an adverse, synergistic, or inhibitory effect from the stimulation of massage
General Drug Effects for Massage Therapy	**Injections/topical/patches**—Absorption rates can be influenced by massage, need to avoid area **Blood clotting medications**—Red flag, release from physician, minimize circulatory massage **Pain medications**—Lower ability to give feedback, caution deep tissue
Common Prescription Medications	*Cardiovascular medications*—Digitalis (Lanoxin) 　Vasodilators—e.g., nitroglycerin, isosorbide 　Beta blockers—e.g., acebutolol, bisoprolol 　Anticoagulants—e.g., Coumadin, Warfarin, Heparin, Lovenox, Pradaxa, Dabigatran *Gastrointestinal medications* 　GERD drugs—Nexium, Prevacid, Protonix 　Antiulcer—e.g., Cimetidine, Peptol, sucralfate *Hormone medications*—Birth control pills 　Antidiabetic—Insulin, glucagons 　Thyroid—e.g., levothyroxine *Central nervous system medications* 　Antianxiety/sedatives—e.g., Diazepam (Valium), clonazepam (Klonopin), alprazolam (Xanax) 　Antidepressants—e.g., selective serotonin reuptake inhibitors: fluoxetine (Prozac), sertraline (Zoloft) 　Amphetamines—e.g., methylphendate (Ritalin) *Respiratory medications* 　Expectorants—e.g., guaifenisin (Robitussin) and Mucinex 　Decongestants—e.g., ephedrine, pseudoephedrine 　Antihistamines—e.g., diphenhydramine
Analgesics	Used to relieve pain 　Narcotic—Causes deep analgesia and drowsiness; Oxycontin, Morphine, Demerol, Tylenol #3, Percocet 　Nonnarcotic—Aspirin, acetaminophen, naproxen
Recreational Drugs	• Alcohol—Widely used • Tobacco and nicotine—Widely used • Caffeine—Widely used • Cocaine • Heroin

	• Lysergic acid (LSD) • Marijuana—Most widely used illicit drug • Anabolic steroids—Enhances performance
Anti-Inflammatory Medications	Reduce body's inflammatory response 　Nonsteroidal (NSAIDs)—Ibuprofen, naproxen 　Steroidal—Cortisone medications; prednisone
Herbs	Medicinal plants that act in similar ways as pharmaceutical medications 　Commonly used herbs: aloe, chamomile, cranberry, echinacea, eucalyptus, gingko, ginseng, green tea, peppermint, senna, St. John's wort, tea tree, and valerian root
Natural Supplements	Vitamins and minerals found naturally in food 　Commonly used supplements: A, B complex, C, D, E, F, and calcium

CHAPTER

18

200 Questions with Answers and Rationales on General Pathology, Pathology of Body Systems, and Pharmacology

OBJECTIVES

Major areas of knowledge/content included in this chapter are based on most of the NCETMB, NCETM, and MBLEx exam topics that cover general pathology and pathology of body systems.

Exam Content Percentages:

NCETMB: 13%

NCETM: 13%

MBLEx: 13%

➤ General Terms of Pathology

➤ Etiology

➤ Disease Risk Factors

➤ Disease Transmission

➤ Terminal Illness

➤ Abuse

➤ Addictions

➤ Stress Related Illnesses

➤ Psychological State

➤ Healing Methods

➤ Factors that Contribute to Disease

➤ Basic Pharmacology

➤ Pathology of Body Systems

DIRECTIONS

Each of the questions or statements below is followed by four suggested answers or completions. Select **one answer** that is best in each case.

1. Which muscle would be paralyzed if the sciatic nerve were severed?
   A. Trapezius
   B. Biceps femoris
   C. Gluteus maximus
   D. Erector spinae

2. Senile lentigo or liver spots on the skin
   A. Are not contraindicated for massage
   B. Are contraindicated for massage
   C. Should be referred to a dermatologist
   D. Can be a symptom of cancer

3. If massage is used in early stages of fracture healing, it should be given particularly on the area
   A. Proximal to the actual site
   B. Distal to the actual site
   C. Medial to the actual site
   D. Lateral to the actual site

4. Contraindicated fungal skin infections include
   A. Herpes simplex
   B. Warts
   C. Athlete's foot
   D. Moles and tags

5. Which condition is present when there is an injury of the ulnar nerve at the elbow?
   A. Inability to flex fingers fully
   B. Spasticity
   C. Flaccidity
   D. Spasms

6. In treating a patient with kyphosis, which muscle(s) should the massage therapist try to stretch and relax?
   A. Pectorals
   B. Rhomboids
   C. Erector spinae
   D. Trapezius

7. If a client has skin damaged by the burns of fire, chemicals, or radiation and requires grafting
   A. Massage can be done after the graft heals
   B. This is a 3rd-degree burn
   C. Gentle range of motion (ROM) can increase mobility
   D. All of the above

8. Which technique is recommended for rheumatoid arthritis?
   A. Effleurage
   B. Gentle friction
   C. Kneading
   D. Tapotement

9. Massage can be beneficial for a headache with symptom(s) of
   A. Sinus pressure
   B. Vascular disruption
   C. Release of toxins
   D. All of the above

10. Thorough assessment of a client's medical intake reveals
    A. Addictions
    B. Emotional problems
    C. Personal information
    D. Contraindications for massage

11. Herpes simplex is a(n) _____ infection of the skin.
    A. Bacterial
    B. Viral
    C. Noncontagious
    D. Autoimmune

12. Adhesion development and excessive scarring following trauma can be prevented or reduced with
    A. Joint movements
    B. Petrissage
    C. Friction massage
    D. Passive movements

13. Most muscle strains occur on the
_____.
   A. Tendon
   B. Antagonist muscle
   C. Tight, spasmed muscle
   D. All of the above

14. Techniques to avoid using on a pregnant client are heavy percussion and
   A. Deep tissue massage
   B. Tapotement
   C. Petrissage
   D. Lymph stimulation

15. Which of the following is a virus-induced mass produced by uncontrolled epithelial skin cell growth?
   A. Moles
   B. Cyst
   C. Carbuncle
   D. Warts

16. If a client has a hernia, the best approach is
   A. Clearance from a physician
   B. Local contraindication around affected area
   C. To reschedule appointment
   D. Start the massage in a prone position

17. In order to evaluate projected pain it is necessary to know the
   A. Portion of the brain involved
   B. Proximal nerve that is compressed
   C. Distal nerve that is compressed
   D. Parasympathetic involvement

18. When a client has fibromyalgia, it is best to
   A. Avoid giving a massage due to the pain
   B. Assess the "tender points" and tailor the treatment
   C. Wait until the disease is in remission
   D. Refer to a reflexologist

19. A sprain with extensive swelling is caused by an injury to the
   A. Muscle
   B. Wrist
   C. Ligament
   D. Tendon

20. Massage can be beneficial if a client is recovering from pneumonia because
   A. Tapotement and vibration on the back can help drain the secretions
   B. The client is no longer contagious
   C. The client can resume normal activity
   D. Antibiotics cannot be used

21. Injuries that have a gradual onset or reoccur often are called
   A. Sprains
   B. Occupational
   C. Acute
   D. Chronic

22. A disease of the nervous system that is contraindicated for massage is
   A. Multiple sclerosis
   B. Meningitis
   C. Sciatica
   D. Parkinson's disease

23. A muscle strain that involves a partial tear of 10-50% of the muscle fibers is classified as
   A. Grade I
   B. Grade II
   C. Grade III
   D. Parietal

24. Which nerve is affected in carpal tunnel syndrome?
   A. Axillary
   B. Median
   C. Medial pectoral
   D. Radial

25. The popliteal fossa is an endangerment site because of the
   A. Lymph nodes
   B. Tibial and peroneal nerves
   C. Median cubital vein
   D. Kidney

26. What client information is critical in the history intake process?
   A. Previous massage history
   B. Personal information
   C. Diet
   D. All medical conditions, surgeries, and illnesses

27. To reduce adhesions and fibrosis, which of the following movements is used?
    A. Cross-fiber friction
    B. Wringing
    C. Pressing
    D. Squeezing

28. Massage interfaces with the effects of many medications; therefore, it is important to reference drugs in the
    A. *Gray's Anatomy*
    B. *Physicians' Desk Reference*
    C. Webster's dictionary
    D. Medical dictionary

29. Massage therapists should be able to assess the effects of medications that alter muscle tone, cardiovascular function, and
    A. Anticoagulants
    B. Personality
    C. Analgesics
    D. Contraindications

30. Why is it important to have the illnesses and/or medical conditions available before a massage?
    A. The state requires this
    B. For the purpose of assessing any potential contraindication
    C. If you are giving a relaxation massage, it is not necessary
    D. It is not necessary to do an intake unless you are a nurse

31. Pathogenic organisms cause the development of many disease processes and include
    A. Virus and bacteria
    B. Fungi
    C. Protozoa
    D. Virus, bacteria, fungus

32. Severe strain of the trapezius and deltoid muscles is called
    A. Racquetball shoulder
    B. Tennis elbow
    C. Skier's snap
    D. Bowler's break

33. Overstretching of the gracilis and adductor muscle on the inner thigh results from
    A. Soccer
    B. Tennis
    C. Horseback riding
    D. Bowling

34. The client may react to pain with
    A. Fear and anxiety
    B. Ischemic response
    C. Active movement
    D. Passive movement

35. Severe varicose veins are a(an) _____ for massage.
    A. Indication
    B. Taboo
    C. Embolus
    D. Contraindication

36. Sciatic nerve damage diminishes the ability to
    A. Flex the hip
    B. Flex the knee
    C. Adduct the hip
    D. Abduct the hip

37. Swelling of one entire leg is usually caused by pathology in
    A. Heart muscle
    B. A blood vessel
    C. Kidney
    D. Liver

38. In a patient with subdeltoid bursitis, the pain is worse if the arm is
    A. Abducted
    B. Adducted
    C. Hyperextended
    D. Laterally rotated

39. Arthritis is a(an)
    A. Vitamin D deficiency
    B. Vitamin C deficiency
    C. Inflammation of the joints
    D. Bone fracture

40. Facial paralysis can be due to a lesion in which cranial nerve?
    A. III
    B. VI
    C. VII
    D. VIII

41. With chronic swelling around the patella, what massage technique do you use on the thigh?
    A. Kneading of the thigh
    B. Friction of the knee
    C. Effleurage proximal to knee
    D. Effleurage distal to knee

42. Inflammation of the walls of a vein is called
    A. Aneurysm
    B. Phlebitis
    C. Varicose vein
    D. Atherosclerosis

43. When treating swelling due to a dislocated knee, which technique is valuable?
    A. Effleurage
    B. Kneading
    C. Tapotement
    D. Friction

44. Most stress and pain patterns that respond to therapeutic massage involve the
    A. Circulatory and nervous system
    B. Nervous and endocrine systems
    C. Muscle system
    D. None of the above

45. To treat the 7th cranial nerve palsy (Bell's palsy), brisk friction kneading should be done
    A. From the mandible to hairline vertically
    B. From the hairline to maxilla
    C. Transversely with both hands
    D. Not at all

46. According to Cyriax, which stroke is best for tenosynovitis?
    A. Effleurage
    B. Transverse friction
    C. Percussion
    D. Vibration

47. Muscular dystrophy is characterized by degeneration and wasting of
    A. Muscle tissue
    B. Nervous tissue
    C. Epithelial tissue
    D. All of the above

48. Massage is helpful with medical supervision for
    A. Rheumatoid arthritis
    B. Lupus
    C. Ankylosing spondylitis
    D. All of the above

49. A term that means an abnormally low level of WBCs is
    A. Leukopenia
    B. Leukocytopenia
    C. Leukocytosis
    D. Leukophoma

50. Tight hamstrings contribute to back pain due to
    A. Limited lumbar movement
    B. Ischial origin
    C. Limited hip flexion
    D. All of the above

51. Carpal tunnel syndrome affects the
    A. Volar aspect of the wrist
    B. Dorsal wrist
    C. Anterior forearm
    D. Forearm extensors

52. When there is damage to the ulnar nerve with the inability to flex the fingers strongly, which condition would be present?
    A. Flaccidity
    B. Spasticity
    C. Spasm
    D. All of the above

53. Cutting the median nerve results in the inability to
    A. Flex the thumb
    B. Extend the wrist
    C. Extend the elbow
    D. Supinate the arm

54. Which is an example of a fungus infection?
    A. Athlete's foot
    B. Furuncle
    C. Typhoid
    D. Dysentery

55. Fusiform swelling in the fingers and joint calcification of the hand are seen in
    A. Gout
    B. Arthritis
    C. Polio
    D. Rheumatoid arthritis

56. Loss of function of the wrist and outer fingers is due to an injury to the
    A. Brachial plexus
    B. Radial nerve
    C. Median nerve
    D. Ulnar nerve

57. A survivor of abuse can benefit from massage by
    A. Feeling a sense of safety
    B. Releasing or letting go
    C. Retrieving memory
    D. All of the above

58. Sciatic nerve injury may include symptoms of
    A. Constipation
    B. Cervical pain
    C. Osteoarthritis
    D. A dislocated hip, lumbar pain

59. Shin splint syndrome affects the
    A. Lateral malleolus
    B. Periosteum around the tibia
    C. Fibula
    D. Medial malleolus

60. Our emotions can lead to disease with the excess use of
    A. Food
    B. Nicotine
    C. Alcohol and drugs
    D. All of the above

61. Somatic pain arises from the stimulation of
    A. Organ receptors
    B. Noxious material
    C. Receptors of the skin, muscles, or joints
    D. Referred areas

62. In pregnancy, a contraindication for prenatal massage is
    A. Spider veins
    B. Overdue date
    C. Too much weight gain
    D. Toximia, varicose veins, early gestation

63. The following deviations that suggest the need for evaluation and referral for cardiovascular clients are
    A. Pulse over 90 or under 60
    B. Hard veins
    C. Tenderness of extremities
    D. High/low pulse, pressure, or chest pain

64. Flaccid paralysis can be benefited by the
    A. Decrease in metabolic heat production
    B. Increase in heart rate and blood pressure
    C. Deep stroking and kneading massage
    D. Relaxation of muscle tissue

65. Myofascial pain syndrome is also known as
    A. Myofascitis
    B. Fibromyositis
    C. Myofascitis trigger points
    D. All of the above

66. Pain sensations are modified by the release of neurochemicals from the CNS, including
    A. Adrenaline
    B. Endorphins and enkephalins
    C. Thyroxin
    D. Prostaglandins

67. Massage therapy is used for pain control in
    A. Labor and delivery
    B. Neuritis and neuralgia
    C. Whiplash
    D. All of the above

68. A systemic inflammatory disease is a chronic condition such as
    A. Arthritis
    B. Bronchitis
    C. Asthma
    D. All of the above

69. The intake history of a client suffering from childhood abuse is very important because
    A. You can act as a psychotherapist
    B. It defines client boundaries and assures protection
    C. It is easy for a client to receive a massage
    D. You will be able to make a diagnosis

70. A massage therapist needs to know that the mechanism of pain includes
    A. A genetic history
    B. Social aspects
    C. Level of exercising
    D. Physiological and psychological aspects

71. A 1st-degree burn is characterized by
    A. Involvement of the dermis and epidermis
    B. Blisters
    C. Severe pain
    D. A typical sunburn

72. A 2nd-degree burn is characterized by
    A. Involvement of the entire epidermis and possibly some of the dermis
    B. No loss of skin functions
    C. Damage to most hair follicles and sweat glands
    D. Never scarring

73. What is the name of the fracture of the distal end of the radius in which the distal fragment is displaced posteriorly?
    A. Stress fracture
    B. Spiral fracture
    C. Pott's fracture
    D. Colles' fracture

74. Which of the following is defined as the degeneration of cartilage allowing the bony ends to touch, usually associated with the elderly?
    A. Osteoarthritis
    B. Osteogenic sarcoma
    C. Osteomyelitis
    D. Osteopenia

75. Limitation due to the stretching of fibrous tissues is called
    A. Hard end feel
    B. Springy end feel

C. Soft end feel
D. Acute inflammation

76. Which ligament is stretched or torn in about 70% of all serious knee injuries?
    A. Anterior cruciate
    B. Arculate popliteal
    C. Lateral collateral
    D. Medial collateral

77. When injured by trauma or infection, neurons of CNS
    A. Repair slowly
    B. Don't repair
    C. Require transplants
    D. Self-destruct

78. Symptoms of the skin marked by an elevation with clear fluid from contact with poison ivy is called a
    A. Cyst
    B. Vesicle
    C. Macule
    D. Laceration

79. Cancer is a disease that can be spread through the
    A. Genes
    B. Lymphatic and blood system
    C. Endocrine system
    D. Digestive system

80. Weak thumb movements, pain in the palm and fingers, and an inability to pronate the forearm is characteristic of an injury to which nerve?
    A. Median
    B. Medial pectoral
    C. Musculocutaneous
    D. Radial

81. Massage is not performed on an area that is
    A. Too fatty
    B. Hairy
    C. Dry
    D. Bruised, burned, or swollen

82. Local anesthetics, such as procaine (Novocain), block pain and other sensations by
    A. Distracting the signal to the brain
    B. Numbing the blood vessels next to the cut

C. Preventing the voltage leakage channels from leaking

D. Preventing the opening of voltage-gated sodium channels

83. Epilepsy is characterized by
   A. Short, recurrent periodic attacks of motor, sensory, or psychological malfunction
   B. Epileptic seizures, which are initiated by abnormal, synchronous electrical discharges from the brain
   C. Contracting skeletal muscles involuntarily
   D. All of the above

84. Which of the following is true about headaches?
   A. Analgesic and tranquilizing compounds are generally effective for migraine headaches
   B. Migraines have been found to be helped by drugs that dilate the blood vessels
   C. Sunlight relieves the tension
   D. Tension headaches classically occur in the occipital and temporal muscles

85. Loss of function of an entire arm is due to injury of the
   A. Ulnar nerve
   B. Median nerve
   C. Radial nerve
   D. Brachial plexus

86. A ringing, roaring, or clicking in the ears is known as
   A. Keratitis
   B. Mydriasis
   C. Scotoma
   D. Tinnitus

87. A lower-than-normal number of RBCs is termed
   A. Hypoxia
   B. Erythropoietin
   C. Normoblastin
   D. Anemia

88. A rapid resting heart or pulse rate over 100 beats per minute is termed
   A. Bradycardia
   B. Myocardia
   C. Pericardia
   D. Tachycardia

89. The artificial cleansing and excretion of waste products from the blood is properly termed
   A. Hemodialysis
   B. Blood clearance
   C. Kidney evacuation
   D. Membrane indwelling

90. Cardiac conditions, diabetes, lung disease, and high or low blood pressure are examples of contraindications for
   A. Hydrotherapy
   B. Hot stone massage
   C. Swedish massage
   D. Both A and B

91. Dysfunction caused by physical trauma or strain is associated with the
   A. Autonomic nervous system
   B. Sympathetic nervous system
   C. Pain-spasm-pain cycle
   D. Parasympathetic nervous system

92. Which of the following causes an increase in body temperature?
   A. Progesterone
   B. Increased body production of epinephrine and norepinephrine into the blood
   C. Contraction of skeletal muscles
   D. Both B and C

93. Acquired immune deficiency syndrome (AIDS) is caused by HIV, which is an acronym for
   A. Having the immune virus
   B. Hapten immune virus
   C. Hepatic immune virus
   D. Human immunodeficiency virus

94. Which term means an exaggeration of the lumbar curve of the vertebral column?
   A. Hyperlordosis
   B. Kyphosis
   C. Scoliosis
   D. Spina bifida

95. The symptoms of an upper respiratory infection including bronchitis, cold, and sinusitis can benefit from
   A. Light massage to area
   B. Tapotement on the chest
   C. Friction to the pectoral muscles
   D. Slapping on the back

96. A chronic, inflammatory disorder that produces sporadic narrowing of airways with periods of coughing, difficult breathing, and wheezing is called
   A. Asthma
   B. Bronchitis
   C. Emphysema
   D. Tuberculosis

97. All of the following are local (regional) contraindications for massage except
   A. Recent burn
   B. Undiagnosed lump
   C. Open sore
   D. Shock

98. Somatic pain arises from stimulation of receptors in the skin or from stimulation of receptors in the
   A. Viscera
   B. Peritoneum
   C. Brain
   D. Muscle, joints, tendons, and fascia

99. Acute inflammation is a massage
   A. Side effect
   B. Contraindication
   C. Indication
   D. Benefit

100. Dr. Travell and Dr. Chaitow agree that gentle stretching to reset the normal resting length of the muscle must follow therapy using
   A. Polarity
   B. Kinesiology
   C. Trigger points
   D. Meridians

101. In difficult joint movement, the main objective is
   A. Active assistive joint movement
   B. Passive joint movements
   C. Active resistive joint movement
   D. ROM

102. In runner's cramp, the massage treatment is
   A. Ice application only
   B. Rest only
   C. Shaking calf
   D. RICE and cross-fiber friction

103. Skin conditions contraindicate massage because
   A. They might be contagious to the practitioner
   B. They can interfere with the massage
   C. The client may be on medications
   D. The client has an infection

104. Psoriasis, a chronic skin disease,
   A. Produces scaly, pink, itchy patches, and is contagious
   B. Is contraindicated
   C. Needs a referral
   D. Is not contagious or contraindicated

105. Massage is contraindicated for the following skin disorders:
   A. Incision
   B. Wound related to diabetes
   C. Bedsores
   D. All of the above

106. Gout is a disease that
   A. Is an inflammatory arthritis caused by uric acid around the joint
   B. Affects the liver and pancreas
   C. Is completely contraindicated
   D. Cannot be corrected by diet

107. In the 1st trimester of pregnancy
   A. Any massage is contraindicated
   B. Deep abdominal work is contraindicated
   C. All prenatal massage is indicated
   D. Massage therapist needs a referral from an OB/GYN

108. Massage therapy of the breast in breast cancer patients
   A. Is still considered untouchable
   B. Has been beneficial in cases
   C. Should not be attempted to prevent metastasis
   D. Is contraindicated

109. A client who reports hepatitis on the medical history
   A. Can be contagious and should avoid massage
   B. Has an inflammation of the gallbladder
   C. Must be cleared by a physician for massage
   D. Both A and B

110. Diverticulitis can be defined as
   A. Colon cancer
   B. A hernia in the esophagus
   C. Small pouches that protrude from the colon
   D. Polyps in the sigmoid colon

111. Massage is indicated in subacute
   A. Common cold
   B. Influenza and Pneumonia
   C. Heart disease
   D. Both A and B

112. In the case of a client with HIV/AIDS
   A. Massage is indicated
   B. Massage is contraindicated
   C. The massage therapist must wear latex gloves
   D. A massage is only indicated in the final stages

113. Paths of infection of a pathogen include
   A. Pathogen transmission by broken skin
   B. Pathogen transmission by inhalation
   C. Pathogen transmission by contact of mucous membrane
   D. All of the above

114. When should the massage therapist use gloves?
   A. If the client has a break in the skin
   B. If the client requests the use of gloves
   C. Temporomandibular Joint Disorder (TMJ) massage
   D. If there is a risk of contamination

115. In which of the following medical condition(s) would massage be contraindicated?
   A. Scoliosis
   B. Contact lenses
   C. Arthritis
   D. None of the above

116. The most important risk factors for breast cancer are
   A. Genetic predisposition and age
   B. Hormonal factors and the female sex
   C. Diet and exercise
   D. Both A and B

117. Palpatory assessment of body temperature is significant
   A. To detect decreased circulation in toes and fingers
   B. To detect fever/infection or inflammation
   C. To warn of restriction in tissues
   D. All of the above

118. A gait assessment of a client's walking pattern can detect
   A. Areas of posture imbalance
   B. Areas of pain
   C. Flat feet
   D. Both A and B

119. If a client indicates hypoglycemia on the medical intake,
   A. Massage is contraindicated
   B. Deep muscle treatment is important for better circulation
   C. Massage is fine but the client should eat after massage
   D. Refer the client for a glucose test

120. If a client indicates diabetes mellitus on the medical intake,
   A. Massage is contraindicated
   B. A massage should only be given by a nurse or medical practitioner
   C. A relaxing and gentle massage is indicated
   D. Be sure the client drinks eight glasses of water before getting a massage

121. If a client has emphysema, the muscles to address include
   A. Deltoid and trapezius
   B. Sternocleidomastoid, scalenes, and pectoralis minor
   C. Erector spinae and rhomboids
   D. Diaphragm and pectoralis major

122. Refer a client with subluxation to a
    A. Chiropractor
    B. Podiatrist
    C. Urologist
    D. Endocrinologist

123. Torticollis is a condition of the
    A. Back
    B. Neck
    C. Shoulder
    D. Hip

124. A client reports having pain across the middle of her back. Which muscle may be involved?
    A. Quadratus lumborum
    B. Supraspinatus
    C. Teres minor
    D. Rhomboids

125. The nerve entrapped in carpal tunnel syndrome is the
    A. Radial
    B. Median
    C. Ulnar
    D. Femoral

126. Which two muscles are involved in a lateral ankle sprain?
    A. Peroneus longus and brevis
    B. Tibialis anterior and posterior
    C. Flexor and extensor digitorum longus
    D. Gastrocnemius and soleus

127. A Colles' fracture would involve which bone?
    A. Ulna
    B. Radius
    C. Fibula
    D. Tibia

128. A Pott's fracture would involve which bone?
    A. Ulna
    B. Radius
    C. Fibula
    D. Tibia

129. The correct medical nomenclature for a heart attack is
    A. Cerebrovascular accident
    B. Transient ischemic attack
    C. Myocardial infarction
    D. Hemiplasia

130. Excessive accumulation of fluid in the interstitial space is known as
    A. Diastole
    B. Edema
    C. Hyperemia
    D. Ischemia

131. While massaging someone with osteoporosis, the Massage Therapist (MT) should be cautious of
    A. Friction
    B. Petrissage
    C. Deep pressure on the bones
    D. The kidneys

132. A client reports having broken his ankle two weeks ago. You should
    A. Proceed with the massage; healing has already begun
    B. Proceed with the massage using deep transverse friction to ligaments and tendons
    C. Proceed with the massage doing range of motion to the ankle
    D. Proceed with the massage, avoiding the area until full bony union is accomplished

133. A client presents with a bruise on the leg. What question should you ask before the massage?
    A. Do you have any other pain?
    B. Where did this occur?
    C. Have you put heat on it?
    D. Did you pinch yourself?

134. A client writes on the intake form that he suffers from rheumatoid arthritis. What symptoms should you expect?
    A. Uric acid buildup with inflamed big toe
    B. Red, white, and blue fingers and toes
    C. Bone growth in ear with loss of hearing
    D. Deformation of joint, pain, and inflammation

135. Kyphosis is defined as an exaggeration of the
    A. Lumbar curvature of the spine
    B. Thoracic curvature of the spine

C. Lateral curvature of the spine

D. Curvature of L1–L4

136. What should you do during a massage when you realize you have come in contact with a fungal infection?

A. Stop massaging the area and continue on with the rest of the body

B. Stop the massage and wash your hands

C. Fungal infections are not contagious

D. Wash the area

137. Deficiency in lipid digestion is related to which organ?

A. Spleen

B. Small intestine

C. Gallbladder

D. Stomach

138. Indicators of gout include

A. Uric acid crystals/inflammation of the big toe

B. Headache/inflammation of the thumb

C. Astigmatism/rosacea

D. Color blindness/hearing loss

139. A client reports having epilepsy. During the massage, she has a seizure. What should you do?

A. Put something in her mouth so she doesn't swallow her tongue

B. Put her into a seated position

C. Remove all objects around her so she doesn't get hurt

D. Hold her down on her back so she doesn't move around

140. Which pigmentation should you report to your client?

A. Moles all over the body

B. Moles with different color, shape, and size

C. You do not report any suspicious moles because you don't want to scare your client

D. Moles are not something to worry about

141. Paralysis of this muscle causes drop foot

A. Tibialis anterior

B. Tibialis posterior

C. Popliteus

D. Plantaris

142. Which anterior muscle would you work for a client who suffers from lordosis?

A. Pectoralis major

B. Vastus medialis

C. Iliopsoas

D. Diaphragm

143. A client reports having whiplash and the brachial plexus is impinged. Which muscle is likely to be involved?

A. Deltoids

B. Pectoralis minor

C. Rhomboids

D. Triceps

144. A client presents with chronic low back pain. Which muscle would be weak?

A. Rectus abdominis

B. Quadratus lumborum

C. Latissimus dorsi

D. Rhomboid

145. Which muscle can entrap the brachial plexus?

A. Scalenes

B. Temporalis

C. Triceps

D. Deltoids

146. Peroneal nerve damage diminishes the ability to

A. Evert the foot

B. Invert the foot

C. Pronate the arm

D. Supinate the arm

147. Lack of oxygen to the muscle causes

A. Ischemia

B. Myositis

C. Cyanide poisoning

D. Halitosis

148. A progressive loss of muscle fibers without any nervous system involvement is caused by

A. Multiple sclerosis

B. Muscular dystrophy

C. Huntington's disease

D. Cerebral palsy

149. The condition in which the tendon sheath is inflamed is called
   A. Shin splints
   B. Sprain
   C. Tendonitis
   D. Tenosynovitis

150. Your 1st client of the day tells you she has a low-grade fever this morning, but she isn't worried because she feels fine. You should
   A. Go ahead with the deep tissue massage she is scheduled for
   B. Give her a massage, but make it Swedish so it isn't that deep
   C. Reschedule the appointment
   D. Call her doctor

151. A client with extremely high blood pressure disagrees with her doctor about whether massage is contraindicated and informs you she is going against his advice because she wants the massage. You are going to
   A. Send her home without the massage
   B. Call the doctor before making a decision
   C. Put her on the table and use gentle holding techniques and/or energy work
   D. Have her sign a release relieving you of any responsibility and give her a massage

152. Thrombosis is another term for a
   A. Blood clot
   B. Thyroid disorder
   C. Sore throat
   D. Lung inflammation

153. A client who has had recent radiation therapy may be contraindicated for deep tissue massage because of the effect of radiation on
   A. The digestive system
   B. The skeletal system
   C. The integumentary system
   D. All systems

154. Endangerment sites are places on the body that should be avoided because
   A. The veins are too close to the heart
   B. Organs in the area are subject to inflammation if massage is performed

   C. Veins, arteries, and/or nerves are superficial
   D. A benign tumor is present

155. A regular client confides to you that she recently has had a mental illness diagnosed and has been experiencing intermittent psychotic episodes. Your best course of action is to
   A. Refuse to treat her any more
   B. Be prepared to subdue her in case she gets violent
   C. Call her doctor (with her permission) to be able to make a more informed decision
   D. Call her doctor (without her permission) to be able to make a more informed decision

156. The most common bacterial sexually transmitted disease is
   A. Syphilis
   B. AIDS
   C. Herpes
   D. Chlamydia

157. Genital herpes is caused by
   A. Bacteria
   B. Fungi
   C. Parasites
   D. Viruses

158. The abnormal growth of the fetus somewhere other than the uterus is called a(n)
   A. Ectopic pregnancy
   B. Myopic pregnancy
   C. Endopic pregnancy
   D. Toxemic pregnancy

159. A lack of oxygen in the blood is caused by
   A. Addison's disease
   B. Jaundice
   C. Cyanosis
   D. Carotemis

160. *Candida albicans* is a
   A. Bacterium
   B. Microphage
   C. Virus
   D. Fungus

161. Scleroderma is
    A. Skin that has flaked off
    B. Skin that has turned yellow
    C. Skin that has turned blue
    D. Skin that has hardened

162. A genetic condition that results in a lack of clotting factors in the blood is
    A. Hypochondria
    B. Sickle-cell anemia
    C. Hyperion anemia
    D. Hemophilia

163. Hypertension is the condition of
    A. Attention-deficit disorder
    B. Low blood pressure
    C. Heart murmur
    D. High blood pressure

164. An excessively rapid heartbeat is known as
    A. Nascardia
    B. Brachycardia
    C. Angina
    D. Tachycardia

165. A progressive narrowing and hardening of the arteries caused by age, high cholesterol levels, smoking, and/or other factors is called
    A. Cerebrovascular accident
    B. Cyanosis
    C. Atherosclerosis
    D. Scleroderma

166. An inflammation of the veins is called
    A. Varicose veins
    B. Necrosis
    C. Phlebitis
    D. Bursitis

167. Which is a contagious skin condition?
    A. Dermatitis
    B. Eczema
    C. Athlete's foot
    D. Acne

168. What disease is caused by a change of estrogen in menopausal women?
    A. Rheumatoid arthritis
    B. Osteoarthritis
    C. Fibromyalgia
    D. Osteoporosis

169. What disease is known for the body's attacking its own tissues, specifically the cartilage and joint linings?
    A. Rheumatoid arthritis
    B. Osteoarthritis
    C. Fibromyalgia
    D. Multiple sclerosis

170. Which of these conditions is contraindicated and will present with a great deal of inflammation?
    A. Fibromyalgia
    B. Osteoarthritis
    C. Multiple sclerosis
    D. Rheumatoid arthritis

171. Varicose veins are caused by
    A. High blood pressure
    B. Lymph pooling
    C. Weak valves
    D. Low blood pressure

172. Which muscles are affected in frozen shoulder?
    A. Supraspinatis, infraspinatis, teres minor, subscapularis
    B. Teres major, latissimus dorsi, triceps brachialis, biceps brachialis
    C. Levator scapula, subscapularis, deltoids, trapezius
    D. Coracobrachilais, infraspinatis, brachialis, pectoralis minor

173. Which muscles are worked on to address TMJ dysfunction?
    A. Biceps brachialis
    B. Masseter
    C. Pterygoids
    D. Both B and C

174. Most headaches come from the muscles of the
    A. Face
    B. Neck and shoulder
    C. Cranium
    D. Back

175. It is necessary to treat which muscle for thoracic outlet syndrome?
   A. Masseter and scalenes
   B. Scalenes and pectoralis minor
   C. Pectoralis minor and deltoid
   D. Trapezius

176. A partial or incomplete dislocation is referred to as a(an)
   A. Subluxation
   B. Sprain
   C. Strain
   D. Luxation

177. Fainting may be caused by compression on which vessel?
   A. Carotid
   B. Subclavian
   C. Subscapular
   D. Vertebral

178. Inflammation, pain, and swelling of a vein is a condition called
   A. Varicose veins
   B. A thrombus
   C. Phlebitis
   D. Hematoma

179. Which type of client would benefit most from a heat application?
   A. A person suffering from fibromyalgia
   B. A person with cancer
   C. A person with tendonitis
   D. A person with acute inflammation

180. Sciatic pain may be caused by pressure from which muscle?
   A. Obturator internus
   B. Superior gemellus
   C. Gluteus maximus
   D. Piriformis

181. What is the name of the disease in which the myelin is destroyed, causing problems in neural transmission?
   A. Muscular dystrophy
   B. Multiple sclerosis
   C. Lupus
   D. Fibromyalgia

182. A malfunction of homeostasis in the body is also known as
   A. Stress
   B. Pain
   C. Disease
   D. All of the above

183. Which nerve is affected when a client has Bell's palsy?
   A. Cervical
   B. Facial
   C. Phrenic
   D. Trigeminal

184. While treating the quadratus lumborum muscle for back pain, you must be cautious of which plexus?
   A. Cervical
   B. Brachial
   C. Lumbar
   D. Sacral

185. The worst type of burn is
   A. Sunburn
   B. Moderate
   C. 2nd degree
   D. 3rd degree

186. The skin of a person who is suffering from heat stroke will feel
   A. Normal
   B. Cold and clammy
   C. Hot and dry
   D. Sweaty

187. A client presents with a subacute ankle sprain. What stroke would be most effective in treating the sprain?
   A. Vibration
   B. Friction
   C. Petrissage
   D. Tapotement

188. A client presents with edema in the ankles. The order of massage should be
   A. Foot, ankle, leg, hip
   B. Hip, leg, ankle, foot
   C. Toes, foot, ankle, leg
   D. Ankle, foot, toe, leg

189. Too little insulin production is typical of
    A. Type I diabetes
    B. Type II diabetes
    C. Leukemia
    D. Anemia

190. Lack of blood flow to an area is defined as
    A. Hyperemia
    B. Atrophy
    C. Ischemia
    D. Hypoxia

191. While pressing on a tender point in the deltoids, the client reports feeling pain in another area of the body. What is this called?
    A. Phantom pain
    B. Cramp
    C. Sprain
    D. Referred pain

192. In which endangerment site is the carotid artery found?
    A. Anterior triangle of the neck
    B. Posterior triangle of the neck
    C. Femoral triangle
    D. Posterior femoral triangle

193. What nerve do you have to be careful of when you are working on the sartorius?
    A. Sciatic
    B. Femoral
    C. Ulnar
    D. Tibial

194. Which structure is not found in the anterior femoral triangle?
    A. Sciatic nerve
    B. Obturator nerve
    C. Femoral nerve
    D. Great saphenous vein

195. Which type of skin cancer is the slowest growing?
    A. Basal cell carcinoma
    B. Squamous cell carcinoma
    C. Malignant melanoma
    D. They all grow very quickly

196. Which disease is most indicated for massage?
    A. Systemic lupus
    B. Lymphoma
    C. Parkinson's disease
    D. Malignant melanoma

197. What muscle is the primary cause of shin splints?
    A. Tibialis anterior
    B. Gastrocnemius
    C. Tibialis posterior
    D. Peroneus longus

198. Idiopathic means
    A. Inflammation of colon
    B. Response different from that which would be normal
    C. Mentally unstable
    D. Cause unknown

199. The effects of histamine on the cardiovascular system include?
    A. Vasoconstriction
    B. Vasodilation
    C. Arterial occlusion
    D. Interstitial restriction

200. Massage is contraindicated for which of the following conditions?
    A. Constipation
    B. Athletes foot
    C. Thrombophlebitis
    D. Pregnancy

ANSWERS AND RATIONALES

1. **B.** The biceps femoris would be paralyzed if the sciatic nerve were severed, since it controls the flexion of the posterior thigh and leg.

2. **A.** Massage is fine for clients with liver or age spots, since they are only brown patches of skin in older people due to excessive sun exposure.

3. **A.** Massage to the proximal area of a fracture promotes healing by stimulating circulation.

4. **C.** Athlete's foot is a fungal skin infection that has rings of red tissue that can bleed, break, and ooze. Local massage is contraindicated because the infection is contagious.

5. **C.** The sensation and motion that is eliminated from the elbow to the fingers due to nerve damage is called flaccidity.

6. **A.** Massage to the pectorals of the chest, by stretching and relaxing, can aid the exaggerated convex curve of the thoracic spine.

7. **D.** Massage should be done when skin is healed or grafts are healed. Massage and range of motion are indicated to increase circulation and prevent adhesions from forming.

8. **B.** Gentle friction helps to milk out body fluids from the inflamed joint. It also softens the massed ground substance between layers of tissue.

9. **D.** Massage can benefit a pain or dull ache in the head or neck causing sinus pressure, muscle tension, release of toxins, or vascular disruption.

10. **D.** Contraindications should be revealed when the client's history is taken. They can include past/present diseases, disorders, and psychological problems.

11. **B.** Herpes simplex or fever blister is a viral infection that lies dormant and appears when there are stimuli such as radiation, hormonal changes, or emotional upset.

12. **C.** Adhesions and scarring can be relieved by regular friction massage. Constrictions can be reduced as the muscle tissue heals.

13. **D.** Muscle strains are the injury of a muscle and tendon due to a violent contraction, forced stretching, or spasm of the antagonist muscle.

14. **A.** Massage during pregnancy should be soothing and relaxing, never deep tissue massage, abdominal kneading, or deep abdominal massage.

15. **D.** Warts are known to be caused by viruses causing the skin to grow in an uncontrolled fashion.

16. **B.** Local massage is contraindicated; general massage is fine unless client is in pain.

17. **B.** Pain is perceived in the tissue supplied by the proximal nerve to the location.

18. **B.** Fibromyalgia is a myofascial syndrome, which is a chronic inflammatory disease that affects muscle and related connective tissue. It is best to assess the condition and trigger points before giving a massage.

19. **C.** An injury to a joint with a tearing or stretching of the ligament and swelling is considered a severe sprain.

20. **A.** Tapotement and vibration on the back help to drain the secretions that build up in the alveoli.

21. **D.** Chronic injuries occur over time or are long lasting and can benefit from gentle massage, depending on the injury.

22. **B.** Meningitis is contraindicated to massage because it is an infection and inflammation of the meninges that causes severe headaches, vertigo, elevated temperature, pulse, and respiration.

23. B. Grade II muscle strain has pain, some loss of function, and some tissue bleeding.

24. B. The median nerve of the brachial plexus is injured in carpal tunnel syndrome by the compression of the nerve through the carpal tunnel.

25. B. Endangerment sites on the body represent areas that can be injured due to exposure of vessels, organs, and nerves to deep massage. The tibial and peroneal nerves are endangered in the fossa of the knee.

26. D. It is important in the assessment of a new client that all medical history, physical and emotional, is considered before the 1st massage session.

27. A. Cross-fiber friction is the best stroke to prevent or reduce adhesions, and fibrosis manipulation moves fibers apart from each other.

28. B. The *Physicians' Desk Reference* helps therapists to recognize the indications and contraindications to a client's medication.

29. D. Because many medications have side effects, it is important to be familiar with the various types that could be a contraindication.

30. B. It is important to do an assessment of the medical conditions and illnesses so that the practitioner is aware of any contraindications.

31. D. Many viruses, bacteria, and fungus cause pathogenic diseases, which must be prevented by use of sanitary conditions and are contraindicated for massage.

32. A. The shoulder and back muscles can be strained from sports such as racquetball and tennis.

33. C. The gracilis and adductor muscles are stretched by the action of horseback riding.

34. A. Depending on the level of pain and experience related to an injury, a client's fear and anxiety can vary.

35. D. If a client has varicose veins, it is not recommended to apply massage to the area since it is a local contraindication.

36. B. The sciatic nerve innervates the leg, and damage can limit the mobility of knee flexing.

37. B. Edema, or swelling, can result from phlebitis, a blockage in the venous system.

38. A. Joint mobility, especially abduction, is limited at the bursae due to trauma or repeated irritation.

39. C. An inflammatory condition of the joints and bone damage is characteristic of arthritis.

40. C. The VIIth nerve controls facial muscles and would affect any facial paralysis.

41. C. Effleurage is the best massage technique for moving fluid from the knee and back to the heart and lymphatic ducts.

42. B. Pain, swelling, and inflammation are characteristic of phlebitis of the veins.

43. A. Effleurage around swelling is advantageous for knee injuries.

44. B. The nervous and endocrine systems are responsible for most stress patterns that can be relieved by disrupting the signals of the sensory receptors.

45. A. In Bell's palsy, the paralyzed side of the mouth area is stretched, and massage should be on both sides from the mandible to the hairline in a kneading stroke.

46. B. Deep transverse friction should be used to break up scar tissue from overuse in tenosynovitis.

47. A. The muscle tissue degenerates during muscular dystrophy as a result of muscle atrophy.

48. D. Many diseases cause inflammation of tissue, and massage is beneficial. They include lupus, spondylitis, and arthritis.

49. A. If the level of WBCs becomes lower than normal, the result is leukopenia.

50. D. Back pain and tight hamstrings are the result of limited hip and lumbar movement.

51. A. The volar area of the wrist is affected in carpal tunnel syndrome.

52. A. Lack of muscle movement due to nerve damage is called flaccidity.

53. A. The median nerve in the arm is responsible for motion and sensation of the thumb, index, and middle finger. If it is cut, the thumb does not have the ability to flex.

54. A. Athlete's foot is a fungus infection that attacks the foot and toes.

55. D. Rheumatoid arthritis is a chronic inflammatory disease of the joint with cartilage erosion and eventual immobilization.

56. D. The ulnar nerve travels through the arms, wrists, and fingers. Any injury to this area prevents the function of the wrist or outer fingers.

57. D. Survivors of abuse benefit from the touch of massage because it allows many feelings and emotions to surface.

58. D. Lumbar pain, a dislocated hip, and a herniated disc are all symptomatic of injury to the sciatic nerve.

59. B. Inflammation of the periosteum around the tibia is one symptom of shin splints.

60. D. People use chemical substances to help our feelings and in turn alter our emotions, but the use of excess food, drugs, and nicotine can lead to disease.

61. C. The receptors of the skin, muscles, and joints can cause somatic pain.

62. D. Even though massage is recommended for pregnancy, many contraindications are possible and need a doctor's attention.

63. D. Any client who suffers from a cardiovascular deviation of any type needs a referral.

64. C. Increasing circulation by deep stroking and kneading aids flaccid paralysis in limbs.

65. D. Myofascial pain includes a plethora of terms: myositis, myofascitis, and fibromyositis.

66. B. The neurochemicals, endorphins and enkephalins, relieve pain and act as analgesia.

67. D. Massage therapy is used for many forms of pain such as labor and delivery, neuritis, and neuralgia.

68. D. A systemic inflammation occurs when an irritant spreads through the body and becomes chronic, as in asthma, arthritis, and bronchitis.

69. B. The history intake of an abused client sets up mental and physical limits and reassures the client that you will understand.

70. D. Pain is difficult to explain or describe because it is a complex of symptoms that include psychological, social, and physiological aspects.

71. D. Sunburn has been classified as a 1st-degree burn.

72. A. In 2nd-degree burns, the epidermis and possibly the dermis are damaged.

73. D. When the radius is fractured on the distal end, it is classified as a Colles' fracture.

74. A. Erosion of the articular cartilage resulting in the bones touching is diagnosed as osteoarthritis.

75. B. When assessing passive movement, the springy end feel is the most common. The end feel indicates the presence, type, and severity of lesions in the tissue associated with the joint.

76. A. Damage to the anterior cruciate ligament of the knee is a very common injury in accidents involving the knee joint.

77. B. Neurons do not repair at all when the CNS is injured or traumatized.

78. B. Vesicles are blisters with clear fluid that lie just beneath the epidermis.

79. B. The spreading of cancer or metastasis can occur through the blood or lymphatic system.

80. A. Median nerve damage affects thumb movement and the inability to flex the wrist and pronate the arm.

81. D. There are many contraindications to massage including bleeding, swelling, burns, skin infections, tumors, and bruises.

82. D. Anesthetics block pain by preventing the opening of the sodium channels so that nerve impulses cannot pass the obstructed region.

83. D. Epilepsy can be characterized by short, recurrent periodic attacks of motor, sensory, or psychological malfunction as well as seizures, which are initiated by abnormal, synchronous electrical discharges from the brain. A person with epilepsy oftentimes will contract skeletal muscles involuntarily.

84. D. Headaches generally occur in the occipital and temporal muscle area. Migraines cannot be helped by analgesics but by drugs that can constrict the blood vessels.

85. D. The nerves of the brachial plexus control movement of the arm.

86. D. Tinnitus is described as the ringing or sounds in the ear as a result of high blood pressure or nerve degeneration.

87. D. When the RBCs drop below the normal number, the condition is known as anemia.

88. D. When there is a heartbeat more than 100 beats per minute, the result is tachycardia.

89. A. The blood can artificially be filtered of wastes by a method called hemodialysis.

90. A. Treatment with hot or cold application should not be given if a contraindication is present.

91. C. The pain-spasm-pain cycle is a result of restricted movement caused by trauma, strain, or injury to the bone, muscle, tendon, or joint. The muscle spasm contracts the muscle, which becomes ischemic, and that in turn stimulates the pain receptors in the muscle.

92. D. When the skeletal muscles contract, the body temperature rises.

93. D. The acronym HIV stands for human immunodeficiency virus.

94. A. Hyperlordosis is a lumbar curvature of the spine due to poor posture, pregnancy, obesity, or rickets.

95. A. Only light massage can benefit the ache and mucous secretion associated with the upper respiratory infections.

96. A. Asthma is the disorder that results in the narrowing of the airways as spasms of the smooth muscle close partially or completely (bronchoconstriction).

97. D. Shock is an absolute general contraindication to massage.

98. D. The muscles, joints, tendons, fascia, and related areas have receptors that are stimulated from deep somatic pain.

99. B. Injuries that cause inflammation to an area should not be massaged.

100. C. The therapist palpates small areas of hypertonicity in the muscle associated with myofascial pain, and gentle leg stretches the muscle back to a resting state.

101. A. In difficult ROM by the client, the therapist's moving the body part may provide assistance.

102. D. When the muscle goes into spasm and cramping results, ice, compression, and cross-fiber friction to contracted muscle provide considerable relief, as well as stretching the spasmed muscle.

103. **A.** Any pathogen or open wound on the skin of the client is a contraindication to a massage. There are many contagious skin disorders that can easily be transmitted to the practitioner. A referral to a dermatologist is appropriate.

104. **D.** Psoriasis is a chronic skin disease found on the elbows, knees, and trunk. It is noncontagious with accelerated psoriatic skin cell division, which appears pink and scaly. It is only locally contraindicated in acute stages of the disease.

105. **D.** Any open wound, sore, or incision as well as any skin disorder related to diabetes is contraindicated. The rule that governs the skin is if the intactness of the skin has been compromised in any way, the client is susceptible to infection.

106. **A.** Gout is a type of arthritis that causes inflammation around the joints of the hands and feet. A diet high in purines is the cause of uric acid crystals forming deposits that result in pain.

107. **B.** The 1st trimester is when fetal attachment is most fragile, and massage therapists must avoid deep abdominal work to prevent any danger to the fetus.

108. **B.** Recent studies have shown that breast massage is beneficial to the client, promoting recovery, healing, and ROM.

109. **C.** All hepatitis is contraindicated and should require a note from the physician.

110. **C.** Diverticulitis is a protrusion from the wall of the colon that can become infected. Massage is contraindicated.

111. **D.** As long as the diseases of the common cold, pneumonia, and influenza are in the subacute stage and not the acute stage, massage is not contraindicated.

112. **A.** Massage is indicated for clients in *all* stages of HIV, as long as the practitioner is healthy and does not jeopardize the client's health.

113. **D.** Pathogens are transmitted by mucous membrane, broken skin, ingestion, inhalation, and intact skin contaminated with poison ivy, fungus, or scabies.

114. **D.** A massage therapist should wear gloves if the client has broken skin, open lesions, or herpes.

115. **D.** Scoliosis, contact lenses, and arthritis are not massage contraindications. Massage is beneficial to any curvature of the spine as well as arthritis. However, it is important to know if a client is wearing contact lenses so that pressure around or on the eye is avoided.

116. **D.** The critical risk factors of breast cancer include age, genetic predisposition, the female sex, hormonal factors, presence of other cancer, and race. Although diet and exercise are important to good health, they do not contribute a high risk to cancer.

117. **D.** Palpatory assessment is through touching with purpose and intent. It is a skill that determines muscle location, temperature of the body, and parts of the body for circulation, fever, inflammation, and restriction in the tissue.

118. **D.** By examining the gait of a client, posture, pain, coordination, and muscle weakness can all be assessed and compared to a normal walking pattern.

119. **C.** Hypoglycemia is a condition when there is not enough glucose in the blood. Massage is indicated, but if the client gets light-headed, then assist him or her off the table and have the client eat or drink something containing carbohydrates.

120. **C.** Anyone with diabetes mellitus can get a massage providing the client has taken medication and the massage is gentle.

121. **B.** The accessory muscles of respiration will be especially tight, so focusing on the SCM, scalenes, and pectoralis minor will benefit the client.

122. **A.** Chiropractors adjust the components of the skeleton.

123. **B.** A wry neck of the SCM muscle.

124. D. Back pain can involve the rhomboids.

125. B. Carpal tunnel is caused by the median nerve entrapment.

126. A. The peroneus longus and brevis are lateral muscles that can be involved in a sprain.

127. B. The radius is involved in a Colles' fracture.

128. C. The fibula is involved in a Pott's fracture.

129. C. Myocardial infarction is a heart attack.

130. B. Edema is fluid that fills interstitial space.

131. C. Any deep pressure or tapotement on the bones is contraindicated for osteoporosis.

132. D. Avoid the broken area until fully healed.

133. A. Be sure the client is not in any other pain.

134. D. Joint pain and inflammation.

135. B. Also called humpback curvation.

136. B. Wash your hands after fungal contact as it is contagious.

137. C. The gallbladder stores bile that acts on lipids.

138. A. Pain in the big toe is a symptom of gout.

139. C. In the case of an epileptic seizure, keep the client safe.

140. B. Moles that show a change should be reported by the massage therapist.

141. A. The tibialis anterior causes foot drop and paralysis.

142. C. Iliopsoas for lordosis.

143. B. Whiplash causes impingment on the pectoralis minor.

144. A. The anterior rectus abdominus could be weak if the client complains of back pain.

145. A. The scalenes at rib one can entrap the brachial plexus.

146. A. The peroneal muscle everts the foot.

147. A. Ischemia is lack of oxygen.

148. B. Loss of muscle fiber is muscular dystrophy.

149. D. Tenosynovitis is inflamed tendon sheaths.

150. C. It is always better to reschedule; a fever is a contraindication.

151. B. Call the doctor for a consultation regarding the client's blood pressure.

152. A. Thrombosis can be a blood clot.

153. D. The entire body is affected by radiation. Massage is not recommended until the client has been cleared by the doctor.

154. C. Endangerment sites are areas where massage should not be deep due to superficial nerves and blood vessels.

155. C. Any mental illness needs clearance from a doctor.

156. D. Chlamydia is the sexually transmitted bacteria.

157. D. A virus causes genital herpes.

158. A. An ectopic pregnancy is the abnormal growth of the embryo in the fallopian tube.

159. C. Cyanosis is lack of oxygen.

160. D. A fungus infection is *Candida albicans*.

161. D. Skin that has hardened is called scleroderma.

162. D. Hemophilia is a genetic disease of the blood.

163. D. High blood pressure is the condition called hypertension.

164. D. Tachycardia is a rapid heartbeat.

165. C. Atherosclerosis is hardening of the arteries.

166. C. Phlebitis is an inflammation of the veins.

167. C. Athlete's foot is a fungal and contagious disease that is contraindicated when massaging.

168. D. A typical disease in postmenopausal women is osteoporosis.

169. A. A self-destructive disease of the joint linings is rheumatoid arthritis.

170. D. Rheumatoid arthitis is a contraindication of massage.

171. C. The weak valves of varicose veins cause the blood to back up.

172. A. The SITS muscles are involved in a frozen shoulder.

173. D. TMJ involves the masseter and pterygoid muscles in the cheek.

174. B. Headaches generally involve the muscles of the neck and shoulder.

175. B. Thoracic outlet syndrome is related to the scalenes and pectoralis minor.

176. A. When a bone is partially dislocated, it is called subluxation.

177. A. When the carotid artery is compressed, a client could faint.

178. C. Phlebitis is a vein that is inflamed and painful.

179. A. Fibromyalgia benefits from heat application.

180. D. The piriformis muscle can cause sciatic pain.

181. B. The myelin sheath is destroyed in multiple sclerosis.

182. C. Disease is an imbalance in the body or a lack of homeostasis.

183. B. Damage to the facial nerve seems to be the cause of Bell's palsy.

184. C. The lumbar plexus is involved in back pain.

185. D. A 3rd-degree burn is the most critical.

186. C. Hot, dry skin is a symptom of heat stroke.

187. B. Friction is best stroke for sprain.

188. B. Edema in ankle should have massage from the hip down.

189. B. Type II diabetes is too little insulin.

190. C. Lack of blood is called ischemia.

191. D. Referred pain is felt away from a tender point.

192. A. The carotid is in the anterior triangle of the neck.

193. B. The femoral nerve runs through the sartorius.

194. A. The sciatic nerve goes through the biceps femoris.

195. A. Basal cell carcinoma is the slowest growing of skin cancers.

196. C. It is okay to massage a client with Parkinson's disease.

197. C. The tibialis posterior muscle is the cause of shin splints.

198. D. Idiopathic is when the cause of a disease is unknown.

199. B. Vasodilation can be an effect of a histamine on the circulation.

200. C. Thrombophlebitis is a contraindication of massage.

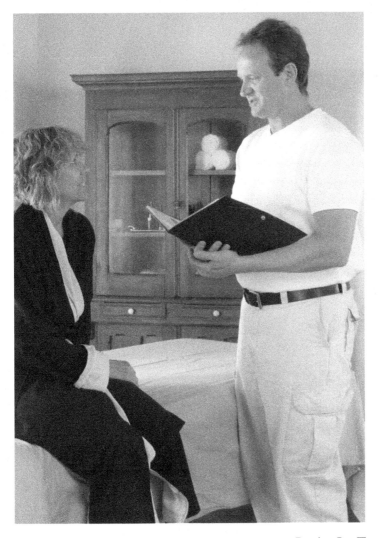

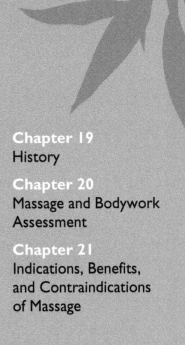

PART

3

History, Therapeutic Massage, and Bodywork Assessment

Part 3 covers the History of Massage to present day, the methods of assessing the clients, the physiological and emotional benefits, and contraindications of massage. The 300 questions make up 16–18% of the content in the NCETMB, NCETM and MBLEx exams.

19 History*

 CONTENTS

*History—MBLEx 5%

HISTORY OF MASSAGE	
Definition	• **Massage is defined as the systemic manual manipulation of soft tissues of the body** • **Movements include kneading, pressing, rolling, slapping, and tapping for therapeutic purposes promoting:** • **Circulation of blood and lymph** • **Relaxation of muscles** • **Relief from pain** • **Restoration of metabolic balance** • **Mental health**
Ancient Times	• Massage has been a major part of medicine and healing for more than 5000 years. • 3000 B.C. Chinese practical massage through acupressure, energy meridians, and acupuncture called *amma*. Today Chinese also refer to the push-pull as *tuina*. • 1800 B.C. The concept of *ayurvedic* medicine was developed by Hindus in India. The physical, emotional, and spiritual environment is energetically required for health. • 300 B.C. Massage was primary to Greek and Roman cultures. Hippocrates (460–380 B.C.), father of medicine, emphasized the value of massage in medicine. • Sixth century A.D. Japanese adopted techniques from Chinese and called the 660 points of stimulation *tsubo*. *Shiatsu* points are pressed to affect *Chi* (life force energy).
Dark Ages	• 476–1450 A.D. The decline of civilization in Western Europe and the Roman Empire is known as the Middle Ages. There was little record of any health practices, and medical institutions abandoned massage.
Renaissance	• 1450–1600 People became interested in art and physical health again. Ambroise Paré, a French surgeon, described the positive effect of massage through movement of friction, flexion, extension, and circumduction of joints. Acceptance of massage for healing and treatment of disease.

(continued)

HISTORY OF MASSAGE (*continued*)	
Modern Massage Techniques	• *Medical Gymnastics* was introduced by Per Hendrick Ling, father of Swedish massage. In 1813, Ling established schools in Sweden, spread into Europe and Russia, and called it Swedish Movements. • *The Swedish Movement Cure* was brought to the United States in 1858 by Charles Taylor, a New York physician who started an orthopedic practice with Swedish Movement cure. • Massage gained public and medical acceptance.

Massage in the United States	• 1960
	
	A renaissance of massage in the United States began and continues today.
	
	Awareness of physical alternatives in healthcare developed a wellness model, which includes massage therapy.
	
	• 1970–1980
	Rise in use of massage as well as other bodywork.
	
	Professional associations formed:
	    American Massage Therapy Association (AMTA)
	    Association of Bodywork and Massage Professionals (ABMP)
	
	• 1992
	Massage therapists were recognized when the National Certification for Therapeutic Massage and Bodyworkers (NCTMB) developed standards and a national certifying exam.
	
	Massage therapists are qualified by education, experience, certification, licensing, and the national exam, National Certifying Exam for Therapeutic Massage and Bodywork (NCETMB).
	
	• 2005
	The National Certification Board for Therapeutic Massage and Bodywork (NCBTMB) changed their format and developed two tests:
	National Certifying Exam for Therapeutic Massage (NCETM), NCETMB
	    FSMTB—Federation of State Massage Therapy Board
	    MBLEx—National licensing exam governed by FSMTB

Contributors to Massage History	• *Per Henrick Ling*—Physiologist who developed the Swedish gymnastics, or Swedish massage. • *Dr. Johann Mezger*—Developed rehabilitation, now called physical therapy. He also codified the French terms of Swedish massage (e.g., effleurage, petrissage). • *Dr. John Kellogg*—Prescribed massage as part of treatment to patients at the Battle Creek Sanitarium of Michigan. • *Elizabeth Dicke*—Developed a connective tissue massage called Bindegewebsmassage. • *James Cyriax*—Developed deep transverse friction techniques to broaden tissue, break down adhesions, and restore mobility.

20 Massage and Bodywork Assessment

 CONTENTS

MASSAGE AND BODYWORK ASSESSMENT	
Definition	***Assessment***—A preliminary evaluation before giving a massage; may include postural, gait, or other physical assessment intended to gain information about the client ***Medical history***—Taking a health history of client (written or verbal) before proceeding with massage in order to be aware of medication, surgeries, or other contraindications
Reason for Assessment	• To design the most appropriate massage session • To refer client to another health care or medical professional, if needed
Assessment Areas	• Soft tissue palpation • Bony landmarks • Endangerment sites • Trigger points • Craniosacral pulses • Lymphatic edema • Energy channel blockage (Asian)
Somatic Holding Patterns	Stimulation of nervous system receptors is interpreted through the somatic reflex arc that helps to maintain homeostasis. Examples include • Guarding muscle • Fascial memory
Assessment Methods	***Visual*** ***Gait or walking pattern***—Is it smooth and balanced? ***Posture***—Symmetrical, distortions, faulty alignment through anterior and posterior ***Basic body structure***—Proper curvature of spine? ***Restrictive range of motion***—At joints, muscles, tendon, or ligaments ***Eyes***—Good eye contact ***Breathing***—Respiration normal, deep, shallow? ***Pathological conditions***—Varicose veins, inflammation, bruises ***Sympathetic or parasympathetic condition***—Anxious, excited, angry, restless, calm, relaxed, or depressed? ***Emotional condition***—State of mind ***Physical condition***—Energetic or tired

Touch

Palpation—Ability to assess qualities of the body through touch, temperature, texture, pulses, tension, pain levels, adhesion, energy flows, and blocks

Focus areas—Anatomical: skin, fascia, tendons, ligaments, muscles, blood vessels, lymph nodes, and bones

Body rhythms—Heartbeat, respiration, cranial

Senses

Auditory—Listen to your client for tone, loudness, and speech articulation as cues to wellness

Olfactory—Notice any abnormal odors including strange or profuse body odor, alcohol, or smoking on client

Energetic—Notice profound energy or fatigue associated with client's behavior

Intuitive—Notice or feel anything that might be different or not quite right about client

21 Indications, Benefits, and Contraindications of Massage

 CONTENTS

INDICATIONS OF MASSAGE	
Definition	**Massage is indicated for treating a condition, injury, or symptom and is not detrimental to the client**
Types of Indications	• Complementary—To enhance any means of healing • Palliative care—To reduce symptoms and discomfort • Direct therapeutic care—Direct muscle relaxation

BENEFITS OF MASSAGE	

Physiological Effects	*General*
	  • Increases joint range of motion
	  • Increases cell metabolism
	  • Increases flexibility and mobility
	  • Reduces pain and inflammation
	  • Promotes hormonal release

Effects on Primary Systems	*Integument system*
	  Increases blood flow to skin
	  Facilitates sebaceous secretions
	  Maintains healthy skin
	
	Muscular system
	  Stretches muscle and promote relaxation
	  Relieves muscle spasms, cramps, and pain
	  Improves muscle tone and athletic performance
	  Relieves inflammation of tendons
	  Promotes healing
	
	Cardiovascular system
	  Improves circulation and delivery of O_2 to cells
	  Removes toxins and metabolic wastes
	  Improves heart rate and blood pressure/hypertension
	
	Nervous system
	  Promotes release of endorphins
	  Relieves pain
	  Promotes homeostasis in parasympathetic and sympathetic systems
	
	Respiratory system
	  Helps to promote deep breathing and relaxation
	  Aids in relieving asthma and COPD patients

(*continued*)

BENEFITS OF MASSAGE (*continued*)	

	Lymphatic system
	     Improves lymphedema
	     Increases lymph circulation
	     Increases toxin removal
	     Increases T cells for autoimmune diseases

Psychological Effects	• Reduces stress from medical conditions • Reduces pain from chronic illnesses • Reduces fatigue and anxiety • Promotes feeling of well-being, healthier, relaxed, energetic, peaceful • Promotes deep relaxation • Increases productivity
Cancer	• Complementary therapy • Aids healing, scarring • Post mastectomy patients
Pediatric Application	• Autistic children • Premature babies • Asthmatic children • Diabetic children
Complement to Chiropractic	• Massage use before or after adjustment relieves tension in muscles and pain

CONTRAINDICATIONS OF MASSAGE	
Definition	• **Treatment that is inadvisable or course of treatment not recommended** • **All pathologies should be considered when deciding to massage a client or not. If unsure about a contraindication, call a client's physician for approval and never work outside your scope of practice** • **Always look for the following life-threatening conditions, contagious and acute conditions, and injuries**
Contraindications (physician release)	***Anemia***—Lack of oxygen ***Aneurysm***—Weakened blood vessel or heart, forms sac-like protrusion ***Arteriosclerosis***—Disease of arteries caused by plaque hardening ***Arthritis***—Inflammation and pain ***Asthma***—Respiratory disease, difficult to breathe ***Athlete's foot***—Fungus ***Bell's Palsy***—7th nerve facial paralysis

Bursitis—Inflammation of bursa, fluid sac at joint

Burns—First, second, third degree open wound of skin

Cancer—Metastasized or lymphatic

Carcinoma—Basal, squamous cell growth

Cirrhosis of the liver—Liver damage

Diabetes—If insulin shock

Fever—High body temperature over 99.6 °F

Heart attack—Blocked coronary arteries

Herniated disc—Rupture or protrusion of nucleus in intervertebral disc

Herpes simplex—Cold sores

High or low blood pressure—Increased pressure on arteries

Infectious skin conditions—Warts, ringworm, bacterial, viral, fungal or parasitic (i.e., scabies)

Influenza—Acute stage, contagious

Inflammation—Pitting edema, pain, heat, redness of area

Intoxication—Heavy alcohol consumption

Hemophilia—Bruises or bleeds easily

Mental disorders—Depression, bipolar, psychosis

Osteoporosis—Bone is weakened

Phlebitis—Vein inflammation, usually in lower limb.

Pneumonia—Respiratory infection

Pregnancy—*Use caution in first trimester (before 14 weeks gestation)*

Sciatica—Severe pain along sciatic nerve

Sprain and Strain—Injury to tendon or ligament

Stroke—Loss of blood to brain, can cause paralysis

Subluxation—Particular incomplete dislocation

Surgery (recent)

Tendinitis—Injury, inflammation to tendon sheaths

TMJ—Tempomandibular joint dysfunction

Torticollis (wry neck)—Deformed neck with tilt

Thrombosis (blood clot)

Varicose veins—Enlarged, protruding veins, poor circulation

Whiplash—Hyperflexion or hyperextension of cervical vertebrae

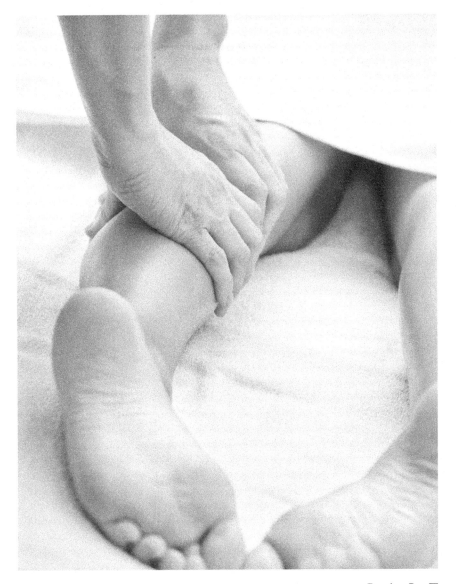

P A R T

4

Therapeutic Massage and Bodywork Application

Part 4 covers the Principles and Methods of massage and includes an understanding of CPR and First Aid, Hydrotherapy, Aromatherapy, Eastern, Western Bodywork, and an overview of Modalities. The 300 questions make up 17–24% of the the content in the NCETMB, NCETM and MBLEx exams.

CHAPTER 22 Massage Application: Basic Principles

 ## CONTENTS

MASSAGE APPLICATION: BASIC PRINCIPLES	
Endangerment Sites	An anatomical area of concern that may contain underlying structures (nerves, blood vessels) that could be damaged by massage: *Anterior triangle*—Carotid, jugular, and vagus nerve *Posterior triangle*—Brachial plexus, subclavian artery *Axilla*—Axillary, median, ulnar nerves, axillary artery, lymph nodes *Ulnar notch*—Ulnar nerve *Lumbar*—Kidney *Femoral triangle*—Femoral artery, nerve, vein, lymph nodes, saphenous vein *Inferior to ear*—Carotid artery, facial nerve, styloid process *Sciatic notch*—Sciatic nerve in gluteus maximus muscle *Cubital*—Median, ulnar, radial arteries *Abdomen*—Aorta, liver, gallbladder, spleen, stomach *Popliteal area (behind knee)*—Popliteal artery, nerve *Medial brachium*—Ulnar, median nerve, brachial artery
Universal Precautions	**Procedures used when conditions require contact with any body fluid (i.e., blood, urine, sweat, tears, saliva, or semen) to prevent spread of infection from healthcare giver to client or vice versa** All are recommended by Centers for Disease Control and Prevention, which include: • *Hand washing* for three minutes to control spread of microorganisms • *Antibacterial hand sanitizer* • *Gloves* for contact with soiled articles or open wounds • *Gown* worn to act as barrier between clothing and body • *Mask* worn to provide a barrier to airborne diseases • *Linens* should be washed separately with chlorine bleach

COMMUNICATION	
Definition	**Communication is a part of the massage treatment; it establishes trust and understanding with the client from the 1st interview throughout the treatment plan.**
Important Facts	• Show courtesy, respect, and professionalism • Assess by observing, interviewing, and palpating • Speak clearly and listen to client's needs • Establish SOAP notes with treatment plan • Plan single and multiple sessions based on conditions of client, goals, and contraindications • Periodically re-evaluate and discuss progress and future plans

(continued)

COMMUNICATION (*continued*)	
Boundaries	There are physical and emotional boundaries during a massage session: *Listen* to build trust *Touch* in a nurturing way that is safe *Empathize* by understanding client's feelings *Ask questions* when appropriate *Do not judge* client personally *Refer* to psychological professional when needed *Care* for a client in a professional way

INTERVIEW AND CONSULTATION	
Definition	**Consultation is an interview process with the client. The practitioner informs the client about the services he or she provides.**
Consult Content	• Greet client and introduce him- or herself • Determine client's needs and expectations • Explain procedures • State policies and fees • Perform a preliminary assessment, verbal, and body movement • Formulate a treatment plan and goals for sessions • Refer to another health professional if needed
Intake and Medical History	*Vital information* in medical history formulates a treatment strategy. *Include in client information:* • Name, address, phone numbers, email • Occupation • General health condition • Serious or chronic illness, accidents, surgery • Medication, blood pressure • Doctor's name or other health practitioner • Why did you come for a massage? • What results are you looking for? • Who referred you? • List of illnesses, pregnancy, alcohol, or smoking • Emergency contact name and number • Cancellation policy • Client's signature and date

Body Diagram	• Use a male or female body diagram to indicate painful spots, trigger points, or stiffness
	• Circle areas of other concern and describe condition
SOAP Charting	To record client and session information, use of SOAP notes is very beneficial to keep and update client records. **S**—*Subjective:* Initial interview, anything the clients tells the therapist **O**—*Objective:* Information the therapist gathers by observation, interview; treatment goals **A**—*Assessment:* Any progress or lack of progress relative to the massage session is documented **P**—*Plan:* Record suggestions for future sessions or homework exercises

23 Massage Assessment: Methods and Techniques

CONTENTS

MASSAGE ASSESSMENT: METHODS AND TECHNIQUES	

Basic Strokes	**Seven strokes are basic to Swedish massage and foundation of other Western bodywork along with stretching and/or joint mobilization:**
	
	Effleurage
	  Long gliding strokes in the direction of the heart
	  Used to warm and relax client, stretch muscles, increase circulation toward heart, used as a transitional stroke
	
	Petrissage
	  Kneading strokes consisting of picking up tissue, kneading, rolling, and lifting
	  Petrissage is used to loosen adhesions, stretch muscles and fascia, increase circulation
	
	Friction
	  Pressure aimed at moving superficial tissue across deep tissue including cross-fiber, circular, and compression applied to fleshy body parts
	  Friction is used to loosen adhesions, fascia and scar tissue, promote flexibility and increase circulation
	  Thumbs, fingers, palms, or elbows can be used
	
	Tapotement—Percussion strokes consisting of slapping, cupping, hacking, and tapping, usually at the end of massage to increase circulation or release phlegm in respiratory tract
	
	Vibration—Shaking or rocking movements, can be slow and sedative or fast and stimulating
	
	Nerve stroke—Referred to as feather stroke at the end of massage
	
	Compression—Gentle pressure into the body to spread tissue against underlying body structure

MASSAGE APPLICATION	
Joint Movements	*Active*—Client participates by contracting and moving the involved muscles of the joint *Active assistive*—Client performs the motion with assistance of therapist *Passive*—The therapist stretches and moves body part while the client relaxes the involved muscles *Resistive*—The client resists movement *Range of motion*—The amount of natural movement within a joint

Stretching	Exercises that promote lengthening of muscle and movement of joint through full range of motion
	
	  Static stretching (assisted)—Stretching until resistance is met, hold to release
	
	  Static stretching (unassisted)—Client stretches into resistance
	
	  Proprioceptive neuromuscular facilitation (PNF)—Assisted stretching technique in which muscle is stretched into resistance, 3 to 4 times

(continued)

MASSAGE APPLICATION (continued)	
	Passive stretching—Slow, steady gentle movement to lengthen muscles when natural resistance is minimal
	Reciprocal inhibition stretching—Contracting the antagonistic muscle to the one being stretched, reduces muscle cramps
	Active isolated stretching (AIS)—Stretching the primary muscle
	Muscle energy technique (MET)—A group of neuromuscular techniques that involve voluntary contraction of specific muscle or muscle group while positioned in a specific direction; contractions can vary in time and intensity as a result of client-active techniques
Postural Integration	To promote *postural balance* through integration of body and mind techniques

DRAPING	
Definition	**The use of linens to keep client covered while performing a massage and at the same time retain comfort, warmth, and modesty. All methods consist of techniques to maintain privacy of client to and from the massage table as well during the massage. The body remains covered with the exposure of each part as it is massaged. Breasts remained covered except for purpose of post operative massage**
Top Cover	A top cover should be large enough to cover the body (72" × 32"), function as the drape, and can be used from and to the dressing area. A sheet or towel is appropriate
Full Sheet	Full-sheet (72" × 80") draping covers the client in a cocoon-like wrap on both top and bottom

TOPICAL APPLICATION	
Definition	**Massage and bodywork use a topical application of lotion, oil, or liniment to enhance their effects, minimize skin friction, or address the pain of sore or sprained muscles**
Oils	Include almond, grapeseed, olive, mineral, or jojoba; regard the hypoallergenic properties and the oil stains on sheets
Lotions	Thinner than oil, good for moisturizing skin, and are water soluble
Gels	A combination of a lotion and oil, hypoallergenic, and popular for use
Creams	A thicker lotion, harder to glide, good for deep tissue work
Liniment	Oil or cream applied for therapeutic purpose of sprained, sore, or bruised muscle; camphor, menthol, or herbs help to relieve pain; not to be used for massage
Hydrotherapy	Wet compresses can be applied to relax muscles or ice to relieve pain
Hot Stone Therapy	Can be applied to body to relax muscles or for massage or trigger point relief

PERFORMING THE MASSAGE	
Environment	• Comfortable temperature • Cleanliness for each client • Sanitized and ventilated room • Lighting subdued • Proper lubricant for client • Room clear of any offensive odor • Professional personal hygiene

Bolsters/Pillows	**Supine**
	    Under knees takes pressure off lower back
	    Under neck to support head and for comfort
	Prone
	    Rolled towel under ankles
	    Under anterior for large breasts
	    Under abdomen takes pressure off lower back
	Side-lying
	    Pillow between legs takes pressure off pelvic joints
	    Pillow under head and under arms for comfort

Body Mechanics	• Proper body mechanics increase length of massage therapist's career and prevents injuries in joints and muscles • The mechanics of muscular activity in the movement of giving a massage • Keep your back straight and knees slightly bent • Work from the center of your pelvis and allow the legs and large muscles do the work • Keep elbows close to body and wrists relaxed • Table at proper height
Routine Procedure	• Complete medical intake • Consultation and client interview • Determine any contraindications • Develop SOAP notes for ongoing massages • Allow client to enter room, disrobe, and get on table supine or prone under sheet or towel • Always drape properly, keeping pelvic and breast areas covered • Use proper body mechanics to prevent injury • Keep talking to a minimum to help client relax • Keep massage within scope of practice; avoid any endangerment sites • If client becomes emotional, stop massage and tell client why you can't continue

(continued)

PERFORMING THE MASSAGE (*continued*)	
	• Treat clients with empathy • Inform client if some pathology is found • Proceed with normal routine to end • Inform client massage is over and he or she can get up slowly and get dressed • Give client cup of water • Ask client how he or she feels and schedule next appointment

MASSAGE AND BODYWORK TOOLS	
Definition	**Any mechanical device (i.e, electric, wood, rubber, plastic) that simulates a stroke or pressure of the human touch to give the therapist alternative options to reduce the physical exertion of the practitioner.**
Types	*Vibrators*—Take the place of rapid percussion. Depending on the rate of vibration, intensity of pressure and duration, a relaxation and release of tension occurs. *Bongers*—Hand-held round rubber-ended massage tools that take the place of tapotement. Used for cellulite reduction. *Acupressure tools*—Wood or plastic tools that apply pressure to a single spot to relieve tight muscles or trigger points.

STRESS MANAGEMENT	
Definition	**Techniques used to relax and combat stress and its harmful physical and emotional effects. The following are to put the body and mind in a state of relaxation, which encourages healing.**
Massage	Promote relaxation through the "touch" of massage therapy
Visualization	Promoting mental images through verbal guidance or meditation. Helps to affect emotional and mental states sometimes called "closed eye processes" or mind "journeys"
Yoga	A system of stretches and exercises for attaining physical, mental, and emotional control and well-being.
Biofeedback	A series of exercises to promote conscious control of or awareness of the physiologic responses to stress, pain, or disease. Involves use of electronic instruments to monitor
Breath Work	Use of breathing exercises designed to promote focus, energy, and physiological responses of relaxation
Exercise	Commonly used stress reducer that creates an endorphin release and promotes physical health

24 CPR and First Aid

 CONTENTS

CPR AND FIRST AID	
Definition	***CPR (cardiopulmonary resuscitation)***—Emergency procedure to artificially return heartbeat and breathing after cardiac arrest by manually compressing chest and forcing air into lungs. ***First Aid***—Actions taken as a first response to injury or sickness, such as applying a tourniquet or administering CPR. Every therapist should be certified in first aid and CPR.
ABC's of CPR	• ***Airway***—Check to see if mouth or throat is clear, sweep finger into the mouth if blocked. • ***Breathing***—Check to see if victim is breathing, if not, start artificial respiration. • ***Circulation***—Check carotid pulse; if no pulse, start CPR.
Heimlich Maneuver	Always call for advanced life support first and then begin intervention. Should be performed if person cannot speak, cough, or breathe due to object lodged in airway. If victim is conscious, stand behind with hands clasped into a fist and place below rib cage and perform five abdominal thrusts until object is coughed up.
Heat-related Injuries	• ***Heat cramps***—Muscular spasms due to loss of salt; give victim sips of saltwater and massage cramps. • ***Heat exhaustion***—Due to extreme sweating without fluid replacement; give victim sips of saltwater, lie down, elevate legs, cold compresses. • ***Heat stroke***—High body temperature (106°F) and lack of sweating; bathe or sponge victim in cold water or rub alcohol to 102°F and then dry and use fans or air conditioner.
Cold-related Injures	• ***Hypothermia***—Body temperature below 90°F; move victim to warm spot, give dry, warm blankets and warm liquid. • ***Frostbite***—Crystals form in fluid of soft tissue of body, usually extremities; cover frostbite with blankets and move to warm environment; give warm drink and lukewarm or room temperature water bath.
Fractures	• A crack in the bone, simple (closed), compound (open) • Swelling, pain, deformity • Protect victim, immobilize break and proximal and distal joints
Strain and Sprain	• Muscle or tendons stretched or torn RICE = Universal Treatment: R = Rest, I = Ice, C = Compression, E = Elevation

CONTENTS

HYDROTHERAPY			
Definition	• **The use of water in a solid state (ice), liquid state (water), or gas state (vapor) for therapeutic purposes; non-toxic, solvent, stones, and transit heat.** • **Water is relaxing, stimulating, and a natural healer used both internally and externally.**		
Types of Heat	*Thermal*—Heat pack, hot stones, hot bath, sauna, steam room *Mechanical*—Sprays or whirlpools *Chemical*—Ingesting or irrigation of water		
Effects to Body	Decrease pain, stiffness, muscle spasm Increase circulation, metabolism, respiration, inflammation		
Cryotherapy	*Ice therapy*—Short application will stimulate (local and systemic); long application will sedate. Used for strains, sprains, fractures, and contusions. The universal treatment for strains and sprains is RICE—Rest, ice, compression, and elevation.		
Application	Ice pack, ice water, cold whirlpool, hydrocolla, or packs, gel pack		
Effects of Cold and Ice	Decreases pain, circulation, digestion inflammation, muscle spasm Increases tissue stiffness, muscle tone		
Contraindication Risks to Hot and Cold	High or low blood pressure Pregnancy Heart or circulatory problems Diabetes Seizures Elderly and young children with care Skin rash Vascular issues Infections Contagious conditions		
Temperature Ranges	Very hot	111°–120°F	Hot pack, sauna
	Hot	101°–110°F	Steam room
	Warm	93°–100°F	Whirlpool
	Tepid	80°–92°F	Warm bath
	Cool	70°–79°F	Cool bath

	Cold	55°–69°F	Cold water
	Very Cold	31°–54°F	Cold pack
	Freezing	32° and below	Ice
Safety Cautions	• Explain treatment • Stay with client during treatment • Thorough case history • Use bathroom before treatment • More is not better; adapt to individual		

AROMATHERAPY	
Definition	**The use of essential oils to promote specific physical and emotional changes and effects (i.e., lavender, sandalwood, peppermint, lemongrass, tea tree).**
How Oils Work	The essential oil enters through inhalation or the skin; enters the blood work quickly or enters the limbic area of the blood brain barrier.
Where Oils Come From	The oils are extracted by various methods including distilling from the leaves, stems, flowers, wood, fruit, or roots of plants. Each oil has a distinct property that affects the body or emotions.
How Oils Are Used	• In massage lubricant • In diffuser • Directly on the body
Guidelines For Safe Use	• Always keep a bottle of mixing oil handy when using essential oils. Vegetable oils are used to dilute essential oils that cause discomfort or skin irritation at full strength. • Keep bottles of essential oils tightly closed and store in a cool location away from light. • Keep essential oils out of reach of children. • Direct sunlight and essential oils. Lemon, bergamot, orange, grapefruit, tangerine, White Angelica, and other citrus oils (marked with an orange drop) may cause a rash or darken when exposed to direct sunlight.

Uses of Essential Oils	Action	Application	Example
	Antiseptic	Cuts, insect bites	Clove, eucalyptus, lavender, lemon, tea tree, thyme, sage
	Anti-inflammatory	Eczema, dermatitis, bruises, infections, strains and sprains	Chamomile, lavender
	Fungicidal	Athlete's foot, thrush/yeast infection (*Candida albicans*)	Lavender, myrrh, marjoram, patchouli, tea tree
	Granulation, stimulation, cicatrizing (healing)	Cuts, burns, scars, stretch marks	Chamomile, frankincense, geranium, neroli, rose
	Deodorant	Perspiration, personal hygiene	Bergamot, cypress, juniper, lemongrass
	Insecticide	Mosquitoes, ticks, fleas, lice	Camphor, cedarwood, citronella, clove, eucalyptus, garlic, geranium, lavender
Contraindications of Essential Oils Use	• Nausea side effects • Skin irritation • Allergies • Pregnancy issues • Some oils contain toxic chemicals		

300 Questions with Answers and Rationales on Therapeutic Massage Assessment and Application

OBJECTIVES

Major areas of knowledge/content included in this chapter are based on most of the NCETMB, NCETM and MBLEx exam topics that cover Therapeutic Massage Assessment and Application.

Exam Content Percentages:

NCETMB 18%

NCETM 17%

MBLEx 16%

➢ History

➢ Assessment
   Reasons for Assessment
   Areas
   Methods

➢ Benefits of Massage

➢ Effects to the System

➢ Contraindications

➢ Applications
   Endangerment Sites
   Universal Precautions
   Topical Applications

➢ Communication

➢ Methods and Techniques
   Basic Strokes
   Joint Movement
   Range of Motion
   Stretching
   Draping and Supports
   Biomechanics
   Medical History
   SOAP Charts
   The Massage Routine
   Stress Management
   First Aid and CPR
   Hydrotherapy
   Aromatherapy

DIRECTIONS

Each of the questions or statements below is followed by four suggested answers or completions. Select **one answer** that is best in each case.

1. Which is a skill for developing an optimal client relationship?
   A. Acceptance
   B. Ignoring
   C. Listening
   D. Humoring

2. When the client reveals sensitive information and honest thoughts and feelings, it is known as
   A. Self-disclosure
   B. Empathy
   C. Consoling
   D. Moralizing

3. The sequences and directions of Swedish massage strokes were adapted to benefit the
   A. Muscle attachments
   B. Subcutaneous adipose tissue
   C. Autonomic nervous system
   D. Lymph drainage and venous return

4. Which best describes the effects of massage therapy?
   A. Increased venous and lymph flow
   B. Increased venous, decreased arterial flow
   C. Decreased venous and lymph flow
   D. Decreased venous, increased lymph flow

5. Some roadblocks to communication between therapist and client include
   A. Giving long-range goals
   B. Criticizing
   C. Interpreting the medical intake
   D. Advising, judging, and analyzing

6. Universal precautions are required when
   A. Handling body fluids
   B. Performing invasive medical procedures
   C. Doing all massage therapy
   D. All of the above

7. When massaging the thigh in the supine position, which is (are) involved?
   A. Hamstrings
   B. Quadriceps
   C. Gluteals
   D. Gastrocnemius

8. The universal precautions were designed by Occupational Safety and Health Administration (OSHA) primarily for
   A. Clinical massage therapists
   B. Practitioners who handle body fluids
   C. Healthcare workers
   D. All of the above

9. In first aid for a choking victim, you want the conscious victim to
   A. Cough
   B. Swallow
   C. Vomit
   D. Inhale

10. In order to control the spread of pathogenic microorganisms, the therapist should
    A. Wash hands often
    B. Disinfect equipment
    C. Massage with gloves
    D. A and B

11. Endangerment sites should be avoided during a massage because
    A. They are bilaterally symmetrical
    B. They are areas that can be easily injured
    C. They are areas that are dysfunctional
    D. They are hard to remember

12. A pregnant client should have pillows under her head and between her knees when she is lying
    A. On her side
    B. Supine
    C. Prone
    D. A and B

13. A pre-event sports massage is shorter with the movements performed
    A. Precisely
    B. Using heat
    C. Slower
    D. Faster

14. Cross-fiber massage must be applied in which direction to the fibers?
    A. Horizontal
    B. Perpendicular
    C. Triangular
    D. Trapezoidal

15. All the following are endangerment sites except
    A. Popliteal artery
    B. Kidney region
    C. Brachial plexus
    D. Transverse colon

16. In the supine position a bolster is placed under the _____ to take pressure off the lower back.
    A. Neck
    B. Ankles
    C. Knees
    D. Sacrum

17. Cold applied for therapeutic purposes is called
    A. Cryptology
    B. Cryotherapy
    C. Ignorance
    D. Cool ice

18. The draping method that covers the entire body is called
    A. Top-cover
    B. Full-sheet
    C. Diaper
    D. Wrapping

19. In the prone position, support is put under the _____ to ease the pressure on the lower back.
    A. Ankles
    B. Abdomen
    C. Shoulders
    D. Chest

20. The draping method that covers the table and wraps the client is called
    A. Top-cover
    B. Full-sheet
    C. Diaper
    D. Wrapping

21. Most current massage styles are based on
    A. Swedish movements
    B. Swiss movements
    C. German movements
    D. Greek movements

22. Nerve trunks and centers are sometimes chosen as sites for the application of
    A. Rolling
    B. Rocking
    C. Pressure
    D. Vibration

23. Support for the cervical area can be provided by a _____ in the supine position.
    A. Triangle
    B. Face cradle
    C. Shoulder cushion
    D. Neck roll

24. A bath with a temperature of 85°–95°F is considered
    A. Cool
    B. Cold
    C. Tepid
    D. Hot

25. The procedure that uses a bouncing movement to improve the flow of lymph through the entire system is called lymphatic
    A. Bounce
    B. Sway
    C. Purging
    D. Pump manipulation

26. The attempt to bring the structure of the body into alignment around a central axis is called
    A. Structural integration
    B. Trauma
    C. Alignment
    D. Adjustment

27. The placement of bolsters in the side-lying position are
    A. Head supported with face cradle
    B. Under bottom leg
    C. Under ankles
    D. Under the head, leg, and arm

28. When you become a massage therapist, you must prepare your _____ and _____.
    A. Lubricant and sheets
    B. Body and feet
    C. Mind and spirit
    D. Balance, stamina, mind, and body

29. Realignment of muscular and connective tissue and reshaping the body's physical posture is called
    A. Adjustment
    B. Centering
    C. Rolfing
    D. Posturing

30. A hyperirritable spot that is painful when compressed is called a(an)
    A. Trigger point
    B. Pain point
    C. Ampule
    D. Rolfing

31. Self-awareness and self-care for a massage therapist is essential to
    A. Balance the body, mind, and spirit
    B. Offer more to the client than normal
    C. Remembering the routine
    D. Maintain balance, strength, and stamina

32. When you are massaging, expose only the
    A. Dorsal side
    B. Ventral side
    C. Area being massaged
    D. Sheet being used

33. Better flexibility is the result of
    A. Sustained stretching
    B. Ballistic stretching
    C. Weight lifting
    D. Bicycling

34. Using too much deep pressure causes the muscles to
    A. Have pain
    B. Go limp
    C. Relax
    D. Cramp

35. The general effects of percussion movements are to tone the muscles by
    A. Vibration
    B. Friction
    C. Kneading
    D. Hacking, cupping, slapping, beating

36. A concern with towel draping is that it
    A. Is too thick to work with
    B. Is more difficult to master
    C. Is not warm enough
    D. Leaves the abdomen exposed

37. The idea that stimulation of particular body points affects other areas is called
    A. Chiropractic
    B. Reflexology
    C. Rolfing
    D. Touching

38. The stance in which both feet are placed perpendicular to the edge of the table is called the
    A. Archer
    B. Horse
    C. Moose
    D. Stirrup

39. Joint mobilization is a passive movement that can be integrated into a massage routine, for example,
    A. Pulling
    B. Friction
    C. Stretching to ROM limit
    D. Tapotement

40. The most difficult part of draping is
    A. Not exposing too much
    B. Covering the body
    C. Turning your client over
    D. Keeping stains off

41. Deep strokes and kneading techniques can cause an increase in
    A. Vasoconstriction
    B. Blood flow
    C. Diastolic arterial pressure
    D. Systolic arterial pressure

42. What best describes the technique of Rolfing?
    A. Reflex zone therapy
    B. German massage
    C. Structural integration
    D. Neuromuscular massage

43. The cupping technique is best suited for
    A. Acute bronchitis
    B. Cancer of the lungs
    C. Bronchiectasis
    D. Acute tracheitis

44. The method of holding the sheets when used to turn a client over is called
    A. Anchor or tenting method
    B. Flip method
    C. Turn over method
    D. Prone method

45. An excellent stroke for assessing tissues is
    A. Effleurage
    B. Petrissage
    C. Friction
    D. Tapotement/percussion

46. Good body mechanics is defined as
    A. Proper use of postural techniques
    B. Biomechanics to decrease fatigue
    C. Making use of the therapist's body weight
    D. All of the above

47. Temperature range for hot immersion baths is best at
    A. 85°–95°F
    B. 100°–110°F
    C. 125°–150°F
    D. 130°–140°F

48. Which of the following are used when applying massage strokes?
    A. No pressure, excursion
    B. Grounding
    C. Speed
    D. Intension, rhythm, sequence

49. The application of force exerted by the massage therapist on the client's body is called
    A. Speed
    B. Depth
    C. Pressure
    D. Excursion

50. In addition to massage, which is most helpful in increasing lymph flow?
    A. Exercise
    B. Heat
    C. Immobilization
    D. Passive movement

51. When applying pressure, it is important to
    A. Not exceed the client's personal pain threshold
    B. Cause muscle relaxation, not contraction
    C. The area on the body where the pressure is applied should be deep
    D. A and B

52. Which ancillary stroke is a light finger tracing over the skin to finish a massage therapy?
    A. Pennate
    B. Nerve stroke
    C. Light friction
    D. Final touch

53. Localized, sensitive ischemic tissue that is hypersensitive to touch but does not cause referred sensations is called
    A. Trigger point
    B. Satellite point
    C. Tender point
    D. Tsubo

54. Stretching that is a combined effort between the therapist and client is known as
    A. Active-passive
    B. Passive-active
    C. Active-assisted
    D. Static-active

55. The therapeutic benefit of friction is
    A. Local hyperemia
    B. Lymphatic drainage
    C. Tonification
    D. Systemic ischemia

56. In body mechanics the horse stance or warrior stance is used to
    A. Perform short, transverse strokes, such as petrissage
    B. Perform long effleurage strokes
    C. Perform chair massage
    D. Adjust the massage table to the correct height

57. The main purpose of deep transverse friction is to
    A. Separate muscle fibers
    B. Lengthen muscle fibers
    C. Shorten muscle fibers
    D. Minimize pain

58. A system of active, passive, and resisted movements of the body's various joints and muscles, most often the presentation of passive ROM, is called
    A. Active stretching
    B. Table gymnastics
    C. Swedish gymnastics
    D. Passive stretching

59. Which stroke most often begins and ends a massage?
    A. Effleurage
    B. Petrissage
    C. Friction
    D. Vibration

60. What is the best massage technique to lift muscles off the bone?
    A. Effleurage
    B. Petrissage
    C. Vibration
    D. Tapotement

61. Joint movements are traditionally categorized as
    A. Free active and passive
    B. Assistive active and passive
    C. Passive and active
    D. All of the above

62. Stretching that involves the therapist's applying gentle resistance while the client is actively engaging in a stretch is
    A. Active-assisted
    B. Ballistic
    C. Resisted or isometric
    D. Static

63. How should you vary massage treatment time with the age of the patient?
    A. Progressively with increased age
    B. Shorter with increased age
    C. Shorter for very old and very young
    D. The same for any age

64. Which massage technique gives the best information about connective tissue structure in ligaments, tendons, and joints?
    A. Effleurage
    B. Friction
    C. Vibration
    D. Tapotement

65. Stretching is a type of _____ joint movement that is performed to the limit of the ROM.
    A. Active
    B. Assistive active
    C. Passive
    D. Resistive active

66. Which stroke is best for breaking down adhesions?
    A. Effleurage
    B. Petrissage
    C. Friction
    D. Vibration

67. In order to challenge the muscles used, practitioners apply _____ movement to a joint.
    A. Resistive
    B. Passive
    C. Free
    D. Assistive

68. Strokes that knead are called
   A. Effleurage
   B. Petrissage
   C. Friction
   D. Vibration

69. Joint mobilization techniques are used to help improve
   A. Body re-alignment
   B. Hip replacement
   C. Muscle relaxation
   D. Alignment, posture, muscle memory

70. What is the best stroke for massaging the intercostals?
   A. Compression
   B. Tapotement
   C. Vibration
   D. Petrissage

71. In order to generally assess the degree of flexibility at a joint, the practitioner should have a knowledge of the
   A. Stretch capacity
   B. Normal ROM and end feel
   C. Resistive movement
   D. Counterstrain

72. How should pressure be administered during effleurage?
   A. Evenly
   B. Deep to lighter
   C. Like nerve stroke
   D. Light to deeper

73. Careful joint movement is important in cases of
   A. Prosthetics
   B. Young children
   C. Menopausal women
   D. Hip replacement, elderly, and metal in joints

74. Biofeedback is useful in
   A. Relieving pain through autogenic training
   B. Controlling voluntary processes
   C. A therapeutic program
   D. All of the above

75. Guided imagery and meditation techniques
   A. Remove blocks and stimulate healing
   B. Are used to prevent healing
   C. Subliminally reinforce the mind
   D. A and C

76. Static stretching can be defined as
   A. A stretch performed for 10 to 15 seconds
   B. Passive movements
   C. A stretch that moves to the point of pain
   D. All of the above

77. Massage can relieve pain without the use of
   A. Imagery
   B. Stimulation
   C. Drugs, alcohol, or narcotics
   D. Endorphins

78. Yoga is a form of meditation for
   A. Good appetite
   B. Muscle balance and relaxation
   C. Dancing
   D. Religion

79. The relaxing action of a muscle is obtained by the application of
   A. Cold
   B. Heat
   C. Neutral
   D. Electric stimulation

80. It is best to stretch a muscle on _____ of the breath.
   A. Exhalation
   B. Holding
   C. Inhalation
   D. Meditation

81. In which massage technique should the fingers move tissue under the skin but not the skin itself?
   A. Tapotement
   B. Effleurage
   C. Vibration
   D. Friction

82. For which type of tissue is vibration the most unsuitable?
    A. Major nerve course
    B. Reduce muscle spasm
    C. Bony prominences
    D. Skeletal muscle

83. In order to stretch the posterior cervical muscles, use the _____ technique with the neck in forward flexion.
    A. Hyperextension
    B. Horizontal flexion
    C. Cross-arm
    D. Finger pushup

84. Which is the first step in beginning massage treatment?
    A. Apply lubricant
    B. Effleurage
    C. Determine contraindications
    D. Diagnose the patient

85. Joint mobilization of the pectoral girdle with the client in the supine position includes all but the following:
    A. Shaking
    B. Tapotement
    C. Horizontal flexion
    D. Scissoring

86. First aid for acute soft tissue injuries involves RICE, which means
    A. Ice
    B. Rest and elevation
    C. Compression
    D. All of the above

87. Which aims most specifically to passively stretch muscle?
    A. Effleurage
    B. Friction
    C. Petrissage
    D. Tapotement

88. Massage benefits lymph flow best when strokes are
    A. Away from heart
    B. Toward heart
    C. Heavy in both directions
    D. In certain local areas

89. For which condition is abdominal massage most beneficial?
    A. Pregnancy
    B. Appendicitis
    C. Constipation
    D. Enteritis

90. In order to create mobility at the hip joint _____ is used on the leg.
    A. Cupping
    B. Shaking
    C. Rocking
    D. Percussion

91. When the heel of the foot is brought toward the buttocks the _____ muscles are stretched.
    A. Calf
    B. Gluteal
    C. Hamstrings
    D. Quadriceps

92. Which is best to prevent adhesions in muscle tissue?
    A. Friction and effleurage
    B. Friction and petrissage
    C. Friction and tapotement
    D. Friction only

93. In tapping a large area of the body, which massage maneuver is used?
    A. Percussion
    B. Friction
    C. Effleurage
    D. Petrissage

94. To mobilize the hip through its full ROM,
    A. Hold for 30 seconds and abduct
    B. Adduct diagonally, extend, abduct diagonally
    C. Circumduct the flexed hip
    D. B and C

95. When applying palmar kneading to calf muscles, with the client in supine position, place a pillow or bolster
    A. Under the sacrum
    B. Under the lower back
    C. Under the knees
    D. Under the ankles

96. Which condition is always a contraindication for massage?
    A. Muscle spasm
    B. Phlebitis
    C. Rheumatoid arthritis
    D. Edema

97. In order to mobilize the ankle joint of the tibia and fibula,
    A. Use a scissoring motion between metatarsals
    B. Dorsiflex the calcaneus
    C. Press the heel of the hands and apply rapid alternate movement of the ankle
    D. Plantarflex the calcaneus

98. In massaging the anconeus, the massage practitioner is working in the area of the
    A. Upper extremity
    B. Lower extremity
    C. Abdominal wall
    D. Face

99. For insomnia, which is best?
    A. Heavy effleurage
    B. Light effleurage
    C. Tapotement
    D. Pickup

100. A scissoring motion can mobilize the joints of the
    A. Metatarsals
    B. Tarsals
    C. Carpals
    D. Phalanges

101. The main purpose of deep transverse friction is to
    A. Separate muscle fibers
    B. Lengthen muscle
    C. Shorten muscle fibers
    D. Minimize pain

102. Which is characteristic of a pressure stroke?
    A. It's of no consequence
    B. Follows venous flow
    C. Follows arterial flow
    D. Follows force

103. When stretching the intrinsic tissue of the foot,
    A. Plantarflex the foot
    B. Interlock fingers between toes
    C. Pull sides of foot away from each other
    D. All of the above

104. A client complains of and requests massage for severe low back pain. Which condition may produce this pain and is a contraindication for massage?
    A. Phlebitis
    B. Postural deviation
    C. Herniated disc
    D. Torticollis

105. To massage the hand, use
    A. Effleurage and petrissage
    B. Compression
    C. ROM and circular friction
    D. All of the above

106. The areas of the body for which passive joint movements are effective are
    A. Neck and shoulder girdle
    B. Wrists and hands
    C. Knees, ankles, and feet
    D. All major joints

107. To massage the elderly, which stroke would you use?
    A. Tapotement
    B. Gentle effleurage
    C. Deep pressure
    D. Friction over pressure area

108. Practitioners use joint movements primarily to
    A. Stimulate production of synovial fluid
    B. Induce muscle relaxation and kinesthetic awareness
    C. Increase joint ROM and muscle strength
    D. All of the above

109. It is essential that the practitioner be knowledgeable about the personal interaction and psychosocial implications of
    A. Structural integration
    B. Touch
    C. Anger
    D. Confidence

110. When palpating the midline of the back, what is being touched?
    A. Transverse process
    B. Vertebral body
    C. Spinal process
    D. Articular joint

111. Mild stimulation of the vagus nerve results in
    A. Irregular heartbeat
    B. No change
    C. Increased heartbeat
    D. Decreased heartbeat

112. Touch by the practitioner is especially important to many special groups of people that include
    A. Elderly
    B. Disabled
    C. Victims of physical need
    D. Victims of traumatic stress and abuse

113. Massage therapy is used in pain management for
    A. Terminal cancer patients
    B. Trauma patients
    C. Post-surgical patients
    D. A and C

114. The use of cold to depress the activity of pain receptors in the treatment of myofascial pain
    A. Maintains skin temperature of 13.6°C
    B. Increases nerve conduction velocity
    C. Permits passive stretching and exercise
    D. Decreases the general activity of patient

115. Because of the use of touch and the interpersonal nature of massage, the gender issue(s) to be aware of is (are)
    A. Cultural background
    B. Age
    C. Sexual orientation
    D. Cross-gender situations

116. The primary physiological effect of massage therapy includes all except
    A. Delivery of oxygen to cells
    B. Clearance of metabolic waste and by-products of tissue damage
    C. Increased blood and lymph circulation
    D. Increased interstitial fluid and hydrostatic pressure

117. Vodder's manual lymph drainage (MLD) was developed for the specific purpose of
    A. Promoting lymph flow from tissue
    B. Eliminating the pneumatic cuff
    C. Decreasing urine output
    D. Increasing erythrocyte count

118. When touch occurs in a sensitive area,
    A. It is not a problem
    B. Additional permission is needed
    C. Have a consent form signed
    D. Professional boundaries are violated

119. The analgesic effect of ice massage is to
    A. Block pain impulse conduction
    B. Reroute pain
    C. Decrease ROM
    D. Eliminate pain

120. Correct lymph massage begins from the
    A. Left thoracic duct
    B. Right arm
    C. Groin
    D. Right thoracic duct at the clavicle

121. Sometimes a recipient's body stores suppressed emotions that may be released in a massage session as
    A. Sighing
    B. Sleeping and snoring
    C. Crying
    D. A and C

122. Conversation between practitioner and recipient during a session should be kept
    A. To a minimum
    B. Continuous
    C. Silent
    D. At a whisper

123. The confidential information about the receiver can include
    A. Information during a session
    B. Observations made by the practitioner about physical or emotional condition
    C. Health history
    D. All of the above

124. If a session starts with the recipient in the prone position, a commonly used sequence is
    A. Legs, back, buttocks
    B. Back, buttocks, leg
    C. Buttocks, legs, back
    D. None of the above

125. The purpose of a lubricant when massaging is to
    A. Keep the body greasy
    B. Prevent blisters from forming
    C. Cleanse the body for relaxation
    D. Avoid uncomfortable friction between the therapist's hand and the patient's skin

126. One of the primary purposes of effleurage in massage is to
    A. Promote relaxation
    B. Increase ROM
    C. Spread lubricant
    D. A and C

127. A light compressive force applied to the skin with one hand to release a dysfunction in the connective tissue is associated with
    A. Myofascial releases
    B. Craniosacral therapy
    C. Amma
    D. MET

128. If the session starts with the recipient in the supine position, a commonly used sequence is
    A. Head, neck, shoulders and arms, chest, legs, feet
    B. Head, legs, feet, shoulders and arms
    C. Feet, legs, head, chest and arms
    D. Head, arms, chest, legs and feet

129. Neck mobilization in a lateral flexion helps to stretch the cervical muscles and the
    A. Trapezius
    B. Deltoid
    C. Occipital
    D. Rhomboids

130. The all-purpose cleanup of bodily fluids is
    A. 2% bleach solution
    B. 10% bleach solution
    C. Distilled water
    D. Concentrated bleach

131. After the massage is complete, the therapist will
    A. Escort the client to the bathroom
    B. Withdraw from the client by using body language
    C. Help dress the client
    D. Ask the client if he or she did a good job

132. If the session starts with the recipient in the supine position, then after turning the recipient over, the generally accepted sequence is
    A. Back, buttock, legs, feet
    B. Legs, buttock, end at the back and neck
    C. Back, legs, buttock, feet
    D. Buttock, back, legs

133. A thorough preliminary client assessment includes
    A. Client history
    B. Client observation
    C. Client examination
    D. All of the above

134. The Trager method uses movement exercises called
    A. Gymnastics
    B. Mentastics
    C. Spirals
    D. Athletics

135. The advantage of starting in the prone position is it
    A. Is warmer
    B. Feels safer to the recipient
    C. Is more comfortable
    D. Is more modest

136. Practitioners use joint movements for a variety of reasons, including
    A. To stretch surrounding tissue
    B. To increase range of motion
    C. To increase kinesthetic awareness
    D. All of the above

137. Perform _____ pressure when using effleurage along the tensor fascia latae.
    A. Light
    B. Moderate
    C. Very deep
    D. All of the above

138. When you are turning a client and anchoring the sheet,
    A. Have the client turn away
    B. "Tenting" is commonly done
    C. Avoid tangling
    D. Have the client turn towards practitioner

139. The various anatomical landmarks for which caution is recommended are
    A. Fragile structures that lie near the surface of the skin
    B. Superficial nerves and blood vessels
    C. Endangerment sites
    D. All of the above

140. A reflex response to massage is that the
    A. Body and nerves respond to stimuli of the sympathetic nervous system
    B. Blood vessels contract
    C. Blood pressure stays the same
    D. Parasympathetic nervous system reacts

141. Attentive nurturing touch can be a significant therapeutic factor in treating aging or ill because of its _____ benefits.
    A. Psychosocial
    B. Physical
    C. Mental and emotional
    D. All of the above

142. After cancer surgery, patients may benefit from massage for
    A. Promoting healthy appearance
    B. Relieving pain and insomnia
    C. Stress reduction and relaxation
    D. B and C

143. Connective tissue massage (CTM) is a useful technique for
    A. Preparing for surgery
    B. Improving psychoemotional status
    C. Loosening tissue following surgery or trauma
    D. Controlling pain

144. Massage is indicated for all but the following:
    A. Headaches
    B. Swelling due to lymphedema
    C. Fever
    D. Conditions of nerve entrapment

145. The endangerment sites located at the lateral and medial epicondyle of the humerus include the _____ nerves.
    A. Tibial and radial
    B. Radial and median
    C. Axillary and musculocutaneous
    D. Ulnar and radial

146. Skeletal muscle is affected by massage for which of the following symptoms?
    A. Increased muscle hypertrophy
    B. Muscle ischemia
    C. Spasm or cramp
    D. Muscle tension, injury, or spasm

147. What is the term used to describe an observable reddening of the skin resulting from increased blood flow?
    A. Anemia
    B. Hypoxia
    C. Hyperemia
    D. Ischemia

148. The reflex effects of massage are the stimulation of
    A. Motor neurons
    B. Sensory receptors of skin and subcutaneous tissues
    C. Synovial fluid at each joint
    D. Chemotransmitter

149. Ice massage is effective for local pain and
    A. Swelling
    B. Relaxed muscles
    C. Fever
    D. Systemic pain

150. A decrease in blood supply to an organ or tissue is referred to as
    A. Hyperemia
    B. Hypoxia
    C. Anemia
    D. Ischemia

151. Nutrition is an important component to the therapist's wellness training because
    A. Food dictates a work schedule
    B. Without sugar, therapy is not possible
    C. Diet affects the behavior and mood changes
    D. Without fat in a diet the therapist can't stay warm

152. Planning single and multiple client sessions
    A. Is not easy to accomplish initially
    B. Depends on the client history and interview
    C. Depends on the emotional status of the client
    D. Can only be effective after six visits

153. Massage is an indication to the integument or skin layer
    A. Stimulating sebaceous and oil glands
    B. To stimulate melanocytes
    C. Help to reduce scar tissue
    D. A and C

154. The adhesions of a well-healed scar can be broken down between skin tissues by applying
    A. Vibration
    B. Petrissage
    C. Friction
    D. Effleurage

155. To help tone weak muscles by increasing muscle spindle activity, _____ is indicated.
    A. Percussion
    B. Effleurage
    C. Tapotement
    D. Friction

156. Massage assists the ease of emotional expression through
    A. Love
    B. Stimulation
    C. Relaxation
    D. Fatiguing the nervous system

157. Reflexology of the hands and feet is based on
    A. Polarity
    B. Trager
    C. Zone therapy
    D. Hydrotherapy

158. A first-aid procedure designed to clear the air passageways of obstructing objects is known as
    A. Pneumonectomy
    B. Cheyne-Stokes
    C. Cardiopulmonary resuscitation
    D. Heimlich maneuver

159. Massage benefits the nervous system by
    A. Improving skin tone
    B. Eliminating waste material
    C. Relieving pain
    D. Stimulating muscles

160. The application of water (in any form) to the body for therapeutic purposes is called
    A. Floating
    B. Hydrotherapy
    C. Therapy
    D. Washing

161. Massage is indicated for conditions of nerve entrapment that occur when soft tissue constricts the nerve, such as
    A. Carpal tunnel syndrome
    B. Sciatica
    C. Thoracic outlet syndrome
    D. All of the above

162. To ensure a safe and comfortable massage, consider the following:
    A. Partial or relative contraindications
    B. Endangerment sites
    C. Absolute contraindications
    D. All of the above

163. During the interview and health history, the therapist may discover a pain area and find a need to evaluate the _____ before the massage, in order to enhance the therapeutic goals of the client.
    A. Gait
    B. Posture
    C. SOAP
    D. A and B

164. A mildly stimulating effect is produced by
    A. Standard massage oils
    B. Effervescent tablets
    C. A salt rub
    D. Lavender bath salts

165. Prolonged use of cold applications has which effect?
    A. Stimulating
    B. Energizing
    C. Depressing
    D. Heating

166. Expansion of blood vessels following cold application is called a(an)
    A. Primary effect
    B. Secondary effect
    C. Afterthought
    D. Energizer

167. A full-body steam bath for the purpose of causing perspiration is called a
    A. Swedish bath
    B. Japanese spa
    C. Greek soak
    D. Russian bath

168. A palpatory assessment is essential for documentation of tissue to
    A. Feel difference between muscles
    B. Locate origin and insertion of muscle
    C. Assess muscle flexibility, tightness, and tone
    D. All of the above

169. An informed consent contains information from which the clients
    A. Can judge the practitioner
    B. Can state the right to reschedule the treatment
    C. Are advised of undesirable effects from the massage
    D. Have decision-making rights

170. Prolonged application of cold leads to a physical condition called
    A. Iglooism
    B. Hyperthermia
    C. Hypothermia
    D. Freezer burn

171. Which is a type of dry heat?
    A. Dry ice
    B. Steam bath
    C. Sauna
    D. Fogging

172. Inform the client that a therapist does not _____ medical conditions.
    A. Judge
    B. Assess
    C. Diagnose
    D. Prognose

173. To integrate the structure and functionality of the client, a _____ assessment helps to evaluate balance and alignment.
    A. Mental
    B. Postural
    C. Ergonomic
    D. B and C

174. Abnormalities in gait are found throughout the postural chain by assessing which of the following body landmarks?
    A. Top of the iliac crests
    B. Top of the fibular heads
    C. Rami of mandible and ears
    D. All of the above

175. Spray showers are effective means of
    A. Calming nerves
    B. Cryotherapy
    C. Moist heat and mild compression
    D. A and C

176. Universal precautions are used when administering first aid because
    A. You have to assume that anyone receiving first aid potentially has infectious diseases
    B. HIV is transmitted by exposure to blood and other body fluids
    C. Hepatitis and other pathogens are transmitted by exposure to blood and other body fluids
    D. All of the above

177. Application of cold should be of short duration to prevent tissue
    A. Pain
    B. Thawing
    C. Damage
    D. Heat

178. To increase circulation to an injured area and promote healing, a therapist can alternate applications of
    A. Vibration and friction
    B. Feathering and kneading
    C. Heat and cold
    D. Percussion and feathering

179. The immediate first-aid actions required in treating an injured person are
    A. Talk to the individual; determine if he or she is responsive
    B. If possible, position the individual on the back (unless vomiting)
    C. Call 911 or other EMS, giving the exact location with identifying landmarks, your phone number, nature of the injury, the condition of victim, what is being done, and any other circumstances
    D. All of the above

180. Instead of using a commercial ice pack, put ice cubes into a
    A. Washcloth
    B. Dish towel
    C. Plastic bag
    D. Bathtub

181. Abnormalities in gait are found through assessing the walking pattern of a client to observe
    A. Placement of the feet
    B. Movement of the hands
    C. Movement of the hips and knees
    D. All of the above

182. When administering first aid, your goal is to obtain all the necessary information related to the injury. You should conduct a primary survey of the situation, which includes
    A. Checking the ABCs (airway, breathing, circulation) and hemorrhaging
    B. Using universal precautions when administering any first aid
    C. Assessing the victim's immediate condition and any unforeseen problems
    D. All of the above

183. Itching, inflammation, sensitivity, or stinging sensations are considered
    A. Normal
    B. Reasonable
    C. Allergic reactions
    D. Safe

184. A massage table should be stable, firm, and
    A. Tall
    B. Short
    C. Wide
    D. Comfortable

185. The height of a massage table is determined by the
    A. Height of the client
    B. Weight of the client
    C. Practitioner's arm length with fist on table
    D. Practitioner's elbow height on table

186. Avoid using which type of oil in massage?
    A. Sunflower
    B. Mineral
    C. Avocado
    D. Canola

187. In rescue breathing, which of the following is done?
    A. Tilt the head back and lower chin
    B. Nose open
    C. Seal lips around mouth with five full breaths
    D. Tilt head, pinch nose, mouth to mouth, two breaths

188. An appropriate hypoallergenic oil combination is
    A. Sesame and almond
    B. Sunflower and canola
    C. Apricot and olive
    D. Peanut and walnut

189. Considerations for designing home therapy for clients with demonstration and return demonstration by the client includes all of the following except
    A. Simple use of only those exercises that are beneficial and necessary
    B. Fitting the client's time, energy, and means
    C. Challenging the client
    D. Providing immediate noticeable results

190. Body areas where caution should be used to avoid damaging underlying anatomical structures are called
    A. Contraindications
    B. Endangerment sites
    C. Off limits
    D. Inferior

191. In adult CPR, the pulse is
    A. Not checked
    B. Checked at the wrist
    C. Checked at side of neck
    D. Checked behind knee

192. If a person is suffering from heat cramps,
    A. Liquid with caffeine or alcohol is permitted
    B. Give any medication needed
    C. Wet compresses at neck, groin, and armpits
    D. Do not give medication, caffeine, alcohol, and cool the body

193. The ideal Fahrenheit temperature for a massage room is
    A. 75°
    B. 60°
    C. 90°
    D. 85°

194. Avoid lighting that
    A. Is too dark
    B. Is too bright
    C. Shines into the client's eyes
    D. All of the above

195. When working close to an affected area, the circulation is stimulated and promotes
    A. Healing
    B. Blood pressure
    C. Blood sugar
    D. Respiration

196. The first-aid treatment for a seizure is aimed at
    A. Actively restoring consciousness
    B. Protecting victim from injury as it occurs
    C. Calming through massage
    D. Calling for help

197. Direct physical effects of massage techniques on the tissues they contact are called
    A. Reflex effects
    B. Pressure points
    C. Physiological effects
    D. Mechanical effects

198. Which of the following is a local effect of cold therapy?
    A. Vasodilation
    B. Increased circulation
    C. Vasoconstriction
    D. Increased local metabolism

199. The first sign of a person choking is
    A. Pupils dilated
    B. Shallow breathing
    C. Victim cannot answer
    D. Coughing

200. To administer CPR, the victim must
    A. Not be breathing or have a pulse
    B. Be awake
    C. Be able to talk
    D. Be standing

201. The most beneficial use of alternate hot/cold (contrast) treatments is with
    A. Acute muscle spasm
    B. Chronic muscle spasm
    C. Insulin-dependent diabetes
    D. Acute fibromyalgia

202. Alternative methods of stress reduction and relaxation techniques include
    A. Breathing techniques
    B. Visualization
    C. Biofeedback
    D. All of the above

203. In CPR performance, always
    A. Close the eyes
    B. Keep the head up
    C. Watch for the victim's eyes to open
    D. Tilt head, pinch nose, breathe, watch chest rise

204. The therapist may refuse to massage in part or in total a client based upon
    A. The physical appearance or behavior of the client
    B. Information gleaned through the health history and interview process
    C. Inappropriate language or behavior of a sexual nature
    D. All of the above

205. With an unconscious victim, always
    A. Get a chair
    B. Leave in any position
    C. Check vital signs
    D. Put pillow under head

206. A method to aid stress-related activities is
    A. Wet compresses
    B. Aerobics
    C. Sleep
    D. Deep breathing exercises

207. Massage can enhance
    A. Muscular contraction
    B. Breathing reduction
    C. An attitude of euphoria
    D. Muscle control and relaxation with yoga

208. Meditation is a useful treatment for
    A. Stimulating the flow of natural healing forces
    B. Preventive treatment
    C. Critical thinking
    D. A and B

209. The universal distress signal for choking is
    A. Pointing to neck
    B. Rotating neck
    C. Clutching the neck between thumb and index finger
    D. Nodding the head

210. The points to check while practicing massage are
    A. Good body positioning and height
    B. Comfort and relaxation of the patient
    C. Even pressure throughout each stroke
    D. All of the above

211. Variations of effleurage include
    A. Knuckling and stroking
    B. Backstroke and friction
    C. Pressure and brushing
    D. Wide angling and stroking

212. Variations of petrissage include
    A. One-handed petrissage
    B. Open and closed "C" position
    C. "V" hand position
    D. All of the above

213. In the application of the universal precautions issued by the CDC in 1991, massage therapists should avoid contact with
    A. All liquids
    B. The patient and sheets
    C. All solids
    D. Blood, vomit, urine, and feces

214. The muscle or group that is not included in a massage of the back is the
    A. Trapezius
    B. Rhomboids
    C. Pectoralis
    D. Erector spinae

215. During a massage of the abdomen, the patient should
    A. Have hip flexors and abdominal muscles relaxed over bolster
    B. Be on his/her side to relax
    C. Be draped completely
    D. Have the bolster removed

216. In massaging the upper extremity,
    A. Omit ROM
    B. Popping of joints is beneficial
    C. Draping is unnecessary
    D. Stroke from distal to proximal along the brachioradialis

217. Massage to the popliteal area requires
    A. Firm deep friction
    B. Gentle working of the gastrocnemius tendon heads
    C. Complete avoidance of space
    D. Petrissage only

218. The Bindegewebsmassage is a variation of massage technique that is based on
    A. Massaging the connective tissue under the skin
    B. Cross-fiber friction
    C. Polarity
    D. Reiki

219. In massage, it is important to
    A. Break touch with the client
    B. Apply oil over the entire body
    C. Maintain contact with the client throughout
    D. Prepare the client in a prone position

220. In massaging the body, it is important to
  A. Drape all parts of the body
  B. Expose only the part to be massaged
  C. Cover the entire body with a sheet
  D. Stand still while delivering technique

221. The Heimlich maneuver is performed by
  A. Pressing the fist into the abdomen with inward thrust standing behind victim
  B. Sternum thrusts
  C. Standing in front of victim with arms around waist
  D. Tilting head, and breathing mouth to mouth two times

222. Which stroke is used to reduce adhesions, separate muscle fibers, promote hyperemia, and milk the tissue of metabolic wastes?
  A. Effleurage
  B. Petrissage
  C. Friction
  D. Vibration

223. Active assistive joint movement requires
  A. Client only moving the extremity
  B. Therapist only moving the extremity
  C. Client and therapist moving the extremity together
  D. That the joint be immobilized

224. A treatment protocol using passive positioning is
  A. Polarity
  B. Strain-counterstrain
  C. MET
  D. Rolfing

225. This stroke creates the most heat in the tissue:
  A. Effleurage
  B. Petrissage
  C. Friction
  D. Vibration

226. Dr. Janet Travell was the founder of
  A. Trigger point therapy
  B. Rolfing
  C. Hellerwork
  D. Shiatsu

227. The plantarflexor that crosses both the knee and ankle is the
  A. Soleus
  B. Gastrocnemius
  C. Peroneus brevis
  D. Tibialis posterior

228. The best way for a client to get off the table after the massage is
  A. Roll onto his or her side and slowly sit up
  B. Rock back and forth until he or she sits up
  C. Roll onto the back and drop one leg over the table
  D. Rock from side to side until he or she reaches the side of the table

229. The most effective hydrotherapy treatment for chronic injuries is
  A. Ice
  B. Heat
  C. Paraffin
  D. Contrast application of cold/heat

230. The proper stance for giving a massage is
  A. Knees bent, shifting body weight from front to back foot, and elbows close to the body
  B. Knees and elbows locked with arms outstretched
  C. One foot perpendicular to the other, with weight on the back foot
  D. Feet parallel to the table with weight on the front foot

231. Your client is obese and has a hard time breathing in the supine position. What might you do?
  A. Place a pillow under her knees
  B. Place a pillow under her low back
  C. Place the client in the side-lying position
  D. Place the client in the prone position

232. The structure located in the lumbar region that makes it an endangerment site is the
  A. Sacrum
  B. Coccyx
  C. Kidney
  D. Bladder

233. The application of heat is contraindicated for
    A. Chronic muscle strain
    B. Subacute muscle strain
    C. Edema
    D. Fibromyalgia

234. The relaxation response is activated by the
    A. Sympathetic nervous system
    B. Parasympathetic nervous system
    C. Integumentary system
    D. Digestive system

235. While performing passive ROM on a client, he reports pain. You can safely assume that the injury/restriction involved is
    A. Muscular
    B. Ligamentous
    C. Tendinous
    D. Articular

236. A client reports having hurt her ankle yesterday. Upon examination, you find it is swollen and she cannot move it. What should you do?
    A. Passive ROM
    B. Lymph drainage to eliminate the swelling
    C. Friction the tendons and ligaments
    D. Encourage client to contact her physician or visit the emergency room

237. Which massage stroke is most effective for post-fracture care?
    A. Friction
    B. Effleurage
    C. Vibration
    D. Petrissage

238. Massage reappeared during the
    A. Renaissance Period
    B. Middle Ages
    C. Dark Ages
    D. Second World War

239. In the side-lying position, a pillow/bolster should be placed between the knees and under the
    A. Head
    B. Ankles
    C. Shoulder
    D. Leg

240. What is the main purpose of performing post-event massage?
    A. Stimulate the muscles
    B. Reduce swelling in sprains/strains
    C. Rid the body of metabolic waste buildup
    D. Treat adhesions

241. In which position would you massage a pregnant client who was in her 3rd trimester?
    A. Inverted
    B. Prone
    C. Side-lying
    D. Massage in the 3rd trimester is contraindicated

242. What is the best modality for a client who states she is not in pain and just wants relaxation massage?
    A. Structural integration
    B. Visceral manipulation
    C. Soft tissue release
    D. Swedish massage

243. Upledger and Sutherland are both known for their work in which modality?
    A. Reflexology
    B. Touch for health
    C. Trigger point therapy
    D. Craniosacral therapy

244. Which modality would be best for a client who desires energy work instead of massage?
    A. Pilates
    B. Structural integration
    C. Myotherapy
    D. Therapeutic touch

245. A client comes in and reports that her lower back has been hurting ever since she mowed her lawn yesterday. In which section of the SOAP notes is this information recorded?
    A. S
    B. O
    C. A
    D. P

246. SOAP is the acronym for
    A. Structure, objective, assessment, protocol
    B. Subjective, objective, assessment, practice
    C. Subjective, observation, action, plan
    D. Subjective, objective, assessment, plan

247. Your client is experiencing pain in the arm, wrist, and hand. You are pretty sure he has carpal tunnel syndrome. You should take the following action.
    A. Share your diagnosis with the client
    B. Apply a heating pad for a short time followed by cryotherapy
    C. Tell him to take a couple of aspirin for the pain, and give him some exercises to do at home
    D. Suggest that he see his doctor for a diagnosis

248. Touching and feeling the muscles for signs of tautness or trauma is referred to as
    A. Effleurage
    B. Palpation
    C. The Knapp's technique
    D. Nerve stroking

249. When a client experiences an emotional release on the table, you should
    A. Tell her what happened when you were confronted with the same situation
    B. Act as if nothing unusual is happening
    C. Be present with her and act the part of a concerned listener
    D. Stop the massage; you can't deal with this

250. Subjective information is obtained by
    A. Assessing the way the client walks
    B. Palpation
    C. Standing the client on the plumb line
    D. Listening to the client

251. You should wash your hands
    A. Before and after you have your lunch break
    B. After handling the laundry at the office
    C. Before and after each client
    D. All of the above

252. It is wise for massage therapists to be trained in CPR and First Aid because
    A. The National Board requires it
    B. They might have to be a first responder
    C. They can't get licensed if they don't
    D. It makes them appear more credible and professional

253. The purpose of proper draping is
    A. To respect the modesty of the client
    B. To protect the therapist
    C. To keep the client from getting cold
    D. Keep the massage table covered

254. To get the client acclimated to your touch and to warm up the muscle, you should begin bodywork sessions with
    A. Effleurage
    B. Friction
    C. Petrissage
    D. Tapotement

255. A client who has an area of inflammation because of a torn muscle would benefit from
    A. A heating pad
    B. Cryotherapy
    C. Vigorous friction on the inflamed area
    D. Stretching the muscle

256. Ballistic stretching would be the best technique as a treatment for a
    A. Torn rotator cuff
    B. Dislocated patella
    C. Hyperextended neck
    D. None of the above

257. The active assisted technique, in which the muscle is stretched into resistance and then held for 10 seconds, followed by the client's holding an isometric contraction for 5 seconds, is the
    A. PNF technique
    B. CNS technique
    C. PNS technique
    D. MET technique

258. The technique that involves pumping is
    A. Compression
    B. Effleurage
    C. Petrissage
    D. Vibration

259. The technique that could be used to loosen congestion in the respiratory tract is
    A. Rocking
    B. Petrissage
    C. Nerve stroking
    D. Cupping

260. You are gently applying stretch to the leg of a client who is lying supine. This is an example of
    A. Active stretching
    B. Passive stretching
    C. Ballistic stretching
    D. Counterstrain

261. The therapist's applying an unassisted stretch to the client would be equivalent to a(an)
    A. Passive static stretch
    B. Ballistic stretch
    C. Passive active stretch
    D. Active static stretch

262. You should never massage someone who is under the influence of drugs or alcohol because the client
    A. May not be in control of him- or herself
    B. May say or do something inappropriate
    C. May accuse you of saying or doing something inappropriate
    D. All of the above

263. One example of an endangerment site is
    A. Just below the medial malleolus
    B. The axillary area
    C. The maxilla
    D. The occipital ridge

264. Which endangerment site contains the median nerve?
    A. Ulnar notch of the elbow
    B. Posterior triangle of neck
    C. Anterior triangle of neck
    D. Cubital area of elbow

265. What is an effect of a cold application?
    A. Increase of local circulation
    B. Decrease of local circulation
    C. Increase of vasodilation
    D. Move more WBCs to area

266. What is an effect of a heat application?
    A. Vasodilation of capillaries
    B. Decrease of WBCs to area
    C. Decrease of cellular metabolism
    D. Produces numbness

267. In massage, we heat up the fascia surrounding the muscle, causing
    A. A thixotropic effect
    B. Critical interfiber distance
    C. Thermogenesis
    D. A flushing effect

268. Massage affects the immune system by
    A. Decreasing the production of T cells
    B. Slowing down the movement of lymph
    C. Increasing to the production of T cells
    D. Causing autoimmunity

269. The proper order for client progress notes is
    A. Subjective, plan, assessment, objective
    B. Subjective, objective, assessment, plan
    C. Objective, assessment, plan, subjective
    D. Plan, subjective, objective, assessment

270. After performing tapotement on a person's back, you notice that the back is red. This result is called
    A. Heat
    B. Hyponemia
    C. Hyperemia
    D. Ischemia

271. Adhesion reduction may be best achieved by performing which of the following treatments?
    A. Vibration
    B. Percussion
    C. Effleurage
    D. Deep transverse friction

272. Which form does a massage therapist return to the referring physician?
    A. SOAP notes
    B. Progress notes
    C. Insurance notes
    D. Name and address

273. What movements are best used before sports?
    A. Friction and petrissage
    B. Effleurage and friction
    C. Tapotement and effleurage
    D. Friction and tapotement

274. How do you position a pregnant woman?
    A. Sitting up
    B. On her side
    C. Prone
    D. Supine

275. When is diaper draping used?
    A. While treating the back
    B. While doing ROM of the lower appendages
    C. While treating a pregnant woman in a laterally recumbent position
    D. Both B and C

276. What are the best massage strokes to break up areas of fibrosis (scar tissue)?
    A. Effleurage
    B. Petrissage
    C. Deep vibration or friction
    D. Tapotement

277. When a client is lying prone with the arm abducted to 90 degrees and the forearm off of the table, which of the following muscles is most prominent to be worked on?
    A. Triceps brachialis
    B. Pectoralis major
    C. Subscapularis
    D. Biceps brachialis

278. The primary goal of pre-event sports massage is to
    A. Reduce anxiety of athlete
    B. Warm up muscle tissues/increase circulation
    C. Stretch muscles
    D. All of the above

279. What strokes are good for bronchitis?
    A. Tapotement
    B. Petrissage
    C. Deep friction
    D. Effleurage

280. Which stroke is defined as a slight trembling of the hand?
    A. Friction
    B. Tapotement
    C. Vibration
    D. Petrissage

281. What is the first thing a massage therapist does during a session?
    A. Turn on the music
    B. Meditate
    C. Calm the client
    D. Wash hands

282. When a client does not want to disrobe, what should a massage therapist say?
    A. That he or she will work through the clothes
    B. That the session cannot be conducted
    C. That the client should take them off anyway
    D. That the client should at least take off the shirt and pants

283. As a therapist, you injure your wrist. What should you do?
    A. Cancel appointments
    B. Wear a splint
    C. Join a gym
    D. Correct body mechanics with strengthening exercises

284. Massage of paralyzed limbs is beneficial because
    A. It helps reduce the flaccidness
    B. It helps restore nerve activity to limb
    C. It improves blood circulation to the limb
    D. All of the above

285. Deep compressive strokes result in
    A. Increased circulation and hyperemia
    B. Reduction of lactic acid
    C. Stimulation
    D. Improved muscle tone

286. Endangerment sites are
    A. Areas that warrant special precautions
    B. Areas with underlying anatomical structures that may be damaged by massage
    C. Areas of major nerves, vessels, arteries, and organs that are exposed
    D. All of the above

287. Your client complains of constipation. What is the best massage technique to use?
    A. Gliding strokes that follow the ascending, transverse, and descending colons
    B. Compression over the upper abdomen

C. Vibration over the stomach

D. Tapotement over the low back area

288. Select the most desirable stress reduction techniques for a relaxation massage.
   A. Deep breathing and stretching
   B. Meditation and visualization
   C. Deep breathing and active movement
   D. Deep breathing and visualization

289. Massage tools can include
   A. Rolling pin
   B. Exercise balls
   C. Percussion instruments
   D. Acupressure stones, bongers and vibrators

290. The best lubricants to use are
   A. Oils
   B. Hypoallergenic
   C. Creams
   D. Gels

291. An example of an assessment area is (are)
   A. Bony landmarks
   B. Palpation of soft tissue
   C. Inguinal lymph nodes
   D. A and B

292. The reason for a client assessment is
   A. To see if you want to develop a relationship
   B. To refer client to someone else
   C. To design an appropriate massage session
   D. To decide if you want to work on this person

293. What would you do if your client was scheduled to have surgery in two weeks?
   A. Postpone massage
   B. Do a lymph drain to prepare for surgery
   C. Have dinner with client
   D. Request that the client postpone surgery

294. The emotional effects of massage include
   A. Increasing relaxation
   B. Decreasing stress

C. Promoting feeling of well-being

D. All of the above

295. An example of an endangerment site is the
   A. Sciatic notch
   B. Mastoid process
   C. Axilla
   D. A and C

296. When your client leaves the session
   A. Discuss your SOAP notes
   B. Ask to schedule another appointment
   C. Tell them to call when they get home
   D. Ask them out for coffee

297. The boundaries of massage is (are)
   A. Breasts
   B. Genital area
   C. Feet
   D. A and B

298. Which stroke encompasses skin rolling?
   A. Kneading
   B. Friction
   C. Vibration
   D. Petrissage

299. How do you stretch the pectoral muscles?
   A. Adduction and medial rotation
   B. Adduction and lateral rotation
   C. Abduction and medial rotation
   D. Abduction and lateral rotation

300. A stroke that would not be beneficial to a competitor in a post-event massage would be
   A. Tapotement
   B. Effleurage
   C. Petrissage
   D. Kneading

ANSWERS AND RATIONALES

1. **C.** Effective listening means that you understand the emotional state of the client and that you are focusing on them.

2. **A.** Disclosure of private, sensitive client information without rebuttal and/or judgmental response of the therapist is called self-disclosure.

3. **D.** The principle of Swedish massage is always to massage toward the heart in order to move venous blood and lymph back to the thoracic duct and right atrium.

4. **A.** All circulation is improved by massage of muscles stimulating blood back to the heart and circulating lymph through elimination organs.

5. **D.** Roadblocks to communication that can cause problems are many, including questioning, analyzing, advising, giving solutions, or interpreting.

6. **D.** Precautions to protect the client and therapist include protective eyewear, vinyl gloves, and disinfectants when handling any body fluids or performing an invasive medical procedure.

7. **B.** The quadriceps are the muscles of the anterior thigh in the supine position.

8. **D.** OSHA supported and helped to pass federal legislation that requires all healthcare workers who may be exposed to body fluids/waste to use the protection of universal precautions.

9. **A.** It is best for the choking victim to cough first to attempt removal of obstruction.

10. **D.** Transmission of pathogens can be controlled by having good hygiene with clothing, linens, washing hands, and disinfecting equipment. Gloves are used for lesions or the terminally ill.

11. **B.** Endangerment sites contain certain anatomical structures that are prone to injury to the client (i.e., blood vessels, nerves, and organs).

12. **A.** Pillows under the head and between her knees as she lies on her side are more comfortable for a pregnant woman.

13. **D.** A pre-event sports massage is a faster, shorter, and more intense technique to prepare the athlete's body for better performance.

14. **B.** For cross-fiber massage to be effective on the muscle fibers, application must be perpendicular to spread them apart.

15. **D.** Many nerves, blood vessels, and organ areas are endangerment sites, except the colon area is safe to massage for constipation problems.

16. **C.** To minimize the pressure under the lower back place a bolster under the knees.

17. **B.** Cryotherapy is a cold therapy to eliminate pain and allow for massage treatment.

18. **A.** A top cover allows the client to be fully covered by a sheet as well as using a sheet to cover the table.

19. **A.** Placing a support under the ankles helps to relieve pressure on the lower back.

20. **B.** The client can be draped using the sheet on the table by lifting it up over the body.

21. **A.** Swedish massage is classified as using the fundamental manipulation of massage used today. Most treatments combine one or more of these movements.

22. **D.** Vibration treatment follows the path of the nerve: gentle, rhythmical, and fine vibration to the nerve trunk.

23. **D.** In order to support and protect the cervical vertebrae, a neck roll is the most functional bolster.

24. **C.** A tepid (slightly warm) bath is soothing and relaxing, good for nervous or excited people.

25. **D.** The lymphatic pump manipulation enhances the flow of lymph and can be done with the lymph drainage massage.

26. **A.** Structural integration is done by manipulating the fascia of the structural muscles resulting from poor posture and binding of connective tissue.

27. D. In the side-lying position, support should be provided for the superior leg and arm and under the head to keep the client stationary and comfortable.

28. D. A massage therapist must prepare him- or herself through mind and body first, then work on strength, stamina, balance, flexibility, and grounding to become a better therapist.

29. C. Rolfing is a method of structural integration intended to correctly align the spine and body segments by the use of heavy pressure of knuckles, fist, or elbow into the muscle and connective tissue.

30. A. Palpating muscles effectively locates tender points and trigger points that are associated with soft tissue pain and dysfunction.

31. D. Massage therapists need to take care of themselves by balancing the mind and body and maintaining strength and stamina in order to provide more to clients.

32. C. Only the area to be massaged should be exposed for privacy as well as warmth to the client. Exposure also depends on massage therapy legislation, if any.

33. A. The mechanical effect of massage is the stretching of superficial tissue, which encourages better flexibility.

34. A. Deep pressure techniques such as Rolfing must be done with caution to avoid too much pain.

35. D. Hacking, cupping, slapping, and beating are all forms of quick percussion to tone muscles.

36. B. Due to its size and what it can cover, it is more difficult to work with a towel over the body. Practice is required to develop this skill.

37. B. Organs and functions of the body can be affected by pressing reflex zones on the hands and feet. This technique is reflexology.

38. B. The foot positions in posture and stances aid balance and allow a more direct delivery of massage strokes. The horse is a common one in which both feet are placed perpendicular to the table.

39. C. Stretching is used to mobilize and increase the flexibility at the joint as it elongates the muscle and connective tissue.

40. C. The greatest challenge to a massage therapist is keeping the drape securely in place when turning the client over, since this is when accidental exposure can take place.

41. B. Any deep pressure strokes stimulate the circulation and therefore blood flow.

42. C. Rolfing aligns the major body segments through fascia manipulation to establish structural integration.

43. C. Congestive lung conditions are treated with the cupping technique of percussion.

44. A. The anchor or tenting method allows for the privacy of the client while turning; the therapist holds the top sheet up to his or her shoulders and anchors the bottom of the sheet against the table with the thighs.

45. A. Effleurage is the first and most frequently used Swedish stroke. Its gliding movements are excellent for assessing the client's body and tissue.

46. D. Good body mechanics include postural techniques, biomechanics, and the therapist's body weight.

47. B. The temperature best for nervous tension, insomnia, and aching muscles is 100°–110°F. This induces relaxation and relieves nervous tension.

48. D. The elements involved in applying a skillful massage are a blend of strokes, biomechanics, your intention, pressure, rhythm, and sequence.

49. C. Pressure is the application of force exerted by the massage therapist. The pressure should start light and gradually increase until the desired effect is achieved. The return stroke should be all light.

50. A. Exercise stimulates lymph flow by muscles contracting on the lymph vessels, forcing the movement of the lymph.

51. D. The sensation of pressure by the compression of the body's surface can be very beneficial and cause relaxation.

52. B. The touch over an area that has just been massaged ends with light nerve stroke.

53. C. A tender point is not considered a trigger point because the site causes no referred sensations.

54. C. Therapeutic stretching is performed by changing the joint position in order to lengthen the specific muscle. Active-assisted stretching is between the therapist and client actively.

55. A. A form of friction called compression increases circulation and lasting hyperemia in the tissue. The pumping action brings blood to deep muscles for long periods.

56. A. The Warrior or house stance is used for petrissage transverse strokes.

57. A. To separate muscle fibers from an injury or scar, transverse friction is the recommended therapy.

58. C. Swedish gymnastics includes the artful and fluid presentation of passive ROM that includes table stretches and joint mobilization.

59. A. The stroke that usually begins and ends a massage is effleurage.

60. B. Petrissage is the best stroke to lift the muscle off the bones.

61. D. Joint mobilizations are performed within the normal range of joint movement and include active (i.e., free or assistive) and passive movements, which can be integrated into a massage routine.

62. C. The resistance of isometrics enhances flexibility and blood flow, which results in relaxation.

63. C. Treatment to the old and young should be shortened. They are often more fragile and cannot endure a lengthy session.

64. B. Friction allows the fingers to feel the tissues below due to the deeper pressure applied.

65. C. Stretching is a type of passive joint movement that can be performed to move a joint to the ROM limit.

66. C. To loosen adhesion tissue, cross-fiber friction is the best stroke to mobilize the area.

67. A. In resistive movement, practitioners offer resistance to the movement, thereby challenging the muscles used.

68. B. In the petrissage stroke, the tissue is lifted up off the bone in a kneading technique.

69. D. Body alignment, posture, and re-educating the muscles are all assets of joint mobilization.

70. A. Compression is an excellent massage for the intercostal muscles of the ribs. The pumping action provides improvement of breathing.

71. B. Knowledge of the normal ROM or end feel is essential to assess the degree of flexibility at a joint.

72. A. The pressure during effleurage should be done evenly from the beginning to the end of the stroke.

73. D. To ensure safe joint movement in the cases of elderly and joint replacement or metal inserts, it is important to understand the condition from medical records or the recipient's physician.

74. D. Biofeedback has many therapeutic uses, including pain relief through autogenic training and aid in controlling involuntary processes.

75. D. Imagery and meditation are techniques used to remove blocks, stimulate healing, and subliminally reinforce the mind.

76. D. Holding a stretch to a limit to pain is passive movement and a static stretch.

77. C. Massage can relieve pain without the use of drugs, alcohol, or narcotics.

78. B. When yoga is practiced, the result can be muscle balance and relaxation.

79. B. Heat to the muscle area stimulates the muscle to relax.

80. A. Breathing may be used to help the recipient relax during a stretch during the process of exhaling.

81. D. Friction is the massage stroke that moves the fascia and tissue under the skin without moving the skin itself.

82. C. Bony prominences are too sensitive for vibration massage.

83. C. The cross-arm stretch is the best technique for cervical muscles by lifting the head with one hand and placing other hand across it to the shoulder.

84. C. All contraindications should be determined before giving a massage treatment.

85. D. Scissoring motion is used to create movement between the metacarpals of the joints.

86. D. RICE is an acronym for rest, ice, compression, and elevation.

87. A. Effleurage is the massage stroke that passively moves and stretches muscles.

88. B. A benefit of massage is that, when the stroke is toward the heart, blood drains from the venous system and lymph from the lymphatic system.

89. C. A benefit of abdominal massage is alleviating constipation.

90. C. Rocking the leg is a good technique to mobilize the hip joint.

91. D. Stretching the quadriceps muscles is accomplished by bringing the foot to the gluteal area.

92. A. Friction and effleurage can prevent scarring and adhesions to muscle tissue by the action of keeping the fiber separated by either cross-fiber or longitudinal strokes.

93. A. Percussion includes tapping, slapping, hacking, cupping, and beating, all strokes that benefit a large area like the back.

94. D. A full ROM for hip flexion is adduction, extend and abduct the knee diagonally to circumduct the hip completely.

95. C. When the client is in the supine position, a pillow or bolster is placed under the knees so that palmar kneading is possible.

96. B. Phlebitis is always a contraindication for massage. Inflammation in the veins or a possible clot is a dangerous condition.

97. C. With the recipient supine, the ankle can be mobilized by placing the heel of the hands on the foot under the malleoli and pressing in, alternating one side then the other.

98. A. Extending the elbow is the action of the anconeus in the upper arm, which originates on the humerus.

99. B. Light strokes to the forehead are good for nervous headaches and insomnia; gentle gliding strokes are beneficial.

100. A. To mobilize the tissues between the metatarsals, use the scissoring motion by taking the knuckles of two toes and moving them up and down.

101. A. The transverse action of friction is applied across muscle and tendon to separate fibers, allowing greater circulation and increased mobility.

102. D. The slightest pressure is transmitted to deeper muscles by force.

103. D. The intrinsic tissues of the foot can be stretched by interlocking fingers between the toes, pulling the sides of the foot away from each other, and plantar flexing the foot.

104. C. When the fibrocartilage of the intervertebral disc is herniated, lower lumbar pain contraindicates massage in that area of the back.

105. D. A complete massage to the hand is effleurage, circular friction to the back of the hand, petrissage, ROM, and compression to wrist and fingers.

106. D. Passive joint movements are effective on most of the body's major joints including neck, shoulder, chest, wrists, hands, hip, knees, ankles, and feet.

107. B. Gentle massage is beneficial to the elderly, even if they are frail.

108. D. Joint mobilization is used and incorporated into a massage routine to relax muscles, stimulate synovial fluids, increase ROM, and kinesthetic awareness.

109. B. Touch is the number one skill a practitioner giving a massage needs. To touch is to come in contact with and communicate feelings.

110. C. The spinal process runs along the midline of the back when palpating the line of the vertebrae.

111. D. The vagus nerve is the 10th cranial nerve, which acts as a decelerator of the heartbeat.

112. D. Because many men and women have been victims of sexual and physical abuse and traumatic stress, these people need special care regarding touch. The practitioner should make the recipient feel especially safe and comfortable.

113. D. Massage therapy is used for post-trauma and post-surgical patients, as well as for cancer and cardiac patients.

114. C. Cold depresses pain receptors, allowing treatment by passive stretching.

115. D. The gender issues to be aware of are the issues of cross-gender massage.

116. D. Interstitial fluid and hydrostatic pressure increases are not significant physiological effects of massage.

117. A. To shift edema fluid from tissues to blood, Vodder (in 1965) designed MLD.

118. B. "Request the client's consent before touching a sensitive area for therapeutic purposes."

119. A. Ice is used to block pain before massaging an area.

120. D. The right thoracic duct is the correct place to start lymph massage.

121. D. As a recipient relaxes and lets down emotional defenses, he may release a sigh or start crying. This is normal and should not stop a session.

122. A. Conversation should be kept to a minimum so that the body and mind can relax.

123. D. In a professional relationship there is implicit trust that the practitioner will keep confidentiality about medical and health history as well as observations made about the recipient before, during, or after a session.

124. B. The common sequence for the prone position first is the back, buttocks, and legs before the recipient is turned over.

125. D. A lubricant avoids an uncomfortable friction on the skin of the patient.

126. D. Spreading of the lubricant and muscle relaxation results from the flow of the effleurage stroke.

127. A. The movement of connective tissue is known as myofascial therapy used by John Barnes and John Upledger.

128. A. The head and neck are started in the supine position. Then the shoulders and arms, chest and abdomen, and legs and feet are finished before turning the recipient over.

129. A. Only the trapezius is stretched with a lateral flexion of the neck.

130. B. A 10% bleach solution is the cleanup for HIV, hepatitis, and viral organisms. The solution is one cup of bleach to one gallon of water.

131. B. The massage therapist will move away from the client when the massage is complete so that it is understood that the session is over.

132. B. When you start a session supine and turn over to the prone position, the sequence is generally legs, buttocks, ending with the back and neck. Either way you start, you should end at the head.

133. D. Client assessment includes a history, observation, and an examination.

134. B. Mentastics is the gentle rocking or shaking of body parts, called the Trager method.

135. B. It generally feels safer to the recipient to start prone, especially if it is a first time massage.

136. D. Movement of the joints stimulates muscle relaxation, increases ROM and kinesthetic awareness, as well as stretching surrounding tissue and stimulating production of synovial fluid.

137. B. Moderate pressure can be applied to the Illiotibial (IT) band and the tensor fascia latae due to its length and strength.

138. D. "To avoid rolling off the table, the recipient should turn toward the practitioner under a tenting of the sheet."

139. D. Endangerment sites include areas of the body that are fragile to the touch and lie superficially to the surface of the skin such as nerves and blood vessels.

140. A. The sympathetic nervous system responds as a reflex of blood vessel dilation, muscle relaxation, and lowering of the resting blood pressure.

141. D. There are many benefits to treating the aging or dying through touch. It can improve physical, mental, and emotional functioning as well as ease some of the pain and anxiety.

142. D. Although massage is generally contraindicated for cancer patients, it has been found the post-surgery massage has many benefits, including stress reduction and relaxation, relieving pain and insomnia, and increasing ROM.

143. C. Connective Tissue Massage (CTM) improves circulation and post-operative ANS reflexes that increase sympathetic nerve activity.

144. C. Fever is a contraindication for massage therapy because the body is fighting an infection.

145. D. The ulnar and radial nerves of the medial and lateral epicondyles of the humerus are considered nerve endangerment sites because they are superficially located.

146. D. The muscle responds to massage after an injury, spasm, or tension.

147. C. The release of histamines and acetylcholine cause dilation of blood vessels called hyperemia.

148. B. Stimulation of the sensory receptors of the skin is the reflex effect of massage.

149. A. Swelling can be reduced by ice packs.

150. D. Muscle pain is a result of a decreased supply of blood to the tissue or an organ, called ischemia.

151. C. One wellness component is taking care of the body through nutrition to help prevent fatigue and mood changes from cravings.

152. B. After a thorough history intake and verbal interview, the therapist can develop a plan of action.

153. D. Massage improves the skin color, texture, stimulation of oil secretion, and reduction of adhesions or scar tissue.

154. C. Friction of the cross-fibers is an excellent method to break down well-healed scar adhesions.

155. C. Tapotement (a form of vibration) creates minute muscle contractions to help tone weak muscles.

156. C. A psychological effect of massage is relaxation to ease emotional expression.

157. C. Different organs and parts of the body respond to reflex zones in the hands and feet.

158. D. The Heimlich maneuver (abdominal thrust) is the first-aid procedure to force air or water out of the trachea or lungs.

159. C. Massage techniques have an effect on reflex reaction to relieve pain.

160. B. Water in the form of ice, liquid, or steam vapor with massage has a therapeutic effect on the body.

161. D. Conditions of the nervous system that are indicated for massaging areas of nerve entrapment are carpal tunnel and thoracic outlet syndromes and sciatica.

162. D. It is essential to heed caution to ensure that the massage is safe and comfortable, therefore partial or relative contraindications, endangerment sites, and absolute contraindications must all be considered.

163. D. The therapist should examine and evaluate the gait and posture of a client with pain in order to proceed with caution and knowledge.

164. C. Salt rubs are stimulating to the skin and increase some circulation as well.

165. C. Nerve sensitivity is depressed with extensive ice application.

166. B. Blood vessels constrict initially after cold application.

167. D. A steam room for cleansing and relaxing provides a Russian bath.

168. D. A palpatory assessment is important before a massage to document the client's soft tissue. The muscle type, structure, flexibility, and tone all add to the style of the massage session.

169. D. Information in an informed consent helps the client to have knowledge and decision-making rights.

170. C. Extreme cold should be of short duration because the tissue temperature lowers, causing hypothermia.

171. C. Heat in a sauna room is always produced by a dry heat source at 120°F.

172. C. A therapist cannot diagnose any medical condition.

173. D. A postural or economic assessment studies the anatomy and physiology as it relates to the balance and alignment of the client.

174. D. Assess symmetry by placing one finger on a bony landmark and drawing an imaginary line bilaterally across the ears, eyes, shoulders, hips, patella, malleoli, and foot arches.

175. D. Spray showers have many hydrotherapeutic effects.

176. D. Potential disease or infection can be transmitted when administering first aid.

177. C. The tissue is injured if it is too cold too long.

178. C. Heat and cold are the most effective methods of promoting healing through circulation.

179. D. Call 911 or EMS. Talk to the person to get a response.

180. C. A sealable plastic bag makes an excellent ice pack.

181. D. Observe a "normal" walking pattern and notice the movement of the client's hands, hips, knees, and feet to determine any abnormalities in the gait.

182. D. Check ABCs (airway, breathing, and circulation) and hemorrhaging and administer first aid.

183. C. These signs indicate sensitivity to skin, resulting in an allergic reaction.

184. D. A table should be comfortable with padding to absorb pressure applied by practitioners.

185. C. To prevent fatigue, the palm of a hand should be flat on the table with arms straight.

186. B. Mineral oils are not recommended because they are petroleum-based, dry the skin, and clog pores.

187. D. Rescue breathing requires tilting the head, pinching the nose, and breathing into the mouth twice.

188. B. Mild oils, such as sunflower and canola, are appropriate, hypoallergenic, and easy to work with. Oils of nuts can cause allergic reactions.

189. C. It is not good to design a home plan that will challenge the client; the design should be to get results and build confidence.

190. B. Endangerment sites are major nerves, blood vessels, and vital organs that, if exposed to deep pressure, can sustain possible injury.

191. C. In CPR the pulse is checked at the carotid artery at side of neck.

192. D. For heat cramps, never give coffee, alcohol, or medication. Cool the person down at the neck, groin, and armpits.

193. A. The temperature of the room must be warm enough for the client and cool enough for the practitioner.

194. D. Indirect, soft natural light is most desirable, especially for the eyes.

195. A. By working on areas that have been injured or affected by overexercising, healing and circulation are improved.

196. B. First-aid treatment can protect the victim from injury during a seizure.

197. D. The mechanical effects of massage are directly related to the physical strokes and techniques used.

198. C. The initial effect of cold is vasoconstriction, which chills the skin and contracts the blood vessels to limit swelling.

199. C. The first sign that a person is choking is that he or she cannot answer.

200. A. CPR can be administered to a victim who is not breathing or does not have a cardiac pulse.

201. B. For chronic muscle spasms, use alternate hot/cold (contrast) to increase local circulation, relieve chronic pain, and aid healing.

202. D. Biofeedback, breathing for relaxation, and visualization are all stress reducers.

203. D. In CPR it is important to pinch off the nostrils, tilt the head back, and observe the victim's chest.

204. D. Any behavior or language that is inappropriate is a reason for the therapist to refuse massage.

205. C. Always turn an unconscious victim on the back and check vital signs before administering CPR.

206. D. Deep breathing is a method to aid stress-related activities.

207. D. Massage enhances muscle control; breathing and relaxation and can complement a yoga meditation session.

208. D. Meditation is a treatment for stimulating the flow of natural healing forces, providing preventive treatment, as well as receiving subliminal messages.

209. C. Clutching the neck between the thumb and index finger is the universal distress signal of a choking victim.

210. D. Good massage techniques include checking patient comfort, even pressure when stroking, and good body positioning.

211. A. Knuckling and stroking are variations of effleurage.

212. D. The petrissage stroke varies as a "V" hand position, open and closed "C" position, and a one-handed petrissage.

213. D. The universal precautions were issued to prevent the spread of bacteria and virus. Therefore, contact with the client's blood, urine, feces, and vomit should be avoided.

214. C. The back does not contain the pectoralis muscle, which is the primary chest muscle.

215. A. Always relax the hip flexors and abdominal muscles when massaging the abdominal area.

216. D. When massaging the upper limbs, care should be taken with the movement of the joints and strokes should go from distal to proximal along the brachioradialis.

217. B. The popliteal area of the posterior leg should be gently massaged at the gastrocnemius tendon heads due to the presence of blood vessels and nerves in the area.

218. A. The massage that concentrates on the connective tissue under the skin is the Bindegewebsmassage.

219. C. Strokes should be continuous and maintained without breaks in contact. The client can become startled with reestablishing contact.

220. B. Expose the area to be massaged, but keep the rest of body draped for privacy and professionalism.

221. A. The procedure for the Heimlich maneuver is to stand behind the victim and apply subdiaphragmatic thrusts into the abdomen with the fists.

222. B. Petrissage is always a milking stroke.

223. C. The client and therapist move together.

224. B. Strain-counterstrain incorporates passive movements.

225. C. Friction will create heat.

226. A. Dr. Travell developed trigger point therapy.

227. B. The gastrocnemius crosses the knee and ankle.

228. A. Roll on side and get up slowly.

229. D. Contrast cold/heat application.

230. A. Good body mechanics, include knees bent, shifting weight and elbows close to the body.

231. C. An obese client can lie on his/her side.

232. C. The kidney is in the lumbar area.

233. C. Heat for a client with edema is always a contraindication.

234. B. The parasympathetic nervous system relaxes.

235. D. Pain during ROM usually involves the joint.

236. D. Refer the client to a doctor or hospital in the case of an injury.

237. A. Friction is good for post-fracture care.

238. A. The Renaissance was the reappearance of massage.

239. A. A pillow should go under the head in side-lying.

240. C. Post-event massage gets rid of waste buildup.

241. C. A pregnant woman in the 3rd trimester is usually most comfortable in a side-lying position.

242. D. Swedish massage is for relaxation.

243. D. Craniosacral therapy is used by both Upledger and Sutherland.

244. D. Therapeutic touch is energy work.

245. A. A client symptom is reported in the subjective part of SOAP notes.

246. D. Subjective, objective, assessment, and plan is abbreviated to SOAP.

247. D. Clients should see a doctor for a diagnosis, rather than the massage therapist.

248. B. Palpation is feeling the muscle.

249. C. Being concerned is important to a client who has had an emotional release.

250. D. Listening to the client informs the massage therapist of subjective information.

251. D. Washing hands before and after a client, after eating, or handling anything is protocol.

252. B. CPR and first aid are skills that may be used in an emergency.

253. A. Draping is intended to cover the client to respect modesty.

254. A. Effleurage is the best stroke to apply lotion and warm up the client.

255. B. Cryotherapy helps to numb and reduce inflammation.

256. D. Ballistic stretching is not good for any pathology.

257. A. PNF is proprioceptive neuromuscular facilitation.

258. A. Compression is a form of pumping.

259. D. Cupping is good for congestion.

260. B. Passive stretching is applied by therapist.

261. A. A passive static stretch is unassisted.

262. D. Use of alcohol and drugs is contraindicated for massage.

263. B. The axillary area contains many lymph nodes.

264. D. The cubital area of the elbow contains the median nerve.

265. B. A cold application decreases local circulation.

266. A. Heat application promotes vasodilation of capillaries.

267. A. The thixotropic effect is to heat the fascia around the muscle.

268. C. In the immune system there is an increase in T cells.

269. B. SOAP notes are used for client progress.

270. C. When blood enters an area, it is called hyperemia.

271. D. Deep transverse friction helps to reduce adhesion.

272. A. SOAP notes are referring information for a physician.

273. D. Friction and tapotement are used for sports massage.

274. B. A pregnant woman is positioned on her side.

275. D. The diaper draping is used for ROM and treating pregnant women.

276. C. Deep vibration or friction is the best stoke for scar tissue.

277. A. The triceps brachialis is the muscle exposed when the arm is abducted in the prone position.

278. D. Pre-event massage stretches muscles, warms up, and reduces anxiety of athlete.

279. A. Cupping or tapotement is good for bronchitis.

280. C. A slight trembling of the hand is vibration.

281. D. A massage therapist must wash his or her hands before the massage.

282. A. If a client refuses to get undressed, perform the massage through the clothes.

283. D. If your wrist is injured, use RICE, modify body mechanics, and perform strengthening exercises.

284. C. Circulation can be improved to paralyzed limbs.

285. A. Deep compression increases circulation and hyperemia.

286. D. Any anatomical structure that may be damaged by massage is classified as an endangerment site.

287. A. Constipation can be helped by stroking along the ascending transverse and descending colons.

288. D. Deep breathing and visualization are good stress reduction techniques for a relaxation massage.

289. D. Although manual massage is best, other tools can help the therapist.

290. B. It is best to use all hypoallergenic lubricants.

291. D. Palpation of soft tissue and bony landmarks are assessment areas.

292. C. Assessment of the client helps in developing massage treatment.

293. B. A massage is very helpful before surgery.

294. D. Relaxation, stress reduction, and a good mental attitude.

295. D. The sciatic notch and axilla are two of the endangerment sites.

296. A. Always try to schedule another appointment.

297. D. The genitals are massage boundaries and the breasts are usually not touched except for cancer patients.

298. A. Skin rolling is part of the kneading stroke.

299. D. The best way to stretch the pectoral muscles is by abducting and laterally rotating.

300. A. Tapotement is better for pre-event sports massage to increase circulation.

27 Eastern Energy Bodywork

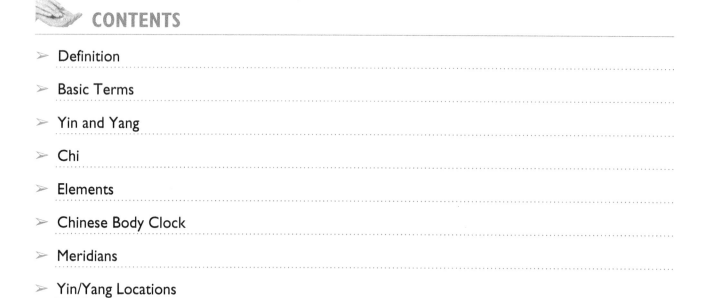

CONTENTS

EASTERN ENERGY BODYWORK	
Definition	• **The body is treated as a whole; the spirit, physical, and mental or mind and body concept.** • **Energy called chi flows throughout the body in channels called meridians.** • **There are 12 (6 pair) and 2 extraordinary vessels. When they are blocked, disease results.**

Basic Terms	***Life force***—Known as chi, ki, qi, prana; chi is the energy that flows throughout the body. Energy flows from superior to inferior and inferior to superior. Disease occurs when there is an imbalance in chi.
	
	 Jitsu—An excess of chi
	
	 Kyo—Deficient chi
	
	 Hara—The center of gravity/point of balance; located four finger-widths below the umbilicus deep in abdomen
	
	 Tsubo—Points along the meridians
	
	 Tsun/cun/sun—Width of the client's thumb; a unit of measurement
	
	 Tao—"The way"; made up of two opposite yet complementary forces: yin and yang; one cannot exist without the other
	
	 Chi—The connection between yin and yang
	
	     Characteristics of yin—Feminine, dark, cold, descending energy, passive, earth, and interior. Yin energy flows from the earth toward the heavens.
	
	     Characteristics of yang—Masculine, light, heat, ascending energy, day, active, heaven, and exterior. Yang energy flows from the heavens toward the earth.
	
	 Amma—Practiced in China for over 4,000 years then moved to Japan; now shiatsu, which is all pressure-point therapy and energy meridian concept.
	
	 Qi-Gong—Chi King: An exercise that is meditative in nature but energizes the body through movement technique, much like tai chi does to promote and maintain health with the movement of chi.
	
	 Acupressure—Acupuncture with needles: Derived from early Chinese theory in which body mapped out as series of *energy meridians*. Energy (chi) flows through channels; digital pressure stimulates or sedates pathways.
	
	 Jin Shin Do—Developed by Iona Teeguarden, it is a blend of shiatsu, acupressure, and breath work that involves local and distal pressure points along meridian-like strange flows to balance the mind, body, and spirit through a clearing of energy between two points held together.
	
	 Shiatsu—The Chinese mapped over 2,000 points on the human body. The Japanese picked 660 points or tsubos and combined with massage as a treatment focused on moving chi within the energy meridians of the body to achieve flow and balance so that the body can heal.

(*continued*)

EASTERN ENERGY BODYWORK (*continued*)	
Yin and Yang	• *Yin and yang* illustrate the connection of all. • The image is a circle composed of a large rounded white area that curves within the circle and gradually becomes thinner and blends with a large black area that curves toward the white, symbolizing the movement and change in the universe. • The Chinese *yin* is the dark side of the mountain with characters of feminine, interior, and cool. The *yang* is the sun side of the mountain, masculine, exterior, moving, warm, and expanding.
Chi	• Everything in the universe • Continuous form of energy, life force • Chi flows through the body in daily cycles, yearly cycles, and lifetime cycles from birth to death • Chi functions are transforming, transporting, holding, protecting, and warming • Disharmony in functions of Chi causes disease to result
Elements	There are five elements with six paired meridians. *Fire*—Heart (yin)/small intestine (yang) and pericardium (yin)/triple warmer (yang) *Earth*—Stomach (yang)/spleen (yin) *Metal*—Lung (yin)/large intestine (yang) *Water*—Bladder (yang)/kidney (yin) *Wood*—Gallbladder (yang)/liver (yin) Extraordinary vessels = governing and conception
Chinese Body Clock	The natural, rhythmic cycles of the body clock are the times the channels flow through the body. 3–5 AM — Lung 5–7 AM — Large intestine 7–9 AM — Stomach 9–11 AM — Spleen 11 AM–1 PM — Heart 1–3 PM — Small intestine 3–5 PM — Bladder 5–7 PM — Kidney 7–9 PM — Pericardium 9–11 PM — Triple warmer

| | 11 PM–1 AM | Gallbladder |
| | 1–3 AM | Liver |

Meridians	• Meridians are "channels" of energy that travels through the body.
	• They are invisible and interconnected.
	• The meridians include:
	Lung	**Lu**
	Large Intestine	**LI**
	Stomach	**St**
	Spleen	**Sp**
	Heart	**H**
	Small Intestine	**SI**
	Urinary Bladder	**Bl**
	Kidney	**K**
	Pericardium	**P**
	Triple Warmer	**TW**
	Gallbladder	**GB**
	Liver	**Liv**
	Governing vessel	**GV**
	Conception vessel	**CV**
Yin/Yang Locations	• Three yin meridians begin in the feet and terminate in the chest: spleen (Sp), liver (Liv), and kidney (K)
	• Three yin meridians begin in the chest and terminate in the fingertips: lung (Lu), pericardium (P), and heart (H)
	• Yin meridians are located on the anterior and medial aspects of the body
	• Three yang meridians begin in the fingertips and terminate in the face: large intestine (LI), small intestine (SI), and triple warmer (TW)
	• Three yang meridians begin in the face and terminate in the feet: stomach (St), bladder (Bl), and gallbladder (GB)
	• Yang meridians are located at the back or lateral aspects of the body, except stomach, which is the only yang meridian at the front of the body
	• The two meridians not associated with an organ are pericardium and triple warmer

MERIDIANS AND THEIR CHARACTERISTICS				
Meridians	**Location**	**Element**	**Yin/ Yang**	**Time**
Lung (Lu); 11 pts.	Begins from chest, up arm, ends at thumb	Metal	Yin	3 AM
Paired with **Large Intestine (LI);** 20 pts.	Begins from index finger, up arm and neck, ends at nose	Metal	Yang	5 AM
Stomach (St); 45 pts.	Begins from eye, down anteriorbody, ends at 2nd toe	Earth	Yang	7 AM
Paired with **Spleen (Sp);** 21 pts.	Begins from big toe, up inside of leg, up anterior body, ends at underarm	Earth	Yin	9 AM
Heart (H); 9 pts.	Begins from underarm, up medial arm, ends at little finger	Fire	Yin	11 AM
Paired with **Small Intestine (SI);** 19 pts.	Begins from little finger, down lateral arm, up the neck, ends in front of ear	Fire	Yang	1 PM
Urinary Bladder (Bl); 67 pts.	Begins from eye, over head down back and posterior leg, ends at little toe	Water	Yang	3 PM
Paired with **Kidney (K);** 27 pts.	Begins from the bottom of foot, up medial leg and torso, ends at chest	Water	Yin	5 PM
Pericardium (P); 9 pts.	Begins from lateral chest, up medial arms, ends at middle finger	Fire	Yin	7 PM
Paired with **Triple warmer (TW);** 23 pts., also as triple heater, triple burner, not paired	Begins from 4th finger, up posterior arm and lateral neck, ends at lateral head	Fire	Yang	9 PM
Gallbladder (GB); 44 pts.	Begins from lateral head, down lateral side of body, ends at 4th toe	Wood	Yang	11 PM
Paired with **Liver (Liv);** 14 pts.	Begins from big toe, up medial leg, ends at 6th intercostal space	Wood	Yin	1 AM
Conception Vessel (CV); 24 pts., not paired	Begins from perineum, up mid-sagittal line of torso, ends at mentolabial groove between chin and lower lip	None	Yin	None
Governing Vessel (GV); 27 pts., not paired	Begins from coccyx, up mid-sagittal line of back and overhead, ends at upper lip	None	Yang	None

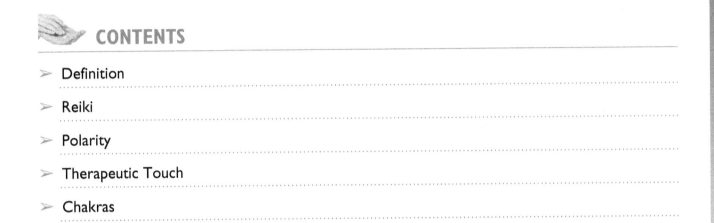

CONTENTS

WESTERN ENERGY BODYWORK	
Definition	• **Human body seems to respond to western bodywork, which supports the health of the body and mind.** • **Physiological response seems to be from peripheral nervous system.** • **The seven chakras are involved in the mechanism, although developed in the East.** • **Recipients frequently report experiencing a different feeling in the mind and body.**
Reiki	• Developed by Dr. Mikas Hsui by applying gentle contact or no contact with the client. • It focuses on chi and clearing the chakras. • Chakras are located over nerve plexuses.
Polarity	• Developed by Randolph Stone; includes life energy, chakras, and elements. • The gunas are the three principles of energy movement: tamas, rajas, and sattra. • There are five electromagnetic currents on each side of the body. • The chakras are root, sacral, solar plexus, heart, throat, 3rd eye, and crown. • The elements are earth, water, fire, air, and ether (only different one to eastern). • The currents relate to organs. • The right side of the body is positive energy and left side is negative.
Therapeutic Touch	• Developed by a nurse, Dolores Krieger, to promote balancing and healing of clients without touch. • It is noninvasive and addresses physical, mental, emotional, and spiritual aspects.

| CHAKRAS AND THEIR ASSOCIATIONS					
Number	**Name**	**Location**	**Color**	**Organs/Body Parts**	**Emotions/ Area of Consciousness**
7th chakra	Crown chakra	Top of head	Violet	Brain, nervous system	Empathy, unity, separation
6th chakra	3rd eye chakra	Center of forehead	Indigo	Forehead, temples	Perception, spirituality
5th chakra	Throat chakra	Base of throat	Sky blue	Throat, neck, upper extremities	Expression, communication, creativity
4th chakra	Heart chakra	Center of chest	Emerald green	Heart, circulatory system, lungs, chest	Love, relationships
3rd chakra	Solar plexus chakra	Solar plexus	Yellow	Muscular system, integumentary system, digestive system, eyes, face	Perception
2nd chakra	Base chakra	Center of abdomen (hara)	Orange	Reproductive system	Sexuality, basic need for food and sex
1st chakra	Root chakra	Perineum	Red	Lymphatic system, skeletal system, excretory system	Trust, survival

29 Modalities: Eastern and Western

 CONTENTS

MODALITIES	
Definition	• **A modality is a system of movements performed in a specific way with the intent of achieving specific results. What separates each modality is the amount of pressure applied, the strokes used, and if it is performed in water.** • **Some bodywork releases muscles and soft tissue; other bodywork is body/mind/spirit work.** • **Most western modalities are based on the five basic strokes of Swedish massage.**
Types of Western Modalities	***Alexander Technique***—Process of movement re-education to identify and rid the body of faulty postures by replacing habit with conscious movement. Developed by Frederick Matthias Alexander. ***Applied Kinesiology***—The use of muscle testing to evaluate strength and weaknesses or imbalances in the body. Developed by George Goodhart. ***Aromatherapy***—The use of essential oils to restore and to heal. ***Aston Patterning*™**—A combination of deep tissue and other massage combined with movement education. Developed by Judith Aston, a student of Ida Rolf. ***Bindegewebsmassage***—The use of dermatomes (areas of innervation) of connective issue to identify problems; based on the theory that imbalance anywhere in the body is imbalance in the total body. ***Connective tissue massage***—A light technique of dragging and pulling the skin to release the superficial fascia. ***Craniosacral***—A technique that focuses on releasing blockages in the flow of the craniosacral fluid and releasing emotional trauma. Upledger, Milne, and Sutherland are all known for their respective craniosacral techniques. ***Deep tissue massage***—Deep pressure massage is applied with the fingers, thumbs, elbows, etc. to release the deeper tissue. ***Esalen***—A body/mind/spirit modality consisting of very light Swedish massage aimed at inducing deep states of relaxation. ***Feldenkrais*™**—A process of unlearning restrictive movement habits and replacing them with efficient, graceful movement. Awareness Through Movement is the movement education part of Feldenkrais. The bodywork part is called Functional Integration, which involves treating the nervous system primarily through the skeletal structure by using hands-on, painless manipulation. Developed by Moshe Feldenkrais. ***Geriatric massage***—A therapy for older adults with attention paid to their specific needs and contraindications. ***Hellerwork***—A type of bodywork consisting of 11 sessions of structural work combined with vocal work aimed at bringing consciousness to posture and movement. Developed by Joseph Heller, student of Ida Rolf. ***Hot stone massage***—Massage performed with heated stones placed and/or rubbed on the body.

(continued)

MODALITIES (continued)

Hydrotherapy—The use of water in any of its forms for relaxation or rehabilitation: ice, heat packs, whirlpool baths, wet or dry saunas. The bigger the variance in temperature from that of normal body temperature, the more intense the effects. Some methods also use water pressure, such as Vichy showers and Scotch douche, to relax sore muscles. Many spas are based on hydrotherapy and may include such modalities as salt glow rubs, mud packs, clay baths, seaweed baths, sugaring, and other therapeutic treatments.

Infant massage—Massage performed on infants with attention paid to their needs and contraindications.

Kinesiology—The study of muscle movement. Also refers to several different modalities of muscle testing to restore health and balance to the body, sometimes incorporating nutrition and other forms of bodywork.

Lymphatic drainage massage—Massage of the lymph nodes and lymph system. Developed by Dr. Hans Vodder.

Medical massage—Bodywork performed for the purpose of injury repair and rehabilitation from pathological conditions.

Myofascial release—Any method directed at treating restrictions or adhesions in the fascia and muscles.

Myotherapy—Trigger point therapy that includes re-education of the muscle. Developed by Bonnie Prudden.

Neuromuscular therapy (NMT)—A technique directed at returning the body to a state of structural balance; also referred to as trigger point therapy. Developed in Europe by Chaitow, popularized in America by Paul St. John and Janet Travell.

On-site/chair massage—Seated massage performed on a fully dressed client, normally in public or corporate settings where full-body massage is inappropriate or impractical.

Orthopedic massage—Massage developed from osteopathic techniques, focusing on rehabilitating connective tissue, tendons, ligaments, cartilage, and soft tissue surrounding a bone injury or insult.

Polarity—Based on the principle that every cell has both negative and positive poles, the use of gentle touch to manipulate the tissue and restore balance; a mind/body/spirit integrative approach.

Postural integration—A body/mind/spirit modality that incorporates breath work, deep fascial work, and emotional work to restore structural balance to the body.

Pregnancy massage—Massage performed during pregnancy, with attention paid to the client's special needs and contraindications of the condition.

Proprioceptive neuromuscular facilitation (PNF)—A technique during which a muscle is stretched to resistance and held for 10 seconds, followed by the client contracting the muscle for 5 seconds.

Reflexology—Treating the reflex zone and points found on the hands, feet, and ears that correspond to a map of the body, internal tissues and organs. Developed by Dr. Fitzgerald and Eunice Ingham.

Reiki—A method in which the practitioner channels universal energy within the chakras directed at the healing of the client. The seven chakras and moving energy are associated with Reiki Chi.

Rolfing—Deep structural realignment that takes place over the course of 10 sessions. Developed by Ida Rolf, it has been used and developed into many other methods by her former students and others.

Rosen method—Breathing and relaxation techniques accompanied by rebalancing alignment and increasing flexibility using nonintrusive touching, verbal interaction, and breathing. Developed by Marion Rosen.

Rubenfield synergy—A body/mind/spirit approach combining psycho-therapy with movements, postures, talk therapy, dreamwork, and other techniques.

Sports massage—The massage of athletes, with attention to their special needs and contraindications.

Strain-counter strain—Also called positional release, is to guide the body into a space where the muscle tension can release on its own from the painful tender point of the strain.

Structural integration—Also referred to as Rolfing; deep structural realignment that takes place over the course of 10 sessions. Developed by Ida Rolf, it has been developed into many other methods by her former students and others.

Swedish massage—Therapeutic massage focused mainly on relaxation; the five basic strokes are the basis of many other techniques. Per Henrik Ling is credited with bringing Swedish massage to the United States.

Therapeutic Touch—Energy work focused on balancing the body's aura through gentle, above-the-body manipulations of the energy field. Developed by Dolores Krieger and Dora Kunz.

Trager™—Gentle rocking and other nonintrusive movements to facilitate the release of deep physical and emotional restrictions. The hook-up, a natural state of being similar to a meditative state, is used to connect the practitioner with the energy of the client. Developed by Dr. Milton Trager.

Trigger point therapy—A technique directed at returning the body to a state of structural balance; also referred to as neuromuscular therapy. Developed in Europe by Leif and Chaitow, popularized in America by Paul St. John and Janet Travell.

Zero Balancing™—Treatments performed with the client fully clothed and in a seated position, progressing to a reclining position; focus on integrating the physical body with the energetic body. Developed by Fritz Smith.

(*continued*)

MODALITIES (*continued*)	
Types of Eastern Modalities	**Acupressure**—Using fingers or other body parts to stimulate points along the meridians to facilitate the flow of energy. **Amma**—Traditional Asian massage, sometimes referred to as amma. Using no oil, amma involves stretching, squeezing, and massaging to stimulate the body to become and/or remain healthy; focuses on improving muscle condition and the circulation of chi, or universal life energy. Amma combines bodywork along the meridians with nutrition, detoxification, herbal therapy, and exercise. **Ayurvedic massage**—Part of the total Ayurvedic philosophy of health and medicine, techniques that focus on detoxification and the restoration of health through the chakras. **Shiatsu**—A form of Japanese acupressure traditionally performed fully clothed on a mat on the floor. **Thai massage**—Work performed on the floor that consists of assisted yoga-like positioning of the body, along with gentle rocking and stretching. **Watsu**—Shiatsu performed in a warm pool of water.

30 100 Questions with Answers and Rationales on Eastern and Western Bodywork

OBJECTIVES

Major areas of knowledge/content included in this chapter are based on the NCTEMB and MBLEx exam topics that cover Eastern and Western Bodywork.

➢ Craniosacral

➢ Energetics

➢ Meridians

➢ Elements

➢ Jin Shin Do

➢ Polarity

➢ Reflexology

➢ Chakras

DIRECTIONS

Each of the questions or statements below is followed by four suggested answers or completions. Select **one answer** that is best in each case.

1. Which one most accurately describes the meridian system?
   A. Energy pathway moving randomly through the body
   B. Energy pathway moving superficially
   C. Energy pathway that doesn't affect organs
   D. 12 meridians and 2 vessels are pathways in which energy moves toward the surface of the body, affecting organs

2. The conception vessel is the confluence of all the
   A. Yin channels
   B. Yang channels
   C. Qi energy
   D. Five elements

3. Grounding exercises in shiatsu are important to prepare you by
   A. Connecting with the ground to remove tension
   B. Breathing correctly
   C. Increasing awareness of your body weight
   D. All of the above

4. Acupuncture, shiatsu, polarity, and reflexology are examples of
   A. Energetic manipulation
   B. Behavioral barometer
   C. Reactive circuits
   D. Systematic massage

5. The finger pressure massage method called *shiatsu* is
   A. Japanese
   B. Chinese
   C. German
   D. French

6. When palming or massaging the medial side of the leg, the following meridians are affected:
   A. Bl, K, LI
   B. Sp, Liv, K
   C. GB, Liv, Sp
   D. St, Sp, Bl

7. The energy of the yin channels flows from
   A. Fingertips to chest to feet
   B. Hand to head downward to the feet
   C. Head to hand downward to the feet
   D. Front of the body and deep organs

8. The tools and techniques of shiatsu include all but the following
   A. Palming
   B. Thumbing
   C. Cross-fiber friction
   D. Stretches and rotation

9. The energy for the stomach meridian is most effective from
   A. 7–9 AM
   B. 7–9 PM
   C. 3–5 AM
   D. 3–5 PM

10. The energy for the spleen meridian is most effective from
    A. 7–9 AM
    B. 7–9 PM
    C. 9–11 AM
    D. 11 PM–1 AM

11. In which directions do yin meridians flow?
    A. Superior to inferior
    B. Inferior to superior
    C. Lateral to medial
    D. Medial to lateral

12. Which meridians are innervated when massaging the medial thigh?
    A. K, Liv, Sp
    B. GB, St, Sp
    C. Liv, St, K
    D. GB, Liv, K

13. Which meridian has a point on the radial side of the little finger?
    A. Small intestine
    B. Triple warmer

C. Heart

D. Pericardium

14. The vascular system is controlled by which meridian?

A. Heart

B. Triple warmer

C. Pericardium

D. Conception vessel

15. Which meridian is involved with a system but does not have a corresponding organ?

A. Spleen

B. Heart

C. Liver

D. Triple heater

16. Which of the following points is located on the nail of the 1st toe?

A. St45

B. K1

C. Liv1

D. Liv3

17. Which meridians transverse the abdomen?

A. Bl, Lu, TW

B. H, HC, Lu

C. GB, SI, CO

D. K, Sp, St

18. Where are the first and last points on the BL meridian?

A. Head and fingers

B. Toes and fingers

C. Head and foot

D. Wrist and finger

19. The triple warmer controls

A. Assimilation, digestion, and elimination

B. Assimilation, digestion, and skin temperature regulation

C. Digestion, elimination, and skin temperature regulation

D. Elimination, digestion, and nervous system

20. Manipulation of the sacral area most directly affects energy in which meridian?

A. Bl

B. GB

C. K

D. St

21. The yin muscle channels of the lung pass through muscles of the chest and arm that include

A. Pectorals

B. Biceps brachii

C. Diaphragm

D. All of the above

22. The governing vessel is the confluence of all the

A. Yin channels

B. Yang channels

C. Chi energy

D. Five elements

23. The chi flowing through the meridians is the

A. Hara breathing meditation

B. Blockage

C. Universal life energy

D. Spirit

24. Jin Shin Do is an oriental therapy that is

A. Preventive rather than symptomatic in nature

B. To strengthen our absorption of life energy

C. Acupressure, breathing, and meditation

D. All of the above

25. The Chinese consider the lung as the delicate organ because

A. It is a delicate tissue

B. It is the 1st organ to be injured by negative substances

C. It cannot work without the heart

D. The diaphragm controls the breathing

26. An energy-balancing therapy that attempts to remove blockages and bring healing energy to the problem area is called

A. Reflexology

B. Therapeutic touch

C. Amma therapy

D. Myofascial release

27. When the dorsum of the foot is massaged, which meridians are stimulated?

A. H and K

B. Liv and Sp

C. Liv and K

D. All Yang meridians

28. The yin and yang comprise a spiral of change that represents

A. Seasons

B. Life in constant flux

C. Rhythms in animals and man

D. All of the above

29. The chi pathways or channels constitute the

A. Shiatsu vessels

B. Amma bioenergy system

C. Chinese meridians

D. All of the above

30. The five elements of fire, earth, metal, water, and wood are associated with

A. Moon phases

B. Heart and lungs

C. Emotions of client

D. A five-pointed star, seasons, and organs of the body

31. The invisible circulation of vital energy is called

A. Chi

B. Regulating channel

C. Hseuh

D. Yin and yang

32. Manipulation of the occipital region primarily affects which meridians?

A. Bl and GB

B. LI and Sp

C. K and TH

D. Liv and Lu

33. To state that a point on the body is jitsu means that it is an area that

A. Is infected

B. Is lacking in energy

C. Has too much energy

D. Is numb

34. In ayurvedic massage, energy points are referred to as

A. Trigger points

B. Dharma

C. Karmas

D. Marmas

35. In Chinese medicine theory, what circulates through the organs every 24 hours?

A. Blood

B. Hormones

C. Chi

D. Fresh oxygen

36. The two meridians that do not have any element associated with them are the

A. Central and lung

B. Lung and liver

C. Circulation sex and governing

D. Conception and governing

37. The meridian that is paired with the lung is the

A. Central vessel

B. Triple warmer

C. Large intestine

D. Kidney

38. The heart meridian is paired with which meridian?

A. Kidney

B. Spleen

C. Triple warmer

D. Small intestine

39. There are _____ primary chakras.

A. 5

B. 7

C. 6

D. 8

40. The chakra associated with communication is the

A. Heart chakra

B. 3rd eye chakra

C. Root chakra

D. Throat chakra

41. Chakras are associated with

A. Points on the spine

B. The pineal gland

C. The rainbow

D. Emotions and colors

42. The root chakra is associated with the sense of

A. Smell

B. Taste

C. Touch

D. Hearing

43. The thyroid gland is affected by the chakra of the

A. Throat

B. 3rd eye

C. Crown

D. Solar plexus

44. Awareness through movement and functional integration are methods for which type of bodywork?

A. Hellerwork

B. Positional release

C. Feldenkrais

D. Rolfing

45. Finger pressure is used primarily in which therapy?

A. Shiatsu

B. Jin Shin Do

C. Polarity therapy

D. Reiki

46. In ayurvedic medicine which dosha is associated with movement in the body?

A. Vata

B. Pitta

C. Kapha

D. Shaman

47. Which type of therapy has massage strokes that follow the direction of dermatomes?

A. Esalen massage

B. Bindegewebsmassage

C. Hellerwork

D. Lomi lomi

48. In reflexology, where is the point that corresponds to the head and neck?

A. Heel

B. Arch of the foot

C. Big toe

D. Little toe

49. Gentle rocking techniques are used in what type of massage?

A. Rolfing

B. Craniosacral

C. Trager

D. Shiatsu

50. What type of bodywork uses tongue and Hara diagnosis?

A. Shiatsu

B. Reiki

C. Craniosacral

D. Applied kinesiology

51. In what type of bodywork does the practitioner apply static pressure with a slow release and a stretch?

A. Touch for health

B. Muscle energy procedure

C. Swedish

D. Neuromuscular

52. A client who is interested in energy work could be referred to whom?

A. An acupuncturist

B. A reflexologist

C. A reiki practitioner

D. A and C

53. In Chinese medicine, which pulse is used for diagnosis?

A. Carotid

B. Radial

C. Ulnar

D. Femoral

54. From where did acupuncture originate?

A. Japan

B. China

C. Germany

D. Russia

55. The governing vessel is

A. A channel down the front of the body to balance energy

B. A channel down the back of the body to balance energy

C. An energy flow through the stomach

D. An energy flow through the gallbladder

56. The conception vessel is

A. A channel down the front of the body to balance energy

B. A channel down the back of the body to balance energy

C. An energy flow through the stomach

D. An energy flow through the gallbladder

57. Which statement is incorrect?
    A. Yin and yang are opposite but complementary forces
    B. Yin is located on the posterior body and yang on the anterior
    C. GB21 is located midway between shoulder and C7
    D. LI20 is a point you would work for sinus and allergy conditions

58. In Eastern medicines, the organs are associated with certain elements. The organs associated with Earth are
    A. Spleen and stomach
    B. Gallbladder and liver
    C. Kidney and urinary bladder
    D. Lung and large intestine

59. Connective tissue massage may include
    A. Transverse friction over tendons and ligaments
    B. Holding static pressure on tsubos
    C. Clearing the chakras
    D. Both A and C

60. The stomach meridian is the only
    A. Yin meridian on the anterior aspect of the body
    B. Yin meridian on the posterior aspect of the body
    C. Yang meridian on the anterior aspect of the body
    D. Yang meridian on the posterior aspect of the body

61. This meridian begins on the plantar surface of the foot:
    A. Kidney
    B. Large intestine
    C. Spleen
    D. Stomach

62. The Hara is considered the
    A. Center of Gravity
    B. Way
    C. "Upper burner"
    D. Pericardium

63. Which meridian would you work for a client who complains of heart palpitations?
    A. GB
    B. CV
    C. Bl
    D. H

64. The time associated with the stomach meridian is
    A. 3–5 am
    B. 5–7 am
    C. 7–9 am
    D. 9–11 am

65. What are the chakras?
    A. Energy pathways
    B. Energy channels
    C. Energy centers
    D. Channel pathways

66. Which meridian would you work to treat low back pain, edema, and impotence?
    A. Sp
    B. Bl
    C. GB
    D. K

67. These meridians make up the metal element:
    A. Heart/lung
    B. Lung/small intestine
    C. Large intestine/heart
    D. Lung/large intestine

68. The GV regulates all
    A. Yang
    B. Yin
    C. Tao
    D. Chi

69. The CV regulates all
    A. Yang
    B. Yin
    C. Tao
    D. Chi

70. A client complains of back pain. Which meridian would you work?
    A. GB
    B. Lu
    C. Bl
    D. CV

71. The element water is related to _____ meridians.
    A. Gallbladder/liver
    B. Bladder/kidney
    C. Heart/small intestine
    D. Lung/intestine

72. LI4, LI10, LI20 would be worked to treat
    A. Low back pain
    B. Shoulder/neck pain
    C. Lateral leg pain
    D. Chest pain

73. In the five elements of Eastern medicine, what organ is yang to the earth?
    A. Spleen
    B. Stomach
    C. Heart
    D. Gallbladder

74. In acupressure, which pulse is taken to read the energy fields related to the organs?
    A. Wrist
    B. Neck
    C. Groin
    D. Temple

75. In Eastern theory, what does "yang" represent?
    A. Sunny side of the slope
    B. Inwardness
    C. Shady side of the slope
    D. Cold

76. Yin/Yang relationship indicated the theory of
    A. Five elements
    B. 11 systems
    C. Good/evil
    D. Dynamic balance

77. Which is not a meridian pathway?
    A. Triple burner
    B. Stomach
    C. Pericardium
    D. Pancreas

78. The liver meridian begins at what point?
    A. Nose
    B. Small toe

    C. Sacrum
    D. Big toe

79. The stomach meridian begins at what point?
    A. 4th toe
    B. Pupil of eye
    C. Heel
    D. Sacrum

80. What organ represents fire?
    A. Kidney
    B. Heart
    C. Lungs
    D. Spleen

81. Another name for tsubo would be
    A. Chakra
    B. Channel
    C. Pathway
    D. Pressure point

82. The therapy that is performed with light contact of the body is
    A. Craniosacral
    B. Rolfing
    C. Jin Shin Do
    D. Reiki

83. Which of the following are correctly paired meridians?
    A. Liver and kidney
    B. Heart and stomach
    C. Stomach and spleen
    D. Stomach and large intestine

84. Which meridian has its endpoint on the little toe?
    A. GB
    B. Bl
    C. H
    D. Sp

85. If a client requests an energy massage, whom would you refer him or her to?
    A. Polarity therapist
    B. Neuromuscular Therapy (NMT)
    C. Reflexologist
    D. Rolfer

86. When performing polarity therapy,
    A. The mind and body are treated separately
    B. The mind and body are treated together
    C. The mind is treated, not the body
    D. The body is treated, not the mind

87. The meridian that zigzags around the head and travels down the lateral side of the body ends on the
    A. Little toe
    B. Little finger
    C. 4th toe
    D. 4th finger

88. From where does the conception vessel begin?
    A. Superior aspect of upper lip
    B. Inferior aspect of lower lip
    C. Perineum
    D. Proximal to the umbilicus

89. Which therapy includes acupuncture, acupressure, yoga, and Taoism?
    A. Jin Shin Do
    B. Reiki
    C. Feldenkrais
    D. Rolfing

90. Which chakra is represented by the color green?
    A. Throat
    B. Heart
    C. Sacral
    D. Crown

91. Life force can be known as
    A. Energy that flows throughout the body
    B. Chi
    C. Jitsu
    D. A and B

92. A detailed map of the foot was developed by Ingham as *Zone Therapy* and later called
    A. Reflexology
    B. Polarity
    C. Amma therapy
    D. Shiatsu

93. Strange flows represent
    A. A blend of shiatsu, acupressure, and breath work
    B. A technique developed by Iona Teeguarden

C. Clearing of energy between two points
    D. All of the above

94. The yin and yang circle is composed of
    A. A black area with a white dot
    B. A white area with a black dot
    C. Black and white areas that blend together
    D. All white or black

95. The yin is the dark side of the mountain with _____ characteristics.
    A. Masculine
    B. Exterior
    C. Expanding
    D. Feminine

96. Disharmony in the functions of chi will result in
    A. Dis-ease
    B. A balance of the meridians
    C. Disease
    D. Continuous energy

97. The 660 tsubo points on the human body represent
    A. Jin Shin Do
    B. Shiatsu
    C. Amma
    D. Qi-Gong

98. The yang side of the mountain represents
    A. Cool
    B. Warm
    C. Interior
    D. Darkness

99. Chi can be explained as cycles of
    A. The holidays in a year
    B. Menses
    C. Spring and fall
    D. A day, four seasons and a year

100. The element wood is related to the _____ meridians.
    A. Gallbladder/liver
    B. Governing/conception
    C. Lung/intestine
    D. Stomach/spleen

ANSWERS AND RATIONALES

1. **D.** The 12 bilateral meridians in the body conduct energy along pathways that are related to organs and the chi (energy).

2. **A.** All the yin channels meet with the deep and superficial pathways of the conception vessels at CV1–CV24.

3. **D.** To practice shiatsu well, one should begin by being in touch with the ground and make a connection to relieve tensions through breathing and increase the awareness of body.

4. **A.** There is a force, or vibration, that, when smooth, results in good health. Techniques detect imbalance in the force and through energetic manipulation regain homeostasis.

5. **A.** The Japanese word *shiatsu* means pressure of the fingers: *shi* (finger) and *atsu* (pressure).

6. **B.** The spleen, liver, and kidney meridian pathways are all along the thigh and calf. When palming or massaging the leg with the petrissage stroke or compression all three are affected.

7. **D.** The yin channels are located on the front of the body and the inner surfaces of the limbs and belong to the deep organs of the body, liver, spleen, and kidney.

8. **C.** The principles and techniques of shiatsu include palming to loosen joints, thumbing for pressure, and stretching and rotation to position limbs. Cross-fiber friction is used in massage for trigger points, adhesions, and scar tissue.

9. **A.** The energy for the stomach meridian is most effective from 7 AM to 9 AM.

10. **C.** The energy for the spleen meridian is most effective from 9 AM to 11 AM.

11. **B.** The flow of energy for the yin meridians is from the inferior part of the body to the superior.

12. **A.** The kidney, liver, and spleen are the meridians that pass through the medial thigh area.

13. **C.** The heart meridian has a point on the little finger, and energy flows from the chest to the inside of the arm.

14. **A.** The heart meridian follows the flow of blood from the chest to the arm to the end of the little finger.

15. **D.** The triple heater (warmer) is the meridian that stands for fire and has no corresponding organ along the energy path from the ring finger to the side of the head.

16. **C.** The liver (Liv) meridian is located on the big toe.

17. **D.** The kidney, spleen, and stomach are the meridians that transverse the abdomen.

18. **C.** The bladder meridian energy flow travels on the posterior side, starting on the head, down the back, along the leg to the toe.

19. **C.** The yang meridian triple warmer goes from the ring finger back to the side of the head, controlling temperature, digestion, and elimination.

20. **A.** The bladder meridian is massaged to affect energy as well as for sacral pain.

21. **D.** The yin of the muscle channels passes through the muscles of the forearm, arm, shoulder, and chest.

22. **B.** All the yang channels meet with the deep and superficial pathways of the governing vessel points GV1–GV28.

23. **C.** The chi within the universe is used within our bodies as purification or detoxification for this energy.

24. D. Jin Shin Do developed as a preventive health art to strengthen the absorption of chi through the techniques of acupressure, meditation, and breathing.

25. B. The lung generally is the 1st line of exposure and defense by a negative substance or energy.

26. C. Amma therapy treats the body by assessing energy imbalances and dysfunctional organs and then bringing healing energy to those areas.

27. B. The liver and spleen meridians are stimulated when the dorsum of the foot is massaged.

28. D. To follow the yin-yang principle is to change from season to season, light to dark, warm to cold, and follow the continual rhythm of all life.

29. D. The shiatsu, meridians, and amma bioenergy system are a series of complex chi channels throughout the body and organs.

30. D. The heart, spleen, lung, kidney, and liver, as well as the seasons, and the climate, are all associated with the five-pointed star of the elements.

31. A. Chi is the Chinese word for the energy flow in the meridian.

32. A. The bladder and gallbladder are yang channels that flow down the back of the head and neck and are the two pathways affected by occipital pressure.

33. C. Jitsu is an excess of energy.

34. D. Marmas are the energy points.

35. C. Chi circulates through the organs every 24 hours.

36. D. None of the elements are associated with the governing or conception meridian.

37. C. The lung meridian is paired with the large intestine.

38. D. The small intestine meridian is paired with the heart.

39. B. There are seven chakras.

40. D. The throat chakra is associated with communication.

41. D. Emotions, glands, and colors are associated with chakras.

42. A. The root chakra is associated with smell.

43. A. The thyroid is associated to the throat chakra.

44. C. Rolfing is functional integration.

45. A. Shiatsu is a form of acupressure that uses finger pressure.

46. A. Vata is associated with body movement.

47. B. The Bindegewebsmassage is a connective tissue massage that follows the dermatomes.

48. C. In reflexology, the big toe represents the head and neck.

49. C. Trager is a gentle rocking technique.

50. A. An examination of the tongue and hara are part of the shiatsu intake.

51. B. Muscle energy procedure is applying static pressure.

52. D. A Reiki practitioner, acupuncturist, and zero balancing are energy workers.

53. B. The radial pulse is used in Chinese medicine.

54. B. Acupuncture originated in China.

55. B. The governing vessel goes down the back to balance energy.

56. A. The conception vessel goes down the front to balance energy.

57. B. Yang is located in the posterior body.

58. A. The spleen and stomach are the organs associated with the earth.

59. A. Connective tissue massage includes transverse friction.

60. C. The stomach is the only yang meridian on the anterior of body.

61. A. The kidney meridian starts on the foot.

62. A. The Hara is the center of gravity.

63. D. The heart meridian is related to heart palpitations.

64. C. The stomach meridian is 7–9 AM.

65. C. Chakras are energy centers.

66. B. The bladder meridian is related to low back pain, edema, and impotence.

67. D. Lung and large intestine meridians make up the metal element.

68. A. The governing vessel regulates yang.

69. B. The conception vessel regulates yin.

70. C. Work on the urinary bladder for back pain.

71. B. The bladder and kidney meridians are the yin and yang water element.

72. B. Work LI for shoulder and neck pain.

73. B. The stomach meridian is yang to the earth.

74. A. The pulse is taken at the wrist.

75. A. Yang is the sunny side of the mountain.

76. D. Yin/Yang represents a universal balance.

77. D. The pancreas is not a meridian.

78. D. The liver meridian begins from the big toe.

79. B. The stomach meridian begins from the pupil of the eye.

80. B. The heart meridian represents fire.

81. D. Tsubos are pressure points.

82. A. Craniosacral is performed with little touch.

83. C. The stomach and spleen meridian are paired.

84. B. The bladder meridian ends on the little toe.

85. A. A polarity therapist is for energy.

86. B. Polarity treats the mind and body together.

87. C. The gallbladder meridian ends on the 4th toe.

88. C. From the perineum to the lower lip.

89. A. Jin Shin Do

90. B. The heart chakra is green.

91. D. Forms of energy include Chi and prana throughout the body.

92. A. Ingham developed her method of Zone Therapy called reflexology and started to teach about healing the body by pressing the feet.

93. D. Jin Shin Do, developed by Iona Teeguarden, is a method of clearing energy between two points.

94. C. A black and white circle that blends its edge represents yin and yang.

95. D. Yin represents passive, descending energy, earth, interior, and feminine.

96. C. A lack of balance leads to disease.

97. B. The numbers of points of shiatsu represent 660 tsubos.

98. B. Light, heat, heaven, exterior, and warm are characteristics of yang.

99. D. The cycles of the day, seasons, year, and life are Chi.

100. A. The gallbladder and liver are the yin and yang wood element.

PART

5

Professional Standards, Ethics, Business and Legal Practices

Part 5 covers the ethical guidelines, how therapists and bodyworkers
should conduct themselves in business, and legal parameters with
related questions. The 100 questions make up 12–13% of the content
in the NCETMB, NCETM and MBLEx exams.

CONTENTS

ETHICS OF MASSAGE AND BODYWORK	
Definition	• **Professional ethics is behaving with integrity using a moral and acceptable protocol.** • **Ethical Principles are founded on values (honesty, equality), rights to privacy, and duties (professional boundaries).** • **Standards for ethical behavior defined in the massage industry are regulated by local licensing laws and professional organizations.** • **NCBTMB's code of ethics is to protect and serve the public and the profession; code of ethics of AMTA, ABMP, AOBTA are similar** • **Provide a safe environment; ensure privacy for the client.** • **Be honest in business practice.** **Commercial aspect of massage therapist.** **Treatment of clients as consumers.** **Encompass area of advertisement, payment, procedures.** • **Work within a scope of practice.** **Acknowledge limitations, refer clients to other healthcare practitioner as appropriate.** • **Promote equitable treatment for each client.** **Refrain from discrimination in any way.**
Ethics and the Therapeutic Relationship	• Client seeks well-being through massage from massage therapist. • Massage therapist agrees to provide service. • Transference occurs when client transfers positive or negative feelings toward massage therapist. • Countertransference occurs when massage therapist transfers positive or negative feelings toward client.
The Code of Ethics	• Commitment to provide quality of care to those who seek professional services • Provide only services qualified to perform • Inform clients and other professionals the scope of practice • Recognize limitations and contraindications for massage and bodywork and refer to appropriate health professional • Respect client's right to refuse or terminate treatment • Provide treatment only when a reasonable expectation of success can be reached • Conduct business and professional activities with honesty and integrity • Refuse any gifts or benefits that are intended to influence a treatment for personal gain • Exercise the right to refuse to treat any person or part of body for just cause • Provide draping that ensures privacy, safety, and comfort

(continued)

ETHICS OF MASSAGE AND BODYWORK (*continued*)	
	• Respect client's right to treatment with informed and voluntary consent verbally or in writing
	• Refrain from any sexual conduct or activities with client
	• Maintain professional knowledge and competence through continued education training
	• Avoid interest, activity, or influence that is in conflict with acting in the best interest of client
	• Respect client's boundaries with regard to privacy, disclosure, and exposure
	• Consistently maintain and improve professional knowledge
	• Follow all policies, procedures and guidelines, regulations, codes, and requirements by NCBTMB

STANDARDS OF PRACTICE	
Definition	**The National Board's Standard of Practice is the principles by which massage therapists and bodyworkers should conduct themselves in their business.**
Client Privacy	• Confidentiality is the most important protection to client. • **Health Insurance Portability and Accountability Act (HIPAA)**—Law enacted in 1996 addresses security and privacy of health data by informing client if you need to use records for insurance purposes of to share with another healthcare professional.
Client Consent	• To allow release of records, draping alterations for special types of massage, or situations about which the client should be informed
Scope of Practice	• Do not work outside of scope of practice by diagnosing, prescribing, asking unnecessary questions, or giving unqualified advice.
Client/Therapist Relationship	• It is the responsibility of a therapist to respect *boundaries*, *right of refusal* of client, recognize *power differential*, and maintain a *professional demeanor*.
Communication	• Keep conversation to questions related to massage, and don't get invested in personal problems. • Relate to goals, treatment outcomes, and aftercare
Conflict Management	• Develop skills in conflict management between client and therapist to resolve conflict peacefully
Discrimination	• Treat a client fairly without regard to sex, race, gender, religion, or ethnicity

Education	• Maintain knowledge of massage by taking continuing education to provide more skills to the profession
Referrals	• When in doubt, refer out; if a client has needs or requires medical attention other than massage, refer him or her to the proper source
Transference	• A client's feelings for a massage therapist
Countertransference	• Feelings of the massage therapist; personalization of the professional relationship

PROFESSIONALISM	
Definition	**Professionalism is based on the therapist's overall appearance, environment, and attitude to promote sense of confidence, sincerity, and compassion.**
Guidelines	• Do no harm in any way to your client • Educate yourself and your clients about the therapeutic value of massage • Explain fee scale, client expectations, and therapist expectations before massage • Greet client by shaking hands and introducing yourself in a safe, friendly, and therapeutic environment • Begin screening appointments with 1st phone call and be sure that client is only interested in a massage • Practice truth in advertising • Maintain a professional business card and distribute in the proper locations • Always dress in appropriate clothing, do not wear jewelry, keep hair short or wear up, and avoid too much of makeup and perfume • Keep a medical history and record assessments and update regularly • Never perform a massage without information to provide a safe and effective massage • Do not perform any activities outside your scope of practice • Do not let your client believe that you know more than his or her more highly trained professional or physician

32 Business and Legal Practices

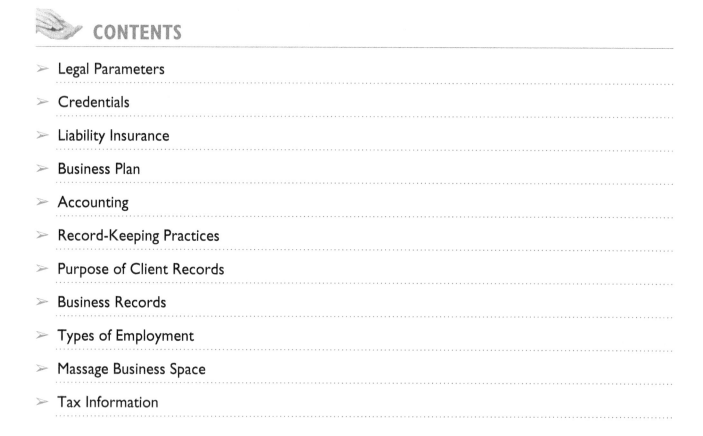

CONTENTS

BUSINESS AND LEGAL PRACTICES	
Legal Parameters	• **To follow all policies, procedures, guidelines, regulations, codes, and requirements regarding the practice and business of massage therapy** • **To follow the laws required by national, state, and local governing bodies** • **To post credentials in plain sight of all clients**
Credentials (may be different according to each states law)	*Licensing (LMT)*—More than 30 states require a professional licensing number based on qualifications, age 18 years, hours of study (500–1000), passing exam (i.e., NCTEMB, MBLEx), no criminal record, code of conduct, fee *Reciprocity*—To practice in another state from your own *Certification (CMT)*—Extensive education, may include NCTMB exam, nongovernmental, voluntary *Registered (RMT)*—Registered Massage Therapist, Canada • Other states have jurisdictions (counties, cities) that regulate the profession (i.e., certification, NCETMB)
Liability Insurance	• All massage therapists should obtain liability insurance for protection against malpractice and accidents. • Insurance can be obtained from AMTA or ABMP.
Business Plan	• Establish a business plan to open your business • Set goals for upcoming year • Create a mission statement about the intent of your business • Determine how you will advertise, spend money • Determine marketing plan: (4 P's) Product, Price, Place, and Promotion • Determine budget, expenses and revenue you expect • Determine expected gross and net income
Accounting	• Bookkeeping, taxes, and accounting can be handled by the massage practitioner or a hired accountant.

Record-Keeping Practices	• Client's files and records must be maintained for good business.
	
	• Client intake forms are essential for initial visit to get personal information and history.
	
	• SOAP notes are used for each client visit.
	    S—*Subjective:* Initial interview, anything the client tells the therapist
	    O—*Objective:* Information the therapist gathers by observation, interview; treatment goals
	    A—*Assessment:* Any progress or lack of progress relative to the massage session is documented
	    P—*Plan:* Record suggestions for future sessions or homework exercises

(*continued*)

BUSINESS AND LEGAL PRACTICES (*continued*)	
Purpose of Client Records	• Record keeping for IRS to validate business and tax returns. • Insurance reimbursement requires all intake and chart notes upon request. • Marketing plan can be from information regarding client trends. • Liability issues require full documentation of clients and their records of treatment.
Business Records	• Establish expenses for starting and maintaining your business. • Monthly budgets includes the expenses of: Rent Electricity Telephone Water (bottled) Advertising Office and janitorial supplies Linen service (if needed) Credit card charges (if needed) • Monthly income includes: Client fees Retail item (if sold) • Net income = gross income − expenses
Types of Employment	***Independent Contractor***—A massage therapist who contracts to work for another person or company with no benefits. ***Sole Proprietor***—A business that has only one owner, the massage therapist. ***Partnership***—A business arrangement between two or more massage therapists. ***Corporation***—A form of doing business characterized by limitations of the owner's liability to the amount invested in the business.
Massage Business Space	• Should be professional, comfortable, and enhance a business. • Business space should provide enough physical space to work comfortably and include a reception area and bathroom. • The following should be part of the treatment room: Massage table Chair Supplies (sheets, lotions) Music source Pleasant smell Proper lighting and heat

Tax Information	Each massage therapist is responsible for filing income tax to IRS based on wages, tips, and barter.

TAX FORMS		
W-2	By employee	Year-end wage and tax statement, submit with 1040
1099	By independent contractor	Year-end wage and tax statement for more than $600 income
Schedule K-1	By partnership members	Year-end wage and tax statement equal to W-2 form
1040	By individual	Year-end tax form
1040 ES	Self-employed	Estimated quarterly tax
Schedule C	Sole proprietor	Business profit and loss for year
Schedule SE	Self-employed	Self-employment tax form attached to 1040

33

100 Questions with Answers and Rationales on Ethics, Professional Standards, Business and Legal Practices

OBJECTIVES

Major areas of knowledge/content included in this chapter are based on most of the NCETMB, NCETM, and MBLEx exam topics, Ethics, Professional Standards, Business and Legal Practices.

Exam Content Percentages:

NCETMB 12%

NCETM 12%

MBLEx 13%

➤ Confidentiality and Client Privacy

➤ Client/Therapist Relationship

➤ Scope of Practice

➤ Referrals

➤ Professional Guidelines

➤ Interprofessional Communication

➤ Income-Reporting Procedures

➤ Business and Accounting Practices

➤ Session Record-Keeping Practices

➤ Legal and Ethical Parameters

➤ Types of Employment

➤ Tax Information

➤ Liability Insurance

DIRECTIONS

Each of the questions or statements below is followed by four suggested answers or completions. Select **one answer** that is best in each case.

1. The purpose of a client-practitioner agreement is to
   A. Develop clarity as to the nature of service
   B. Protect from unrealistic expectations
   C. Act as consent reinforcement
   D. All of the above

2. When screening new clients, it is important to
   A. Design a questionnaire that is personal
   B. Determine if the client has sexual needs
   C. Meet for lunch to get familiar
   D. Be ready and professional

3. A massage therapist is qualified to be employed by
   A. Self only
   B. Hospital operating rooms
   C. Armed forces
   D. Chiropractors, spas

4. When someone calls requesting sexual services,
   A. Hang up and get caller ID
   B. Explain the nature of the profession and the services you provide
   C. Stay centered in your professionalism
   D. B and C

5. Many massage therapists are confronted with obstacles that diminish the drive and motivation of a new business such as
   A. Too many clients to handle
   B. Failing to complete state requirements
   C. Lack of clients
   D. No business knowledge

6. In business, phone etiquette is important because
   A. It gives the caller an impression of who you are ethically and professionally
   B. It conveys how you feel about your practice
   C. The phone call is taped
   D. A and B

7. If a client's condition is outside the massage technician's scope of practice, the technician should
   A. Schedule extra sessions
   B. Refer the client to the proper professional care
   C. Take more training
   D. Read textbooks to learn more

8. Clear written contracts are an integral part of a business relationship because
   A. They provide a predetermined method to resolve problems
   B. They help avoid problems
   C. They keep you focused on your goals
   D. All of the above

9. If you are planning to be an independent contractor,
   A. You are paid in regular intervals (i.e., hour, week, month)
   B. You are reimbursed for travel expenses
   C. You must provide your own table, linens, lotion, etc.
   D. You can be discharged by the employer

10. Reviewing records before a client's visit refreshes your memory and gains the client's
    A. Sympathy
    B. Information
    C. Trust
    D. Dependence

11. If you are planning to be an employee, Internal Revenue Service (IRS) requires that you
    A. Have been trained by the business to perform services
    B. Have investment in the facility
    C. Become an independent contractor
    D. All of the above

12. All client information should be considered
   A. Essential
   B. Important
   C. For the record
   D. Confidential

13. Examples of common ethical dilemmas in the health care profession is (are)
   A. Inappropriate advertising
   B. Breaking confidentiality
   C. Practicing beyond your scope
   D. All of the above

14. The NCTMB code of ethics is designed to
   A. Promote respect for the dignity of persons
   B. Promote integrity in relationships
   C. Promote responsible caring for clients
   D. All of the above

15. A professional code of ethics includes the following:
   A. Keeping policies confidential
   B. Maintaining an open book policy
   C. Design a code of ethics to your needs
   D. Following confidentiality all local requirements for policy and procedures

16. When opening a massage business, helpful resources include
   A. Yellow pages
   B. Keeping a journal
   C. Attorney general
   D. Helpful consultants include SBA, accountant, and chamber of commerce

17. Pricing a service business such as massage therapy is based on
   A. Assets and cash flow
   B. Capitalized earnings
   C. Net present value and future earnings
   D. All of the above

18. If a massage therapist is found guilty of violation of the Massage Practice Act or Rules of Conduct, which action should be taken?
   A. Warning only
   B. Suspension of license only

   C. Revocation of license only
   D. Any action can be taken

19. The major benefit(s) in good interprofessional communication is (are)
   A. Client retention
   B. Referrals
   C. Quality therapeutic results
   D. All of the above

20. Business expenses can include the cost of
   A. A new car
   B. Clothes to keep in style
   C. Homeowner's insurance
   D. License, business cards, advertising, and liability insurance

21. What is the importance of documenting your work and keeping files?
   A. You can't count on your memory
   B. For insurance reasons
   C. Record keeping is necessary for IRS
   D. A and B

22. Client files are important for
   A. Record keeping for the Internal Revenue Service
   B. Keeping well informed of client's needs
   C. Documenting your work on clients
   D. All of the above

23. Techniques to market professional skills include
   A. Publications and presentations
   B. Business cards and brochures
   C. Donation of services
   D. All of the above

24. A typical client intake form should include
   A. Name and address
   B. Name, address, occupation, physician, emergency number
   C. Name, phone, hobbies
   D. Name, marital status, children

25. A massage therapist or bodyworker can claim business deductions on Schedule C for
   A. Cost of massage table, linens, and oils
   B. All vacations

C. Professional convention fees

D. A and C

26. In opening a massage office, it is essential to investigate certain requirements including
    A. Board of Health
    B. Police Department
    C. NCETMB requirements
    D. Zoning and licensing laws

27. SOAP charting is being widely adopted by massage professionals because
    A. Use of a professional reporting system enhances the image of massage as a valuable therapy
    B. Other healthcare professionals cannot understand the language
    C. It can be used in a court of law
    D. Clients want a record of their health

28. A ledger that separates and classifies every business expenditure is called a(an)
    A. Inventory
    B. Disbursement record
    C. Voucher
    D. Tax ID

29. A good way to save on advertising is to
    A. Make up client referral cards with a discount
    B. Use the yellow pages
    C. Send out flyers
    D. Purchase name lists to solicit

30. Many massage therapists and bodyworkers are
    A. Entrepreneurs
    B. Partners
    C. Sole proprietors
    D. Employers

31. If you choose to work for insurance reimbursement,
    A. Thorough documentation is necessary
    B. Your treatment must be medically necessary
    C. You need a letter of referral from the physician
    D. All of the above

32. A record of monies owed to you by others is called
    A. Charges
    B. Accounts receivable
    C. Statements
    D. Liabilities

33. The insurance company(ies) that a massage therapist can submit a claim to is (are)
    A. Workers compensation
    B. Managed care HMO/PPO
    C. Automobile insurance
    D. All of the above

34. In record keeping for tax time it is important to
    A. Record what activity you do hour by hour
    B. Keep track of the names of clients
    C. Keep track of automobile business mileage in a ledger
    D. Know how many clients cancelled

35. If you are in business for yourself, it is important to
    A. Spend the money as you please and use December for taxes
    B. Save money for taxes
    C. Belong to a professional association
    D. Invest your money in the stock market

36. All of the following are retirement plans to help manage your money except
    A. Roth IRA
    B. IRA
    C. NCTMB
    D. 401(K)

37. Business activities directed toward promoting and increasing business are called
    A. Assets
    B. Reputation
    C. Marketing
    D. Goals

38. Developing personal and professional contacts for the purpose of giving and receiving support and sharing information is called
    A. Hotline
    B. Networking

    C. Advertising

    D. Promotions

39. A business that has stockholders is called a

    A. Sole proprietorship

    B. Partnership

    C. Corporation

    D. Subsidiary

40. Professional arrangement(s) available to massage therapists or bodyworkers who work with clients for insurance reimbursement are

    A. The physician pays the therapist

    B. The client pays the therapist

    C. The insurance company pays the therapist

    D. All of the above

41. The current status of insurance reimbursement for massage is

    A. Licensed massage therapists are the only ones to receive payment

    B. Nurses are the only ones to receive payment

    C. Massage has to be done in the doctor's office

    D. Very complicated, and is handled case by case

42. The costs of education are deductible if

    A. They improve your professional skills

    B. You are training in a new field

    C. You are paying for massage school

    D. They are to meet minimal professional requirements

43. The insurance that covers costs of injuries occurring on your property and any resulting litigation is called

    A. Disability

    B. Liability

    C. Homeowner's

    D. Comprehensive

44. To qualify as a deductible home office,

    A. It must be used for personal use

    B. It must be used regularly and exclusively for massage in your practice

    C. You can deduct a portion of all living expenses

    D. It can be used as a den or bedroom as well

45. Massage therapists who are self-employed

    A. Have a business profit if there is money left after deductions

    B. Report on IRS form Schedule C

    C. Pay self-employment tax and income tax

    D. All of the above

46. In a personal service business, hygiene and safety are especially important to

    A. The client

    B. The facility

    C. The practitioner

    D. Everyone concerned

47. Business and personal deductions allowable for income tax purpose include all but the following:

    A. Cost of supplies

    B. Interest on home loan or student loan

    C. Professional association dues

    D. Cost of a car

48. A taxpayer identification number can be defined as

    A. A number given by IRS form SS-4

    B. A social security number

    C. A PIN number chosen and submitted to IRS

    D. A and B

49. It is important for the massage practitioner to know the difference between sensuality and

    A. Sensitivity

    B. Sexuality

    C. Common sense

    D. Sympathy

50. City or municipal governments have the legal power

    A. To require fingerprints

    B. To decide what businesses can operate in the city

    C. To require a physician's clearance to practice

    D. A and B

51. When you consider opening an office, startup costs include

    A. Massage table, phone, rent, ads, music, and sheets

    B. Massage table only

C. Business cards, phone, and table

D. A cost of $500

52. The ability to set positive goals and put forth the energy and effort required to achieve them is
    A. Self-motivation
    B. Self-preservation
    C. Self-indulgence
    D. Selfishness

53. Business enterprises for profit entities include all but the following:
    A. Limited Liability Company
    B. Proprietorship
    C. Membership or trust
    D. Corporation

54. If you have a business name, you must register it with
    A. IRS
    B. City or state clerk's office
    C. AMTA
    D. Insurance company

55. Keep your knowledge current by
    A. Attending seminars
    B. Reading trade journals
    C. Joining professional associations
    D. All of the above

56. To practice good ethics is to be concerned about the welfare of the public and individual clients, as well as your personal and professional
    A. Health
    B. Reputation
    C. Clothing
    D. Lifestyle

57. A well-written business card can be used for
    A. Referrals
    B. Advertising
    C. Promotional coupons
    D. A and B

58. Developing business relationships with people who are also promoting a business is called
    A. Referral
    B. Volunteerism
    C. Networking
    D. A partnership

59. An important part of ethics is to keep client communications
    A. Recorded
    B. Confidential
    C. Written down
    D. Open to the public

60. Good business practice(s) to prevent burnout is (are)
    A. Take time off indefinitely
    B. See a psychiatrist
    C. Eat out more
    D. Relax and get a massage for yourself

61. Which of the following types of insurance provides you with income in the event that you cannot work due to illness or injury?
    A. Professional liability
    B. General liability
    C. Business personal property
    D. Disability insurance

62. Confidentiality of your client's records is required for many reasons. The primary reason is
    A. To protect yourself if sued by the client
    B. To ensure adequate information for insurance billing purposes
    C. Professional ethics
    D. You were told to do so by your instructor

63. Important business resources include a variety of business and civic organizations such as the
    A. Public library
    B. Service Core of Retired Executives (SCORE)
    C. Small Business Association (SBA)
    D. All are important resources

64. You are self-employed. How often do you have to make estimated tax payments?
    A. Once a month
    B. Annually, before December 31 of the tax year
    C. You do not; just pay your taxes before April 15 when the return is due
    D. Quarterly

65. A massage therapist can get professional liability insurance from
    A. Prudential Insurance Company
    B. American Massage Therapy Association (AMTA)

C. U.S. Health Care

D. COBRA

66. When a client discusses personal matters with you, what should you do?

   A. Just listen and be compassionate

   B. Offer the client your advice

   C. Tell the client you'd prefer he didn't talk

   D. Tune out the client

67. A new client has left her bra on. Without saying anything to her about it, you unsnap it while she is in the prone position so you can work on her back. You have just violated

   A. The scope of practice

   B. Her morals

   C. Her boundaries

   D. The rules about sexual misconduct

68. One of your clients starts asking you personal questions about another client that she saw leaving as she was coming in. You should

   A. Answer her questions honestly

   B. Tell her politely that you cannot talk about your clients

   C. Just change the subject

   D. Tell her she is being rude and nosy

69. Another massage therapist has moved into your neighborhood, and you have discovered that she is not licensed. The best course of action is

   A. Send a formal complaint to the licensure board

   B. Ignore the situation; your clients are loyal, and you don't have to worry about it

   C. Change your sign to read "The only licensed therapist in the area"

   D. Call her and inform her that you are going to put her out of business

70. What is the main purpose of a code of ethics?

   A. To satisfy the licensure laws

   B. To provide parameters for a safe scope of practice for a client/therapist

   C. To impress clients

   D. To keep the massage board from revoking your license

71. If a massage practitioner who has a license in one state moves to another state and a license is granted based on the license from the previous state, what is that called?

   A. Reciprocity

   B. Equality

   C. Right to license

   D. Dual licensure

72. If a practitioner receives a referral from a doctor, what follow-up form should she provide to the doctor?

   A. The intake form

   B. 1099

   C. SOAP notes

   D. The insurance form

73. Which of the following would be legitimate tax-deductible business expenses?

   A. The cost of continuing education after you have your license

   B. Training for a new career in massage therapy

   C. An hourly rate for your time while studying for the licensure examination

   D. Car expenses for commuting to massage school

74. If you are working as an independent contractor, the IRS requires that you file quarterly

   A. Sales tax

   B. Self-employment taxes

   C. 1099

   D. 1040

75. If you are a business owner who employs other therapists, pays them by the hour, and provides them with benefits, you will be giving them a form at the end of the tax year called a

   A. W-4

   B. WC

   C. W-2

   D. W-3

76. A written expression of the goals and purpose of a business is referred to as

   A. An advertisement

   B. A business plan

   C. A mission statement

   D. SOAP notes

77. To protect yourself from a lawsuit, you should have the following:
    A. National certification
    B. A state license
    C. Liability insurance
    D. Zoning approval

78. How long should your tax returns be kept on file?
    A. 3 years
    B. 5 years
    C. 7 years
    D. 10 years

79. When two massage therapists begin to work together in the same office, how do they avoid forming a legal partnership?
    A. By both being sole proprietors
    B. By becoming a corporation
    C. By having different accountants
    D. All of the above

80. One of the most powerful sources of advertising is
    A. Yellow pages
    B. Newspapers
    C. Word of mouth
    D. Radio

81. Assuming your regular fee for massage is $40/hr and your client gives you an extra $10 for a tip, how much money from that massage do you need to declare with the IRS?
    A. $10
    B. $40
    C. $50
    D. None of it, as long as the client paid in cash

82. Why do most businesses fail?
    A. Lack of effort
    B. Underestimation of capital and expenses
    C. Too little advertising
    D. Too many massage therapists in one office

83. Client records are confidential except when
    A. Directed by the client
    B. Requested through a subpoena
    C. You don't like the client
    D. Both A and B

84. What is the most important skill during a client intake?
    A. Talking clearly
    B. Listening
    C. Looking at the client's posture
    D. Reading the intake form

85. Who is required to submit a Schedule C tax statement to the IRS?
    A. Contracted employees
    B. Sole proprietor businesses
    C. Corporations
    D. Partnerships

86. Which of the following statements in the code of ethics is accepted in the massage profession?
    A. Inform clients, other healthcare practitioners, and the public of the scope of practice
    B. Insure yourself with liability insurance
    C. Provide treatment only when there is reasonable expectation that it will be long-term care
    D. Conduct your business and professional activities according to strict business procedures

87. Which of the following provides protection against potential lawsuits involving malpractice?
    A. State licensing
    B. Schedule C taxes
    C. K-1 form
    D. Liability insurance

88. Which of the following is a good legal reason to keep client records and files?
    A. Tax purposes
    B. Marketing purposes
    C. Liability
    D. Tracking trends

89. Which of the following tax forms is filed by self-employed individuals?
    A. W-2
    B. 1040
    C. 1065
    D. 1040ES

90. In which of the following situations would it be inappropriate to disclose confidential client information?
   A. At the request of the client's physician
   B. At the request of the client's insurance company
   C. When requested by the IRS
   D. When required by court order

91. Client intake forms are extremely important. The most important reason is that
   A. Careful notes help you assess and develop a treatment plan
   B. Information received gives you medical history and helps recognize any contraindications or precautions
   C. The forms help you to get to know your client and specific needs
   D. Obtaining all necessary client information can help protect the therapist if there is a malpractice suit

92. Confidentiality of your client's records is required for many reasons. The primary reason is
   A. To protect yourself if sued by client
   B. To ensure adequate information for insurance billing purposes
   C. Professional ethics
   D. You were told to do so by your instructor

93. A client is on the table and tells the therapist that he does not want to continue. The client is obviously upset about something. The therapist should do what?
   A. Ask what is wrong and try to counsel him
   B. Immediately stop the massage and try to talk about what bothered the client after he is dressed
   C. Continue with the massage since you are not finished yet
   D. Refuse to work on that client again

94. How does continuing education support professional ethics?
   A. It promotes business
   B. It tests commitment to massage therapy

   C. It is required for membership in professional organizations
   D. It promotes a higher standard in the profession

95. When do you release a client's medical record?
   A. When the insurance company requests a copy of the record
   B. When the attorney calls for it
   C. When the client calls you on the phone and requests it
   D. When the client signs a release of information form

96. What is the most important protocol for documenting progress of your client?
   A. RICE
   B. SOAP
   C. ANS
   D. TXS

97. What type of insurance do massage therapists buy to cover their work in case a client sues?
   A. Malpractice and life
   B. Homeowners
   C. Life
   D. Liability and malpractice

98. As a massage therapist, always practice
   A. Within your scope of practice
   B. Truth in advertising
   C. Beginning your assessment with 1st phone call
   D. All of the above

99. All credentials should be
   A. Posted in plain sight of all clients
   B. Kept confidential
   C. Only shown upon request
   D. Filed away

100. All of the following are needed in a treatment room except
   A. Massage table
   B. Music source
   C. File cabinet
   D. Proper lighting

ANSWERS AND RATIONALES

1. **D.** Client-practitioner agreement and policy statements are important to inform the client and protect the therapist.

2. **D.** When you are screening a client, always have ready questions to ask as well as an understanding of expectations of client or special needs. Being prepared helps the conversation and leaves the client with a sense of your professionalism.

3. **D.** As a massage therapist, there are many employment opportunities in addition to being self-employed.

4. **D.** When a massage therapist is confronted with obscene calls, it is always best to be as professional as possible and explain the services of your business.

5. **D.** Many massage therapists have difficulty and fail in their new businesses due to burnout, lack of funds, or lack of marketing skills.

6. **D.** Communication on the phone is a way of creating an invisible impression to a potential client. It is essential to be as polite and professional as possible.

7. **B.** A client should always be referred to another health practitioner if the treatment required goes beyond massage.

8. **D.** The information in a contract should reflect the specific nature of your business and goals to prevent legal conflict.

9. **C.** All independent contractors supply their own materials and equipment and are paid for their services one time without expecting any expenses to be paid.

10. **C.** Reviewing accurate records prior to massage establishes confidence and trust on the part of the client.

11. **D.** An employee is trained and paid regularly by the company to which they provide a service. IRS outlines these and other factors that determine the definition of an employer.

12. **D.** All personal information regarding a client should be kept in a secure place and confidential.

13. **D.** Ethical concerns of massage therapists include sexual misconduct, practicing beyond your scope, poor advertising, misleading claims of curative abilities, and more.

14. **D.** After obtaining national certification, all massage therapists should follow the NCTMB code of ethics concerning respect, integrity, and caring.

15. **D.** The code of ethics provides for confidentiality, credentials, policies, and government requirements.

16. **D.** Many consultants are available when opening a business including an attorney, the Small Business Administration (SBA), an accountant, and the Chamber of Commerce.

17. **D.** The capitalized earnings, assets, cash flow, and present value and future earnings all are considered as methods for pricing a business.

18. **D.** Violating massage Rules of Conduct can result in a warning, suspension, or revocation of license.

19. **D.** Good communication between therapist and client can ensure client return, referrals, and effective therapeutic sessions.

20. **D.** Business expenses include the costs of license, insurance, cards, linens, professional clothes, and memberships.

21. D. Documenting work and keeping a client file ensures a permanent record for IRS, client needs, and finances.

22. D. Client files document all the work you have done for your use and for the IRS.

23. D. Marketing includes business cards and brochures, publications, and presentations.

24. B. All important information should be included on intake: name, address, phone, and physician.

25. D. Business deductions include anything that helps to develop or maintain your trade including equipment, rent, phone, and any professional fees.

26. D. The office location requires that you meet the local governmental requirements, including application for new business, zoning, and fire and health inspection.

27. A. SOAP charting is an efficient and effective way to document all types of healthcare treatment.

28. B. The disbursement record comes from the checkbook, but columns separate each category of expenditure.

29. A. Clients prefer to have a massage by someone who was referred rather than opening the yellow pages or responding to a flyer.

30. C. Many massage therapists and bodyworkers are sole proprietors in which they are the only one in charge of the business. Renting a space or working from home qualifies this.

31. D. Insurance reimbursement requires a great deal of documentation, a physician referral, and a medical reason for doing the bodywork or massage.

32. B. This is a record of credit extended to clients.

33. D. All kinds of insurance companies can reimburse for massage services, including workers compensation, managed care, liability, and automobile or group health insurance.

34. C. It is important to keep a record of car mileage related to business travel; keep receipts, cancelled checks, and bills for tax time at the end of the year.

35. B. If you are self-employed, the most difficult thing to do is put money aside in a savings account for year-end taxes.

36. C. NCTMB is the National Certification for Therapeutic Massage and Bodywork and it has no retirement plan. The IRAs and 401(K) are ways to save money tax-free or tax-deferred.

37. C. Marketing is advertising, public relations, promotion, and client referrals.

38. B. Networking enhances the extension of the business.

39. C. Stockholders share in profits but are not legally responsible for the actions of the corporation.

40. D. The client, physician, or insurance company can pay the massage therapist or bodyworker for reimbursement. Keep all records of billing for your records for insurance claims.

41. D. The variation of insurance policies, state laws, and licensing make the subject of insurance reimbursement very complicated; each case is individual.

42. A. You can deduct the cost of education, plus travel and meals, if the education maintains or improves your professional skills or is required by law for keeping your professional status.

43. B. Liability insurance is part of a homeowner's policy but may not cover business-related occurrences.

44. B. A home office must be used regularly or exclusively for massage or business book-keeping and cannot be used as another room, guest, or den.

45. D. Self-employed massage therapists always report on Schedule C for IRS and are subject to self-employment tax and income tax. Profits are calculated after business deductions.

46. D. Everyone concerned should be aware that safety and personal hygiene are essential to a healthy atmosphere.

47. D. The cost of a car is not a tax deduction, only the travel expenses, gas, repair, and services.

48. D. A taxpayer number can be a social security number if you are a sole proprietor or have no employees or a taxpayer ID number applied for on IRS form SS-4.

49. B. Good ethics and professional conduct are required for a certified, licensed, or registered massage practitioner.

50. D. Municipal governments have the right to restrict the businesses of massage therapy. They can require photo, fingerprints, educational certifications, or a physician clearance.

51. A. You will need many items to start an office, massage table, sheets, phone, rent and security, music, phone, brochures, and ads, all costing a minimum of about $3,000.

52. A. Self-motivation means to keep working toward goals.

53. C. Membership or trust organizations are business entities that are not for profit and have compliance, tax, and liability consequences that require the assistance of attorneys and accountants.

54. B. When you give your business a name, you must file it with the city or state clerk's office to protect another business from using your name.

55. D. Learning about new aspects of the field of massage as a health science is important.

56. B. Individual ethics become part of the professional code of ethics.

57. D. A good business card can project who you are and what you do and can serve as an advertisement or referral card.

58. C. Networking is a way to learn from others, such as the Chamber of Commerce, civic groups, professional memberships, massage conferences, and conventions.

59. B. Communicate in a confidential and professional manner without exposing personal matters.

60. D. Burnout is being tired and unhappy with one's work. It includes boredom, lack of productivity, and boundaries. Take a vacation, exercise, or get a massage.

61. D. Disability insurance protects your income if you become ill or have a prolonged injury.

62. C. Ethics are standards of acceptable and professional behavior.

63. D. There are many business resources to use for information such as the SBA, public library, SCORE, Rotary Club, or Chamber of Commerce.

64. D. According to the IRS, self-employed individuals must make quarterly tax payments.

65. B. Malpractice insurance is essential for a massage therapist. Professional organizations, such as AMTA, can provide liability protection.

66. A. Listening is the best communication.

67. C. A client's boundaries require you to ask permission to unsnap a bra.

68. B. Refer to confidentiality and consideration.

69. A. Always report someone who does not follow the laws.

70. B. A scope of practice based on a code of ethics protects the client/therapist.

71. A. Reciprocity allows you to work in another state.

72. C. SOAP notes relay to the doctor explanation of treatment.

73. A. Continuing education is a business expense.

74. B. An independent contractor must file self-employment tax.

75. C. The W-2 form is provided by an employer.

76. C. A mission statement is the purpose and scope of a business.

77. C. Insurance is necessary for injury or malpractice.

78. C. Keep tax records for 7 years.

79. A. You can work together as independent contractors.

80. C. The best way to advertise is to give a good massage, and you will get referrals.

81. C. All money for a massage, including a tip, is to be reported as income.

82. B. Before starting a business, make a list of equipment and supplies and a monthly budget to estimate capital and business expenses.

83. D. Client records are released by the client's request or a subpoena.

84. B. Listening to the client is the most important.

85. B. A sole proprietor must submit a schedule C tax form.

86. B. According to the code of ethics, it is important to insure yourself with liability insurance.

87. D. Liability insurance protects against malpractice.

88. C. The legal reason to keep good client records is in case of a liability lawsuit.

89. D. Someone who is self-employed uses a 1040ES tax form.

90. A. Client information is necessary for IRS, court order, or the client's insurance company.

91. B. Contraindications and precautions for massage are information that is part of a good client intake.

92. C. It is professional to keep your clients' records confidential.

93. B. Always listen to the client and honor his or her request to stop if necessary.

94. D. Continuing education helps to promote higher professional standards.

95. D. Medical records must be signed for before they are released.

96. B. SOAP notes are used to document client progress.

97. D. Liability and malpractice insurance is necessary.

98. D. A massage therapist must practice and advertise within the professional boundaries.

99. A. License and insurance certificates should be posted in office.

100. C. There is no need to keep a file cabinet in the treatment room.

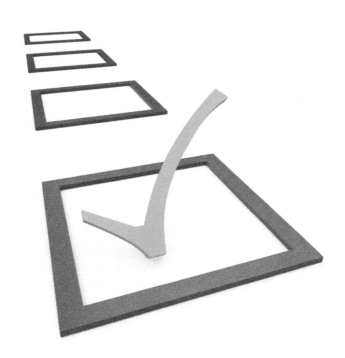

PART

6

Comprehensive Simulated Exams and Answers

34 Comprehensive Simulated NCETMB Exam

This simulated exam contains 125 questions on **Western and Eastern Massage and Bodywork.**

NCETMB Content:

➤ Kinesiology and musculoskeletal anatomy and physiology 19–24%

➤ Systemic anatomy and physiology 13–18%

➤ Pathology, contraindications and cautionary sites 14–19%

➤ Professional standards 11–15%

➤ Massage therapy theory, evaluation and techniques 30–37%

DIRECTIONS

Each of the numbered items or incomplete statements in this chapter is followed by answers or completion of the statement. Select the **ONE** lettered answer or completion that is **BEST** in each case. The maximum time to complete the 160-question exam is two hours and forty minutes. The actual exam also contains 160 questions, including 20 pretest questions not counted in the final score. Answer all the questions!

1. The sequences and directions of Swedish massage strokes are most adapted to which anatomical or physiological situation?
   A. Muscle attachments
   B. Subcutaneous adipose tissue
   C. Autonomic nervous system
   D. Lymph drainage and venous return

2. Good bookkeeping for healing arts professionals can
   A. Eliminate tracking sheets
   B. Decrease bank statements
   C. Increase petty cash funds
   D. Increase legitimate tax deductions

3. When massaging the thigh in the supine position, which muscle is involved?
   A. Hamstring
   B. Quadriceps
   C. Gluteal
   D. Gastrocnemius

4. Massage is contraindicated for which of the following conditions?
   A. High blood pressure
   B. Constipation
   C. Keloid scar
   D. Adhesions

5. The iliopsoas flexes the hip because of its insertion on the
   A. Femur
   B. Greater trochanter
   C. Lesser trochanter
   D. Iliac crest

6. The tricuspid valve is found between the
   A. Right atrium and right ventricle
   B. Left ventricle and aorta
   C. Left ventricle and right ventricle
   D. Right atrium and left atrium

7. Which is a true statement concerning Golgi tendon apparatus?
   A. Found in joint capsules
   B. Detects overall tension in tendon
   C. Originates in Purkinje fibers
   D. Activated by vagal reflex

8. Which muscles are adductors?
   A. Pectoralis and deltoid
   B. Pectoralis and latissimus dorsi
   C. Deltoid and latissimus dorsi
   D. Biceps and deltoids

9. Which muscle would be paralyzed if the sciatic nerve were severed?
   A. Trapezius
   B. Biceps femoris
   C. Gluteus maximus
   D. Erector spinae

10. Which statement most accurately describes the meridian system?
    A. Energy pathway moving randomly through the body
    B. Energy pathway moving superficially
    C. Energy pathway that doesn't affect organs
    D. 12 meridians and 2 vessels are pathways in which energy moves toward the surface of the body, affecting organs

11. What type of insurance do MTs buy to cover their work in case a client sues?
    A. Malpractice
    B. Homeowners
    C. Life
    D. Liability

12. Which condition is present when there is an injury of the ulnar nerve at the elbow?
    A. Inability to flex fingers fully
    B. Spasticity
    C. Flaccidity
    D. Spasms

13. The only joint where the axial skeleton articulates with the appendicular skeleton is
    A. Sternoclavicular
    B. Glenohumeral
    C. Sternoscapular
    D. Scapularclavicular

14. What muscle is not a part of the rotator cuff?
    A. Supraspinatus
    B. Infraspinatus
    C. Teres major
    D. Teres minor

15. When opening a massage business, helpful resources include
    A. Chamber of Commerce
    B. Accountant
    C. Small Business Administration
    D. All of the above

16. Acupuncture, shiatsu, polarity, and reflexology are examples of
    A. Energetic manipulation
    B. Behavioral barometer
    C. Reactive circuits
    D. Systematic massage

17. When massaging the lateral head of the fibula, of which structure should you be careful?
    A. Popliteal endangerment site
    B. Peroneal nerve
    C. Tibial nerve
    D. Femoral nerve

18. Cross-massage must be applied in which direction to the fibers?
    A. Horizontally
    B. At right angles
    C. Triangularly
    D. Trapezoidally

19. With client in the supine position, how do you expose the serratus anterior?
    A. Lateral rotation and adduction of the arm
    B. Medial rotation and adduction of the arm
    C. Horizontal abduction of the arm
    D. Horizontal adduction of the arm

20. Hypercontraction of the pectoralis minor causes rounded shoulders. Which muscle would be weak and overstretched?
    A. Pectoralis minor
    B. Rhomboids
    C. Subclavius
    D. Levator scapula

21. Which share a common attachment?
    A. Biceps brachii, brachioradialis, coracobrachialis
    B. Coracobrachialis, brachioradialis, pectoralis minor
    C. Pectoralis minor, coracobrachialis, brachioradialis
    D. Biceps brachii, coracobrachialis, pectoralis minor

22. Friction, percussion, and vibration are techniques that
    A. Stimulate
    B. Relax
    C. Strengthen
    D. Weaken

23. All of the following dorsiflex the ankle except
    A. Tibialis anterior
    B. Extensor hallucis longus
    C. Peroneus longus
    D. Peroneus tertius

24. The muscles, from medial to lateral, are
    A. Biceps femoris, semitendinosus, semimembranosus
    B. Semitendinosus, semimembranosus, biceps femoris
    C. Semimembranosus, semitendinosus, rectus femoris
    D. Semimembranosus, semitendinosus, biceps femoris

25. We do not massage the SCM bilaterally because of the
    A. Femoral artery
    B. Common carotid artery
    C. Peroneal artery
    D. Tibial artery

26. What is the insertion of the brachioradialis?
    A. Styloid process of radius
    B. Lateral epicondyle of humerus
    C. Medial epicondyle of humerus
    D. Styloid process of ulna

27. What is the origin of the teres minor?
    A. Vertebral border of scapula
    B. Axillary border of scapula
    C. Lesser tubercle
    D. Greater tubercle

28. The attempt to bring the structure of the body into alignment around a central axis is called
    A. Structural integration
    B. Trauma
    C. Alignment
    D. Adjustment

29. What muscle shares an attachment with the deltoids?
    A. Levator scapula
    B. Biceps brachialis
    C. Trapezius
    D. Supraspinatis

30. A hyperirritable spot that is painful when compressed is called a(an)
    A. Trigger point
    B. Pain point
    C. Ampule
    D. Rolfing

31. Which rotator cuff muscle is positioned anterior on the scapula?
    A. Supraspinatis
    B. Infraspinatis
    C. Subscapularis
    D. Teres minor

32. In which directions do yin meridians flow?
    A. Superior to inferior
    B. Inferior to superior
    C. Lateral to medial
    D. Medial to lateral

33. Injuries that have a gradual onset or reoccur often are called
    A. Sprains
    B. Occupational
    C. Acute
    D. Chronic

34. What is the insertion for pectoralis major?
    A. Medial clavicle
    B. Medial bicipital groove
    C. Sternum
    D. Lateral bicipital groove

35. What name may be given to a muscle that acts on the thumb?
    A. Hallucis
    B. Longus
    C. Pollicis
    D. Brevis

36. If a client's condition is outside the massage technician's scope of practice, the technician should
    A. Schedule extra sessions
    B. Refer the client to the proper professional
    C. Take more training
    D. Read textbooks

37. Which erector spinae muscle is the most medial of the group?
    A. Spinalis
    B. Multifidous
    C. Longisimus
    D. Iliocostalis

38. What is the insertion site for the levator scapulae?
    A. Ribs 1-8
    B. Medial border of the scapula
    C. Superior angle of the scapula
    D. C1-C4

39. Which meridians are innervated by massaging the medial thigh?
    A. KI, LIV, SP
    B. GB, ST, SP
    C. LIV, ST, KI
    D. GB, LIV, KI

40. Endangerment sites should be avoided during a massage because they are
    A. Bilaterally symmetrical
    B. Areas that can be easily injured
    C. Areas that are dysfunctional
    D. Hard to remember

41. If you are a self-employed massage therapist, you must file
    A. No returns
    B. Only Schedule C—Profit or Loss form
    C. Form 1040 and Social Security Self-Employment Tax form
    D. B and C

42. The draping method that covers the table and wraps the client is called
    A. Top cover
    B. Full sheet
    C. Diaper
    D. Wrapping

43. Which of the following muscles does not abduct the thigh?
    A. Gluteus maximus
    B. Gluteus medius
    C. Gluteus minimus
    D. Sartorius

44. Cancer is a disease that can be spread through the
    A. Genes
    B. Lymphatic and blood system
    C. Endocrine system
    D. Digestive system

45. Which is a type of dry heat?
    A. Ice cube
    B. Microwave
    C. Sauna
    D. Fog

46. An informed consent contains information from which the client
    A. Can make decisions for his or her own protection
    B. Can state the right to cancel treatment
    C. Is advised of benefits/undesirable effects
    D. All of the above

47. Aligning major body segments through manipulation of connective tissue is the
    A. Rolfing method
    B. Traeger method
    C. Palmer method
    D. Reflexology method

48. Abnormalities in gait are found throughout the postural chain by assessing which body landmarks?
    A. Top of the iliac crests
    B. Top of the fibular heads
    C. Rami of mandible and ears
    D. All of the above

49. Application of cold should be of short duration to prevent tissue injury from
    A. Pain
    B. Thawing
    C. Freezing
    D. Heat

50. To reduce adhesions and fibrosis, which movement is used?
    A. Cross-fiber friction
    B. Wringing
    C. Pressing
    D. Squeezing

51. Massage is not performed on an area that is
    A. Bleeding
    B. Swollen
    C. Burned
    D. All of the above

52. As an alternative to a commercial ice pack, put ice cubes into a
    A. Washcloth
    B. Dishtowel

C. Plastic bag

D. Bathtub

53. When administering first aid, your goal is to obtain all the necessary information related to the injury. You should conduct a primary survey of the situation, which includes
   A. Checking the ABCs (airway, breathing, circulation) and hemorrhaging
   B. Using universal precautions when administering any first aid
   C. Assessing the victim's immediate condition and any unforeseen problems
   D. All of the above

54. Avoid using which type of oil in massage?
   A. Sunflower
   B. Mineral
   C. Olive
   D. Apricot

55. Severe varicose veins is a(an) _____ for massage.
   A. Indication
   B. Circulation
   C. Embolus
   D. Contraindication

56. A survivor of abuse can benefit from massage by
   A. Feeling a sense of safeness
   B. Releasing or letting go some of the abuse
   C. Retrieving memory
   D. All of the above

57. Which meridian is lateral to the midsagittal line of the posterior cervical vertebrae?
   A. Governing vessel
   B. Triple warmer
   C. Stomach
   D. Bladder

58. What forms the outer layer of the lateral abdominal wall?
   A. Rectus abdominis
   B. Transversalis
   C. Serratus anterior
   D. External oblique

59. If a person is suffering from heat cramps,
   A. Do not give liquid with caffeine or alcohol
   B. Do not give any medication
   C. Cool with compresses at neck, groin, and armpits
   D. All of the above

60. A basic pattern of energy for the stomach channel is
   A. 7 – 9 AM
   B. 7 – 9 PM
   C. 3 – 5 AM
   D. 3 – 5 PM

61. Sciatic nerve damage diminishes ability to
   A. Flex the hip
   B. Flex the knee
   C. Adduct the hip
   D. Abduct the hip

62. Deep strokes and kneading techniques can cause an increase in
   A. Vasoconstriction
   B. Blood flow
   C. Diastolic arterial pressure
   D. Systolic arterial pressure

63. What best describes the technique of Rolfing?
   A. Reflex zone therapy
   B. German massage
   C. Structural integration
   D. Connective tissue massage

64. Manipulation of the occipital regions of the neck primarily affects
   A. HT and BL meridians
   B. CO and KI meridians
   C. BL and GB meridians
   D. ST and SP meridians

65. Facial paralysis can be due to a lesion in which cranial nerve?
   A. III
   B. VI
   C. VII
   D. VIII

66. Which muscle elevates and depresses the scapula?
    A. Trapezius
    B. Latissimus dorsi
    C. Rhomboids
    D. All of the above

67. With the elbow flexed, which muscle supinates the palm?
    A. Pronator
    B. Supinator
    C. Quadrator
    D. Brachialis

68. When massaging the body, it is important to
    A. Drape all parts of the body
    B. Expose only the part to be massaged
    C. Cover the entire body with a sheet
    D. Stand still while delivering technique

69. The cupping technique is best suited for
    A. Acute bronchitis
    B. Cancer of the lungs
    C. Bronchiectasis
    D. Acute tracheitis

70. The Heimlich maneuver is performed by
    A. Pressing the fist into the abdomen with inward thrust
    B. Subdiaphragmatic thrusts
    C. Standing behind victim with arms around waist
    D. All of the above

71. The exchange of O_2 and CO_2 takes place in the
    A. Alveoli
    B. Bronchi
    C. Bronchioles
    D. Pleural cavity

72. Active assistive joint movement requires
    A. Client only moving the extremity
    B. Therapist only moving the extremity
    C. Client and therapist moving the extremity together
    D. The joint to be immobilized

73. While performing passive ROM on a client, he or she reports pain. You can safely assume that the injury/restriction involved is
    A. Muscular
    B. Ligamentous
    C. Tendinous
    D. Articular

74. Good client records should include the
    A. Intake form
    B. Intake, health information, treatment, and session notes
    C. Client history
    D. Payments received

75. In the side-lying position, a pillow/bolster should be placed between the knees and under the
    A. Head
    B. Ankles
    C. Shoulder
    D. Leg

76. What is the main purpose of performing post-event massage?
    A. Stimulate the muscles
    B. Reduce swelling in sprains/strains
    C. Rid the body of metabolic waste buildup
    D. Treat adhesions

77. Which is a band of strong, fibrous tissue that connects the articular ends of bones and binds them together?
    A. Membrane
    B. Fascia
    C. Cancellous tissue
    D. Ligament

78. Which stroke most often begins and ends a massage?
    A. Effleurage
    B. Petrissage
    C. Friction
    D. Vibration

79. Which modality would be best for a client who desires energy work instead of massage?
    A. Pilates
    B. Structural integration

C. Myotherapy

D. Therapeutic touch

80. A client comes in and reports that her lower back has been hurting ever since she mowed her lawn yesterday. In which section of the SOAP notes is this information recorded?

A. S

B. O

C. A

D. P

81. Client files are important because

A. The Internal Revenue Service requires record keeping

B. Practitioners must keep well informed of clients' needs

C. You have documented your "work" on clients

D. All of the above

82. Subjective information is obtained by

A. Assessing the way the client walks

B. Palpation

C. Standing the client on the plumb line

D. Listening to the client

83. To get the client acclimated to your touch and to warm up the muscle, you should begin bodywork sessions with

A. Effleurage

B. Friction

C. Petrissage

D. Tapotement

84. An appropriate hypoallergenic oil combination is

A. Sesame and almond

B. Sunflower and canola

C. Apricot and olive

D. Peanut and walnut

85. In which massage technique should the fingers move tissue under the skin but not the skin itself?

A. Tapotement

B. Effleurage

C. Vibration

D. Friction

86. You should never massage someone who is under the influence of drugs or alcohol because the client

A. May not be in control of him- or herself

B. May say or do something inappropriate

C. May accuse you of saying or doing something inappropriate

D. All of the above

87. Which endangerment site contains the median nerve?

A. Ulnar notch of the elbow

B. Posterior triangle of neck

C. Anterior triangle of neck

D. Cubital area of elbow

88. Which is the 1st step in beginning massage treatment?

A. Apply lubricant

B. Effleurage

C. Determine contraindications

D. Diagnose the patient

89. When giving CPR to a 6-year-old child, you use the

A. Heel of one hand

B. Heel of two hands

C. Fingers of one hand

D. Fingers of two hands

90. The popliteus muscle of the leg

A. Adducts

B. Extends

C. Plantar flexes the ankle

D. Medially rotates the tibia

91. First aid for acute soft tissue injuries involves RICE, which means

A. Ice

B. Rest and elevation

C. Compression

D. All of the above

92. Massage treatment of the chest should never be done over the

A. Ribs

B. Heart

C. Female nipples

D. All of the above

93. Which aims most specifically to passively stretch muscle?
    A. Effleurage
    B. Friction
    C. Petrissage
    D. Tapotement

94. Massage benefits lymph flow best when strokes are
    A. Away from the heart
    B. Toward the heart
    C. Heavy in both directions
    D. In certain local areas

95. The nerve that supplies the adductors of the thigh is the
    A. Femoral nerve
    B. Superior gluteal nerve
    C. Tibial nerve
    D. Obturator nerve

96. The thoracic duct drains the
    A. Entire body below the ribs
    B. Head, neck, chest, left limbs
    C. Right side of the body
    D. All are true

97. Which muscle is innervated by the axillary nerve?
    A. Deltoid
    B. Brachial
    C. Pectoralis major
    D. None of the above

98. Which is the best to prevent adhesions in muscle tissue?
    A. Friction and effleurage
    B. Friction and petrissage
    C. Friction and tapotement
    D. Friction only

99. Petrissage beginning just distal to the medial condyle and moving proximal to the gluteal fold affects what muscles?
    A. Anterior adductors
    B. Medial hamstrings
    C. Quadriceps
    D. Deltoids

100. The parasympathetic nervous system causes the body to
    A. Increase heart rate
    B. Increase respiration
    C. Decrease adrenaline and heart rate
    D. Decrease excretory processes

101. Which condition is always a contraindication for massage?
    A. Muscle spasm
    B. Phlebitis
    C. Rheumatoid arthritis
    D. Edema

102. The main purpose of deep transverse friction is to
    A. Separate muscle fibers
    B. Lengthen muscle
    C. Shorten muscle fibers
    D. Minimize pain

103. Which is higher than normal adult body temperature?
    A. 37°C
    B. 98°F
    C. 98.6°F
    D. 39°C

104. A genetic condition that results in a lack of clotting factors in the blood is
    A. Hypochondria
    B. Sickle-cell anemia
    C. Hyperion anemia
    D. Hemophilia

105. Which muscle plantarflexes and everts the foot?
    A. Tibialis anterior
    B. Gastrocnemius
    C. Plantaris
    D. Peroneus longus

106. An excessively rapid heartbeat is known as
    A. Nascardia
    B. Brachycardia
    C. Angina
    D. Tachycardia

107. What is the action for the gluteus maximus?
    A. Rotation of hip, medial rotation
    B. Extension of hip, medial rotation

C. Flexion of hip, medial rotation

D. Extension of hip, lateral rotation

108. Massage therapy is used in pain management for
    A. Cardiac and terminal cancer patients
    B. Post-trauma patients
    C. Post-surgical patients
    D. All of the above

109. Connective tissue massage (CTM) is a useful technique for
    A. Preparing for surgery
    B. Psychoemotional status
    C. Loosening tissue following surgery or trauma
    D. Controlling pain

110. What action does piriformis play?
    A. Abducts and medially rotates
    B. Adducts and medially rotates
    C. Abducts and laterally rotates
    D. Adducts and laterally rotates

111. Vodder's manual lymph drainage (MLD) was developed for the specific purpose of
    A. Promoting lymph flow from tissue
    B. Eliminating the pneumatic cuff
    C. Decreasing urine output
    D. Increasing erythrocyte count

112. How many pairs of cranial nerves are there?
    A. 35
    B. 31
    C. 12
    D. 11

113. The analgesic effect of ice massage is to
    A. Block pain-impulse conduction
    B. Reroute pain
    C. Decrease ROM
    D. Eliminate pain

114. Business expenses can include
    A. Business cards and advertising
    B. Professional clothes and linens
    C. License, insurance, and memberships
    D. All of the above

115. The Amma therapy is a full-body manipulation of the coetaneous regions, 12 organ channels, governing and conception vessels, as well as
    A. Tendino-muscle channels
    B. TS points
    C. Yin-yang
    D. Qi of heaven

116. Which best describes the effects of massage therapy?
    A. Increase venous and lymph flow
    B. Increase venous, decrease arterial flow
    C. Decrease venous and lymph flow
    D. Decrease venous, increase lymph flow

117. In the prone position, support is put under the _____ to ease the pressure on the lower back.
    A. Ankles
    B. Abdomen
    C. Shoulders
    D. Chest

118. Beneficial techniques to market professional skills include
    A. Publications and presentations
    B. Business cards and brochures
    C. Donation of services
    D. All of the above

119. Massage reappeared during the
    A. Renaissance
    B. Middle Ages
    C. Dark Ages
    D. Revolution

120. A typical client intake form should include
    A. Name and address
    B. Name, address, occupation, physician, emergency number
    C. Name, phone, hobbies
    D. Name, marital status, children

121. The Heimlich maneuver is performed by
    A. Pressing the fist into the abdomen with inward thrust
    B. Subdiaphragmatic thrusts
    C. Standing behind victim with arms around waist
    D. All of the above

122. The purpose of a lubricant when massaging is to
    A. Keep the body greasy
    B. Prevent blisters from forming
    C. Cleanse the body for relaxation
    D. Avoid uncomfortable friction between the therapist's hand and the patient's skin

123. The reflex effects of massage are the stimulation of
    A. Motor neurons
    B. Sensory receptors of skin and subcutaneous tissues
    C. Synovial fluid at each joint
    D. Chemotransmitter

124. During a massage of the abdomen, the patient should
    A. Have hip flexors and abdominal muscles relaxed
    B. Be on his or her side to relax
    C. Be draped completely
    D. None of the above

125. Endorphins, which act like morphine for pain relief, are released from the
    A. ANS
    B. Midbrain
    C. Limbic system and brainstem
    D. CNS

Comprehensive Simulated NCETMB Exam

ANSWER KEY

1. D	40. B	79. D
2. D	41. C	80. A
3. B	42. B	81. D
4. A	43. A	82. D
5. C	44. B	83. A
6. A	45. C	84. B
7. B	46. D	85. D
8. B	47. A	86. D
9. B	48. D	87. D
10. D	49. C	88. C
11. A	50. A	89. A
12. C	51. D	90. D
13. A	52. C	91. D
14. C	53. D	92. C
15. D	54. B	93. A
16. A	55. D	94. B
17. B	56. D	95. D
18. B	57. D	96. B
19. C	58. D	97. A
20. B	59. D	98. A
21. D	60. A	99. B
22. A	61. B	100. C
23. C	62. B	101. B
24. D	63. C	102. A
25. B	64. C	103. D
26. A	65. C	104. D
27. B	66. A	105. D
28. A	67. B	106. D
29. C	68. B	107. D
30. A	69. C	108. D
31. C	70. D	109. C
32. B	71. A	110. C
33. D	72. C	111. A
34. D	73. D	112. C
35. C	74. B	113. A
36. B	75. A	114. D
37. A	76. C	115. A
38. C	77. D	116. A
39. A	78. A	117. A

118. D
119. A
120. B
121. D
122. D
123. B
124. A
125. C

35 Comprehensive Simulated NCETM Exam

This simulated exam contains 125 questions on **Western Massage** and excludes Eastern Bodywork.

NCETM Content:

➢ Kinesiology and musculoskeletal anatomy and physiology 19–24%

➢ Systemic anatomy and physiology 13–18%

➢ Pathology, contraindications and cautionary sites 14–19%

➢ Professional standards 11–15%

➢ Massage therapy theory, evaluation and techniques 30–37%

DIRECTIONS

Each of the numbered items or incomplete statements in this chapter is followed by answers or completions of the statement. Select the **ONE** lettered answer or completion that is **BEST** in each case. The maximum time to complete the 160-question exam is two hours and forty minutes. The actual exam also contains 160 questions, including 30 pretest questions not counted in the final score. Answer all the questions!

1. The tricuspid valve is found between the
   A. Right atrium and right ventricle
   B. Left ventricle and aorta
   C. Left ventricle and right ventricle
   D. Right atrium and left atrium

2. Which statement is true about the Golgi tendon apparatus?
   A. Found in joint capsules
   B. Detects overall tension in tendon
   C. Originates in Purkinje fibers
   D. Is activated by vagal reflex

3. Which muscles are major adductors?
   A. Pectoralis and deltoid
   B. Pectoralis and latissimus dorsi
   C. Deltoid and latissimus dorsi
   D. Biceps and deltoids

4. Which supplies the lower limbs?
   A. Dorsal primary rami
   B. Sciatic nerve
   C. Lumbosacral plexus
   D. Femoral nerve

5. Which muscle adducts and medially rotates the femur at the hip?
   A. Gluteus medius
   B. Pectineus
   C. Quadratus femoris
   D. Tensor fascia latae

6. Which of the following factors contribute to muscle fatigue?
   A. Insufficient oxygen
   B. Depletion of glycogen
   C. Lactic acid buildup
   D. All of the above

7. A sudden involuntary contraction of a muscle is called a(an)
   A. Levator
   B. Proximal
   C. Isometric
   D. Spasm

8. Which facial muscle attaches into the mandible, angles of the mouth, and skin of the lower face?
   A. Buccinator
   B. Depressor labii inferior
   C. Levator labii superioris
   D. Platysma

9. What is the spinal nerve contribution that composes the brachial plexus?
   A. C_1–C_4; T_1
   B. C_5–C_8; T_1
   C. C_7–C_8; T_1
   D. T_2–T_{12}; L_1

10. The prefix *macro* means
    A. Little
    B. Big
    C. Death
    D. Bacteria

11. What muscle forms the outer layer of the anterior and lateral abdominal wall?
    A. Rectus abdominis
    B. Transversalis
    C. Serratus anterior
    D. External oblique

12. With the elbow flexed, which muscle supinates the palm?
    A. Pronator
    B. Supinator
    C. Quadrator
    D. Brachialis

13. Which muscle abducts the scapula?
    A. Serratus anterior/pectoralis minor
    B. Rhomboids
    C. Latissimus dorsi
    D. Trapezius

14. Which is (are) not a part of the central nervous system (CNS)?
    A. Cranial nerves
    B. Cerebellum
    C. White tracts
    D. Medulla oblongata

15. Which muscle extends the femur?
    A. Soleus
    B. Gluteus minimus
    C. Gluteus maximus
    D. Peroneus

16. What is the normal systolic pressure?
    A. 80 mm Hg
    B. 90 mm Hg
    C. 120 mm Hg
    D. 140 mm Hg

17. Which of the following innervate the five flexor muscles of the forearm?
    A. Radial nerve
    B. Median nerve
    C. Median and ulnar nerves
    D. Radial and ulnar nerves

18. Which is true of a medial collateral ligament?
    A. Connects the femur to the tibia
    B. Connects the femur to the fibula
    C. Crosses the middle of the knee joint
    D. Attaches to the anterior cruciate ligament

19. Which muscle is not a part of the rotator cuff?
    A. Supraspinatus
    B. Infraspinatus
    C. Teres major
    D. Teres minor

20. Which of the following is true with regard to the humerus?
    A. The olecranon fossa is an anterior depression that receives the ulna's olecranon process

B. The medial and lateral epicondyles are rough projections on either side of the proximal end
C. The radial fossa is a posterior depression that receives the head of the radius when the forearm is flexed
D. Its trochlea articulates with the ulna

21. The prominence felt on the medial surface of the ankle is the
    A. Fibular notch
    B. Medial condyle
    C. Medial malleolus
    D. Tarsus

22. Which of the following joint classifications is described as freely movable?
    A. Amphiarthrosis
    B. Cartilaginous
    C. Diarthrosis
    D. Fibrous

23. Which reflex is essential to maintaining muscle tone and adjusts muscle performance during exercise?
    A. Crossed extensor
    B. Flexor
    C. Stretch
    D. Tendon

24. Which of the following are involved in the abduction of the arm?
    A. Deltoid and subscapularis
    B. Supraspinatus and infraspinatus
    C. Teres major and teres minor
    D. Supraspinatus and deltoid

25. Which of the following muscles does not abduct the thigh?
    A. Gluteus maximus
    B. Gluteus medius
    C. Gluteus minimus
    D. Sartorius

26. Which muscle would be paralyzed if the sciatic nerve were severed?
    A. Trapezius
    B. Biceps femoris
    C. Gluteus maximus
    D. Erector spinae

27. Senile lentigo or liver spots on the skin
    A. Are not contraindicated for massage
    B. Are contraindicated for massage
    C. Should be referred to a dermatologist
    D. Can be a symptom of cancer

28. If massage is used in early stages of fracture healing, it should be given particularly on the area
    A. Proximal to the actual site
    B. Distal to the actual site
    C. Medial to the actual site
    D. Lateral to the actual site

29. Contraindicated fungal skin infections include
    A. Herpes simplex
    B. Warts
    C. Athlete's foot
    D. All of the above

30. Pathogenic organisms cause the development of many disease processes and include
    A. Virus and bacteria
    B. Fungi
    C. Protozoa
    D. All of the above

31. A severe strain of the trapezius and deltoid muscles is called
    A. Racquetball shoulder
    B. Tennis elbow
    C. Skier's snap
    D. Bowler's break

32. Overstretching of the gracilis and adductor muscle on the inner thigh can result from
    A. Soccer
    B. Tennis
    C. Horseback riding
    D. Bowling

33. The client may react to pain with
    A. Fear and anxiety
    B. Ischemic response
    C. Active movement
    D. Passive movement

34. Sciatic nerve damage diminishes ability to
    A. Flex the hip
    B. Flex the knee
    C. Adduct the hip
    D. Abduct the hip

35. Facial paralysis can be due to a lesion in which cranial nerve?
    A. III
    B. VI
    C. VII
    D. VIII

36. Inflammation of the walls of the vein is called
    A. Aneurysm
    B. Phlebitis
    C. Varicose vein
    D. Atherosclerosis

37. Muscular dystrophy is characterized by degeneration and wasting of
    A. Muscle tissue
    B. Nervous tissue
    C. Epithelial tissue
    D. All of the above

38. Carpal tunnel syndrome affects the
    A. Volar aspect of the wrist
    B. Dorsal wrist
    C. Anterior forearm
    D. Forearm extensors

39. In pregnancy a contraindication for prenatal massage is
    A. Varicose veins
    B. Toxemia
    C. Dizziness
    D. All of the above

40. The following deviations that suggest the need for evaluation and referral for cardiovascular clients are
    A. Pulse over 90 or under 60
    B. Red, warm, or hard veins
    C. Pain and tenderness of extremities
    D. All of the above

41. The intake history of a client suffering from childhood abuse is very important because
    A. You can act as a psychotherapist
    B. It defines client boundaries and assures protection

C. It is easy for a client to receive a massage

D. You will be able to make a diagnosis

42. A second-degree burn is characterized by
   A. Involvement of the entire epidermis and possibly some of the dermis
   B. No loss of skin functions
   C. Damage to most hair follicles and sweat glands
   D. Never scarring

43. What is the name of the fracture of the distal end of the radius in which the distal fragment is displaced posteriorly?
   A. Stress fracture
   B. Spiral fracture
   C. Pott's fracture
   D. Colles' fracture

44. Torticollis is a condition of the
   A. Back
   B. Neck
   C. Shoulder
   D. Hip

45. A genetic condition that results in a lack of clotting factors in the blood is
   A. Hypochondria
   B. Sickle-cell anemia
   C. Hyperion anemia
   D. Hemophilia

46. An excessively rapid heartbeat is known as
   A. Nascardia
   B. Brachycardia
   C. Angina
   D. Tachycardia

47. When screening new clients, it is important to
   A. Design a questionnaire to ensure you get information desired
   B. Determine if the client has special needs
   C. Determine the expectations of the client
   D. All of the above

48. The letters SOAP refer to
   A. Scale, office, access, plan
   B. Subjective, open, area, parameter
   C. Social, object, active, plan
   D. Subjective, objective, assessment, plan

49. Business expenses can include the cost of
   A. Business cards and advertising
   B. Professional clothes and linens
   C. License, insurance, and memberships
   D. All of the above

50. SOAP charting is being widely adopted by massage professionals because
   A. Use of a professional reporting system enhances the image of massage as a valuable therapy
   B. Other health care professionals cannot understand the language
   C. It can be used in a court of law
   D. Clients want a record of their health

51. If you choose to work for insurance reimbursement,
   A. Thorough documentation is necessary
   B. Your treatment must be medically necessary
   C. You need a letter of referral from the physician
   D. All of the above

52. In record keeping for tax time, it is important to
   A. Record what activity you do hour by hour
   B. Keep track of the names of clients
   C. Keep track of automobile business mileage in a ledger
   D. None of the above

53. If you have a business name, you must register it with the
   A. IRS
   B. City or state clerk's office
   C. AMTA
   D. All of the above

54. Confidentiality of your client's records is required for many reasons. The primary reason is
   A. To protect yourself if sued by the client
   B. To ensure adequate information for insurance billing purposes
   C. Professional ethics
   D. You were told to do so by your instructor

55. If you are a business owner who employs other therapists, pays them by the hour, and provides them with benefits, you will be giving them a form at the end of the tax year called a
    A. W-4
    B. WC
    C. W-2
    D. W-3

56. The most critical skill for developing an optimal client relationship is
    A. Acceptance
    B. Feelings
    C. Listening
    D. Humoring

57. The sequences and directions of Swedish massage strokes are most adapted to which anatomical or physiological situation?
    A. Muscle attachments
    B. Subcutaneous adipose tissue
    C. Autonomic nervous system
    D. Lymph drainage and venous return

58. Which best describes the effects of massage therapy?
    A. Increased venous and lymph flow
    B. Increased venous, decreased arterial flow
    C. Decreased venous and lymph flow
    D. Decreased venous, increased lymph flow

59. Universal precautions are required when performing
    A. Handling of body fluids
    B. Invasive medical procedures
    C. All massage therapy
    D. All of the above

60. When massaging the thigh in the supine position, which is (are) involved?
    A. Hamstrings
    B. Quadriceps
    C. Gluteals
    D. Gastrocnemius

61. The universal precautions were designed by OSHA primarily for
    A. Clinical massage therapists
    B. Practitioners who handle body fluids

C. Healthcare workers
D. All of the above

62. Endangerment sites should be avoided during a massage because they are
    A. Bilaterally symmetrical
    B. Areas that can be easily injured
    C. Areas that are dysfunctional
    D. Hard to remember

63. In the supine position a bolster is placed under the _____ to take pressure off the lower back.
    A. Neck
    B. Ankles
    C. Knees
    D. Sacrum

64. The draping method that covers the entire body is called
    A. Top cover
    B. Full sheet
    C. Diaper
    D. Wrapping

65. A bath temperature of 85°F to 95°F is considered
    A. Cool
    B. Cold
    C. Tepid
    D. Hot

66. A hyperirritable spot that is painful when compressed is called a(an)
    A. Trigger point
    B. Pain point
    C. Ampule
    D. Rolfing

67. Self-awareness and self-care for a massage therapist is essential to
    A. Balance the body and mind
    B. Offer more to the client
    C. Maintain balance, strength, and stamina
    D. All of the above

68. Cold applied for therapeutic purposes is called
    A. Cryptology
    B. Cryotherapy
    C. Ignorance
    D. Cool ice

69. Which is a type of dry heat?

   A. Dry ice

   B. Steam bath

   C. Sauna

   D. Fogging

70. To integrate the structure and function of the client, a _____ assessment helps to evaluate balance and alignment.

   A. Mental

   B. Postural

   C. Ergonomic

   D. B and C

71. Itching, inflammation, sensitivity, or a stinging sensation is considered

   A. Normal

   B. Reasonable

   C. An allergic reaction

   D. Safe

72. An appropriate hypoallergenic oil combination is

   A. Sesame and almond

   B. Sunflower and canola

   C. Apricot and olive

   D. Peanut and walnut

73. Considerations for designing home therapy for clients with demonstration and return demonstration by the client include all of the following except

   A. Simple use of only those beneficial and necessary

   B. Fitting the client's time, energy, and means

   C. Challenging the client

   D. Providing immediate noticeable results

74. The Heimlich maneuver is performed by

   A. Pressing the fist into the abdomen with inward thrust

   B. Subdiaphragmatic thrusts

   C. Standing behind victim with arms around waist

   D. All of the above

75. A treatment protocol using passive positioning is

   A. Polarity

   B. Strain-counterstrain

   C. MET

   D. CRAC

76. In general, where do the flexors of the wrist originate?

   A. Lateral epicondyle of the humerus

   B. Greater tubercle of the humerus

   C. Medial epicondyle of the humerus

   D. Lesser tubercle of the humerus

77. Which muscle expands the thoracic cavity?

   A. Internal intercostals

   B. Diaphragm

   C. Multifidus

   D. Levator scapula

78. A synergist to the gluteus medius in abduction of the hip is the

   A. Gracilis

   B. Pectineus

   C. Tensor fascia latae

   D. Adductor magnus

79. Contraction of the iliopsoas will cause the pectineus to

   A. Lengthen

   B. Shorten

   C. Spasm

   D. Cramp

80. The action of the deltoid muscles working as a group is

   A. Extension

   B. Adduction

   C. Abduction

   D. Flexion

81. Which muscle stabilizes the scapula by preventing extreme elevation and protraction of the clavicle?

   A. Subscapularis

   B. Subclavius

   C. Supraspinatus

   D. Serratus anterior

82. The muscle that does not attach to the humerus is the

   A. Pectoralis major

   B. Biceps brachii

C. Subscapularis

D. Brachialis

83. Which muscle has no attachments on the scapula?

A. Pectoralis major

B. Subscapularis

C. Rhomboids

D. Pectoralis minor

84. The passage of food throughout the intestinal tract is possible because of

A. Mastication

B. Fermentation

C. Peristalsis

D. Defibrillation

85. The pulmonary veins carry _____ blood from the lungs to the heart.

A. Oxygenated

B. Deoxygenated

C. Carbon dioxide-rich

D. Carbon monoxide-rich

86. The direction of urine output is

A. Bladder, ureters, urethra, kidneys

B. Kidneys, urethra, ureters, bladder

C. Urethra, ureters, kidneys, bladder

D. Kidneys, ureters, bladder, urethra

87. Which of the following carries deoxygenated blood to the lungs?

A. Pulmonary veins

B. Pulmonary arteries

C. Aorta

D. Inferior vena cava

88. Which muscle(s) are involved in forced expiration?

A. External intercostals

B. SCM

C. Internal intercostals

D. Scalenes

89. The origin of the gluteus maximus is

A. Superior gluteal line

B. Middle gluteal line

C. Inferior gluteal line

D. Linea aspera

90. Which muscle crosses two joints?

A. Popliteus

B. Brachialis

C. Soleus

D. Rectus femoris

91. Which tendons make up the Achilles tendon?

A. Gastrocnemius and soleus

B. Plantaris and semitendinosus

C. Semitendinosus and soleus

D. Biceps femoris and gastrocnemius

92. Which muscle stabilizes the humerus in the glenoid cavity and abducts the humerus?

A. Teres major

B. Trapezius

C. Subscapularis

D. Supraspinatus

93. A client comes in for a massage and the scapula is still abducted after the massage. Which muscle do you recommend that the client stretch?

A. Pectoralis minor

B. Rhomboids

C. Subscapularis

D. Latissimus dorsi

94. What do you call the bony prominence at the proximal end of the ulna?

A. Medial epicondyle

B. Lateral epicondyle

C. Olecranon process

D. Styloid process

95. With your client in the supine position, how do you expose the serratus anterior?

A. Lateral rotation and adduction of the arm

B. Medial rotation and adduction of the arm

C. Horizontal abduction of the arm

D. Horizontal adduction of the arm

96. All of these muscles share a common attachment

A. Biceps brachii, brachioradialis, coracobrachialis

B. Coracobrachialis, brachioradialis, pectoralis minor

C. Pectoralis minor, coracobrachialis, brachioradialis

D. Biceps brachii, coracobrachialis, pectoralis minor

97. A bursae sack is usually located
    A. Inside of a joint
    B. Between the bone and a tendon
    C. Between muscle and tendon
    D. Between muscle and bone

98. The name of the joint between the skull and the 1st cervical vertebra is
    A. Atlantoaxial joint
    B. Axioatlantal joint
    C. Atlantooccipital joint
    D. Intervertebral joint

99. How many ribs are there in the body?
    A. 12
    B. 15
    C. 24
    D. 7

100. The shoulder joint is called the
    A. Humeroglenoid joint
    B. Humeroulnar joint
    C. Acromioclavicular joint
    D. Glenohumeral joint

101. Which muscle can rotate the head?
    A. SCM
    B. Splenius capitis
    C. Trapezius
    D. A and B

102. What is the insertion of the brachioradialis?
    A. Styloid process of radius
    B. Lateral epicondyle of humerus
    C. Medial epicondyle of humerus
    D. Styloid process of ulna

103. What is the origin of the teres minor?
    A. Vertebral border of scapula
    B. Axillary border of scapula
    C. Lesser tubercle
    D. Greater tubercle

104. What muscle shares an attachment with the deltoids?
    A. Levator scapula
    B. Biceps brachialis
    C. Trapezius
    D. Supraspinatis

105. What is the insertion site for the levator scapulae?
    A. Ribs 1-8
    B. Medial border of the scapula
    C. Superior angle of the scapula
    D. C1–C4

106. What action does piriformis play?
    A. Abducts and medially rotates
    B. Adducts and medially rotates
    C. Abducts and laterally rotates
    D. Adducts and laterally rotates

107. Which vessel takes the blood from the heart to the lungs?
    A. Pulmonary arteries
    B. Pulmonary veins
    C. Coronary arteries
    D. Coronary veins

108. The parasympathetic nervous system causes the body to
    A. Increase heart rate
    B. Increase respiration
    C. Decrease adrenaline and heart rate
    D. Decrease excretory processes

109. What nerve innervates the quadriceps?
    A. Femoral
    B. Tibial
    C. Superior gluteal
    D. Obturator

110. Where does the lymphatic system drain?
    A. Aorta
    B. Lymph nodes
    C. Subclavian vein
    D. Kidneys

111. Which stroke encompasses skin rolling?
    A. Kneading
    B. Friction
    C. Vibration
    D. Petrissage

112. How do you stretch the pectoral muscles?
    A. Adduction and medial rotation
    B. Adduction and lateral rotation
    C. Abduction and medial rotation
    D. Abduction and lateral rotation

113. A stroke that would not be beneficial to a competitor in a post-event massage would be
    A. Tapotement
    B. Effleurage
    C. Petrissage
    D. Kneading

114. You are gently applying stretch to the leg of a client who is lying supine. This is an example of
    A. Active stretching
    B. Passive stretching
    C. Ballistic stretching
    D. None of the above

115. One example of an endangerment site is
    A. Just below the medial malleolus
    B. The axillary area
    C. The maxilla
    D. The occipital ridge

116. Adhesion reduction may be best achieved by performing which of the following treatments?
    A. Vibration
    B. Percussion
    C. Effleurage
    D. Deep transverse friction

117. Which form does a massage therapist return to the referring physician?
    A. SOAP notes
    B. Progress notes
    C. Insurance notes
    D. Name and address

118. What movements are best used before sports?
    A. Friction and petrissage
    B. Effleurage and friction
    C. Tapotement and effleurage
    D. Friction and tapotement

119. What is the best massage position for a pregnant woman?
    A. Sitting up
    B. On her side
    C. Prone
    D. Supine

120. When a client does not want to disrobe, what should a massage therapist say?
    A. That he or she will work through the clothes
    B. That the session can not be conducted

C. Take them off anyway
D. That the client should at least take off shirt and pants

121. Deep compressive strokes result in
    A. Increased circulation and hyperemia
    B. Reduction of lactic acid
    C. Stimulation
    D. Tone muscle

122. Your client complains of constipation. What is the best massage technique to use?
    A. Gliding strokes that follow the ascending, transverse, and descending colons
    B. Compression over the upper abdomen
    C. Vibration over the stomach
    D. Tapotement over the low back area

123. Select the most desirable stress reduction techniques for a relaxation massage.
    A. Deep breathing and stretching
    B. Meditation and visualization
    C. Deep breathing and active movement
    D. Deep breathing and visualization

124. You should never massage someone who is under the influence of drugs or alcohol because the client
    A. May not be in control of him- or herself
    B. May say or do something inappropriate
    C. May accuse you of saying or doing something inappropriate
    D. All of the above

125. Avoid using which type of oil in massage?
    A. Sunflower
    B. Mineral
    C. Olive
    D. Apricot

Comprehensive Simulated NCETM Exam

ANSWER KEY

1. A	40. D	79. B
2. B	41. B	80. C
3. B	42. A	81. B
4. C	43. D	82. B
5. B	44. B	83. A
6. D	45. D	84. C
7. D	46. D	85. A
8. D	47. D	86. D
9. B	48. D	87. B
10. B	49. D	88. C
11. D	50. A	89. A
12. B	51. D	90. D
13. A	52. C	91. A
14. A	53. B	92. D
15. C	54. C	93. A
16. C	55. C	94. C
17. C	56. C	95. C
18. A	57. D	96. D
19. C	58. A	97. B
20. D	59. D	98. C
21. C	60. B	99. C
22. C	61. D	100. D
23. C	62. B	101. D
24. D	63. C	102. A
25. A	64. A	103. B
26. B	65. C	104. C
27. A	66. A	105. C
28. A	67. D	106. C
29. C	68. B	107. A
30. D	69. C	108. C
31. A	70. D	109. A
32. C	71. C	110. C
33. A	72. B	111. A
34. B	73. C	112. D
35. C	74. D	113. A
36. B	75. A	114. B
37. A	76. C	115. B
38. A	77. B	116. D
39. D	78. C	117. A

118. D
119. B
120. A
121. A
122. A
123. D
124. D
125. B

36 Comprehensive Simulated MBLEx Exam

This simulated exam contains 125 questions on all **Massage and Bodywork.**

MBLEx Content:

➢ Anatomy and Physiology (14%)

➢ Kinesiology (11%)

➢ Pathology, Contraindications, Areas of Caution, Special Populations (13%)

➢ Benefits and Physiological Effects of Techniques that Manipulate Soft Tissue (17%)

➢ Client Assessment and Treatment Planning (17%)

➢ Overview of Massage and Bodywork History/Culture/Modality (5%)

➢ Ethics Boundaries, Laws, Regulations (13%)

➢ Guidelines for Professional Practice (10%)

DIRECTIONS

Each of the numbered items or incomplete statements in this chapter is followed by answers or completions of the statement. Select the **ONE** lettered answer or completion that is **BEST** in each case. The maximum time to complete the 125-question exam is two hours and thirty minutes. Answer all the questions!

1. Which statement is true about the Golgi tendon apparatus?
   A. Found in joint capsules
   B. Detects overall tension in tendon
   C. Originates in Purkinje fibers
   D. Is activated by vagal reflex

2. Which muscles are major adductors?
   A. Pectoralis and deltoid
   B. Pectoralis and latissimus dorsi
   C. Deltoid and latissimus dorsi
   D. Biceps and deltoids

3. Which supplies the lower limbs?
   A. Dorsal primary rami
   B. Sciatic nerve
   C. Lumbosacral plexus
   D. Femoral nerve

4. Which muscle adducts and medially rotates the femur at the hip?
   A. Gluteus medius
   B. Pectineus
   C. Quadratus femoris
   D. Tensor fascia latae

5. Which of the following factors contribute to muscle fatigue?
   A. Insufficient oxygen
   B. Depletion of glycogen
   C. Lactic acid buildup
   D. All of the above

6. A sudden involuntary contraction of a muscle is called a(an)
   A. Levator
   B. Proximal
   C. Isometric
   D. Spasm

7. Which facial muscle attaches into the mandible, angles of the mouth, and skin of the lower face?
   A. Buccinator
   B. Depressor labii inferior
   C. Levator labii superioris
   D. Platysma

8. What is the spinal nerve contribution that composes the brachial plexus?
   A. C_1–C_4; T_1
   B. C_5–C_8; T_1
   C. C_7–C_8; T_1
   D. T_2–T_{12}; L_1

9. What muscle forms the outer layer of the anterior and lateral abdominal wall?
   A. Rectus abdominis
   B. Transversalis
   C. Serratus anterior
   D. External oblique

10. With the elbow flexed, which muscle supinates the palm?
    A. Pronator
    B. Supinator
    C. Quadrator
    D. Brachialis

11. Which muscle abducts the scapula?
    A. Serratus anterior/pectoralis minor
    B. Rhomboids
    C. Latissimus dorsi
    D. Trapezius

12. Which is (are) not a part of the central nervous system (CNS)?
    A. Cranial nerves
    B. Cerebellum
    C. White tracts
    D. Medulla oblongata

13. Which muscle extends the femur?
    A. Soleus
    B. Gluteus minimus
    C. Gluteus maximus
    D. Peroneus

14. Which of the following innervate the five flexor muscles of the forearm?
    A. Radial nerve
    B. Median nerve
    C. Median and ulnar nerves
    D. Radial and ulnar nerves

15. Which is true of a medial collateral ligament?
    A. Connects the femur to the tibia
    B. Connects the femur to the fibula
    C. Crosses the middle of the knee joint
    D. Attaches to the anterior cruciate ligament

16. Which muscle is not a part of the rotator cuff?
    A. Supraspinatus
    B. Infraspinatus
    C. Teres major
    D. Teres minor

17. Which of the following is true with regard to the humerus?
    A. The olecranon fossa is an anterior depression that receives the ulna's olecranon process
    B. The medial and lateral epicondyles are rough projections on either side of the proximal end
    C. The radial fossa is a posterior depression that receives the head of the radius when the forearm is flexed
    D. Its trochlea articulates with the ulna

18. The prominence felt on the medial surface of the ankle is the
    A. Fibular notch
    B. Medial condyle
    C. Medial malleolus
    D. Tarsus

19. Which of the following joint classifications is described as freely movable?
    A. Amphiarthrosis
    B. Cartilaginous
    C. Diarthrosis
    D. Fibrous

20. Which reflex is essential to maintaining muscle tone and adjusts muscle performance during exercise?
    A. Crossed extensor
    B. Flexor

C. Stretch
D. Tendon

21. Which of the following are involved in the abduction of the arm?
    A. Deltoid and subscapularis
    B. Supraspinatus and infraspinatus
    C. Teres major and teres minor
    D. Supraspinatus and deltoid

22. Which of the following muscles does not abduct the thigh?
    A. Gluteus maximus
    B. Gluteus medius
    C. Gluteus minimus
    D. Sartorius

23. Which muscle would be paralyzed if the sciatic nerve were severed?
    A. Trapezius
    B. Biceps femoris
    C. Gluteus maximus
    D. Erector spinae

24. If massage is used in early stages of fracture healing, it should be given particularly on the area
    A. Proximal to the actual site
    B. Distal to the actual site
    C. Medial to the actual site
    D. Lateral to the actual site

25. Contraindicated fungal skin infections include
    A. Herpes simplex
    B. Warts
    C. Athlete's foot
    D. All of the above

26. A severe strain of the trapezius and deltoid muscles is called
    A. Racquetball shoulder
    B. Tennis elbow
    C. Skier's snap
    D. Bowler's break

27. The client may react to pain with
    A. Fear and anxiety
    B. Ischemic response
    C. Active movement
    D. Passive movement

28. Sciatic nerve damage diminishes ability to
    A. Flex the hip
    B. Flex the knee
    C. Adduct the hip
    D. Abduct the hip

29. Facial paralysis can be due to a lesion in which cranial nerve?
    A. III
    B. VI
    C. VII
    D. VIII

30. Inflammation of the walls of the vein is called
    A. Aneurysm
    B. Phlebitis
    C. Varicose vein
    D. Atherosclerosis

31. Muscular dystrophy is characterized by degeneration and wasting of
    A. Muscle tissue
    B. Nervous tissue
    C. Epithelial tissue
    D. All of the above

32. Carpal tunnel syndrome affects the
    A. Volar aspect of the wrist
    B. Dorsal wrist
    C. Anterior forearm
    D. Forearm extensors

33. In pregnancy a contraindication for prenatal massage is
    A. Varicose veins
    B. Toxemia
    C. Dizziness
    D. All of the above

34. The following deviations that suggest the need for evaluation and referral for cardiovascular clients are
    A. Pulse over 90 or under 60
    B. Red, warm, or hard veins
    C. Pain and tenderness of extremities
    D. All of the above

35. The intake history of a client suffering from childhood abuse is very important because
    A. You can act as a psychotherapist
    B. It defines client boundaries and assures protection
    C. It is easy for a client to receive a massage
    D. You will be able to make a diagnosis

36. What is the name of the fracture of the distal end of the radius in which the distal fragment is displaced posteriorly?
    A. Stress fracture
    B. Spiral fracture
    C. Pott's fracture
    D. Colles' fracture

37. A genetic condition that results in a lack of clotting factors in the blood is
    A. Hypochondria
    B. Sickle-cell anemia
    C. Hyperion anemia
    D. Hemophilia

38. When screening new clients, it is important to
    A. Design a questionnaire to ensure you get information desired
    B. Determine if the client has special needs
    C. Determine the expectations of the client
    D. All of the above

39. The letters SOAP refer to
    A. Scale, office, access, plan
    B. Subjective, open, area, parameter
    C. Social, object, active, plan
    D. Subjective, objective, assessment, plan

40. Business expenses can include the cost of
    A. Business cards and advertising
    B. Professional clothes and linens
    C. License, insurance, and memberships
    D. All of the above

41. SOAP charting is being widely adopted by massage professionals because
    A. Use of a professional reporting system enhances the image of massage as a valuable therapy
    B. Other health care professionals cannot understand the language

C. It can be used in a court of law

D. Clients want a record of their health

42. If you choose to work for insurance reimbursement,
   A. Thorough documentation is necessary
   B. Your treatment must be medically necessary
   C. You need a letter of referral from the physician
   D. All of the above

43. In record keeping for tax time, it is important to
   A. Record what activity you do hour by hour
   B. Keep track of the names of clients
   C. Keep track of automobile business mileage in a ledger
   D. None of the above

44. Confidentiality of your client's records is required for many reasons. The primary reason is
   A. To protect yourself if sued by the client
   B. To ensure adequate information for insurance billing purposes
   C. Professional ethics
   D. You were told to do so by your instructor

45. If you are a business owner who employs other therapists, pays them by the hour, and provides them with benefits, you will be giving them a form at the end of the tax year called a
   A. W-4
   B. WC
   C. W-2
   D. W-3

46. The sequences and directions of Swedish massage strokes are most adapted to which anatomical or physiological situation?
   A. Muscle attachments
   B. Subcutaneous adipose tissue
   C. Autonomic nervous system
   D. Lymph drainage and venous return

47. Which best describes the effects of massage therapy?
   A. Increased venous and lymph flow
   B. Increased venous, decreased arterial flow
   C. Decreased venous and lymph flow
   D. Decreased venous, increased lymph flow

48. Universal precautions are required when performing
   A. Handling of body fluids
   B. Invasive medical procedures
   C. All massage therapy
   D. All of the above

49. When massaging the thigh in the supine position, which is(are) involved?
   A. Hamstrings
   B. Quadriceps
   C. Gluteals
   D. Gastrocnemius

50. Endangerment sites should be avoided during a massage because they are
   A. Bilaterally symmetrical
   B. Areas that can be easily injured
   C. Areas that are dysfunctional
   D. Hard to remember

51. In the supine position a bolster is placed under the _____ to take pressure off the lower back.
   A. Neck
   B. Ankles
   C. Knees
   D. Sacrum

52. The draping method that covers the entire body is called
   A. Top cover
   B. Full sheet
   C. Diaper
   D. Wrapping

53. A hyperirritable spot that is painful when compressed is called a(an)
   A. Trigger point
   B. Pain point
   C. Ampule
   D. Rolfing

54. Self-awareness and self-care for a massage therapist is essential to
   A. Balance the body and mind
   B. Offer more to the client
   C. Maintain balance, strength, and stamina
   D. All of the above

55. An appropriate hypoallergenic oil combination is
    A. Sesame and almond
    B. Sunflower and canola
    C. Apricot and olive
    D. Peanut and walnut

56. Considerations for designing home therapy for clients with demonstration and return demonstration by the client include all of the following except
    A. Simple use of only those beneficial and necessary
    B. Fitting the client's time, energy, and means
    C. Challenging the client
    D. Providing immediate noticeable results

57. The Heimlich maneuver is performed by
    A. Pressing the fist into the abdomen with inward thrust
    B. Subdiaphragmatic thrusts
    C. Standing behind victim with arms around waist
    D. All of the above

58. In general, where do the flexors of the wrist originate?
    A. Lateral epicondyle of the humerus
    B. Greater tubercle of the humerus
    C. Medial epicondyle of the humerus
    D. Lesser tubercle of the humerus

59. Which muscle expands the thoracic cavity?
    A. Internal intercostals
    B. Diaphragm
    C. Multifidus
    D. Levator scapula

60. A synergist to the gluteus medius in abduction of the hip is the
    A. Gracilis
    B. Pectineus
    C. Tensor fascia latae
    D. Adductor magnus

61. Contraction of the iliopsoas will cause the pectineus to
    A. Lengthen
    B. Shorten
    C. Spasm
    D. Cramp

62. The action of the deltoid muscles working as a group is
    A. Extension
    B. Adduction
    C. Abduction
    D. Flexion

63. Which muscle stabilizes the scapula by preventing extreme elevation and protraction of the clavicle?
    A. Subscapularis
    B. Subclavius
    C. Supraspinatus
    D. Serratus anterior

64. The muscle that does not attach to the humerus is the
    A. Pectoralis major
    B. Biceps brachii
    C. Subscapularis
    D. Brachialis

65. Which muscle has no attachments on the scapula?
    A. Pectoralis major
    B. Subscapularis
    C. Rhomboids
    D. Pectoralis minor

66. The pulmonary veins carry _____ blood from the lungs to the heart.
    A. Oxygenated
    B. Deoxygenated
    C. Carbon dioxide-rich
    D. Carbon monoxide-rich

67. Which of the following carries deoxygenated blood to the lungs?
    A. Pulmonary veins
    B. Pulmonary arteries
    C. Aorta
    D. Inferior vena cava

68. The origin of the gluteus maximus is
    A. Superior gluteal line
    B. Middle gluteal line
    C. Inferior gluteal line
    D. Linea aspera

69. Which muscle crosses two joints?
    A. Popliteus
    B. Brachialis
    C. Soleus
    D. Rectus femoris

70. Which tendons make up the Achilles tendon?
    A. Gastrocnemius and soleus
    B. Plantaris and semitendinosus
    C. Semitendinosus and soleus
    D. Biceps femoris and gastrocnemius

71. Which muscle stabilizes the humerus in the glenoid cavity and abducts the humerus?
    A. Teres major
    B. Trapezius
    C. Subscapularis
    D. Supraspinatus

72. A client comes in for a massage and the scapula is still abducted after the massage. Which muscle do you recommend that the client stretch?
    A. Pectoralis minor
    B. Rhomboids
    C. Subscapularis
    D. Latissimus dorsi

73. What do you call the bony prominence at the proximal end of the ulna?
    A. Medial epicondyle
    B. Lateral epicondyle
    C. Olecranon process
    D. Styloid process

74. With your client in the supine position, how do you expose the serratus anterior?
    A. Lateral rotation and adduction of the arm
    B. Medial rotation and adduction of the arm
    C. Horizontal abduction of the arm
    D. Horizontal adduction of the arm

75. All of these muscles share a common attachment:
    A. Biceps brachii, brachioradialis, coracobrachialis
    B. Coracobrachialis, brachioradialis, pectoralis minor
    C. Pectoralis minor, coracobrachialis, brachioradialis
    D. Biceps brachii, coracobrachialis, pectoralis minor

76. A bursae sack is usually located
    A. Inside of a joint
    B. Between the bone and a tendon
    C. Between muscle and tendon
    D. Between muscle and bone

77. The name of the joint between the skull and the 1st cervical vertebra is
    A. Atlantoaxial joint
    B. Axioatlantal joint
    C. Atlantooccipital joint
    D. Intervertebral joint

78. The shoulder joint is called the
    A. Humeroglenoid joint
    B. Humeroulnar joint
    C. Acromioclavicular joint
    D. Glenohumeral joint

79. Which muscle can rotate the head?
    A. SCM
    B. Splenius capitis
    C. Trapezius
    D. A and B

80. What is the insertion of the brachioradialis?
    A. Styloid process of radius
    B. Lateral epicondyle of humerus
    C. Medial epicondyle of humerus
    D. Styloid process of ulna

81. What is the origin of the teres minor?
    A. Vertebral border of scapula
    B. Axillary border of scapula
    C. Lesser tubercle
    D. Greater tubercle

82. What muscle shares an attachment with the deltoids?
    A. Levator scapula
    B. Biceps brachialis
    C. Trapezius
    D. Supraspinatis

83. What is the insertion site for the levator scapulae?
    A. Ribs 1-8
    B. Medial border of the scapula
    C. Superior angle of the scapula
    D. C1–C4

84. What action does piriformis play?
    A. Abducts and medially rotates
    B. Adducts and medially rotates
    C. Abducts and laterally rotates
    D. Adducts and laterally rotates

85. Which vessel takes the blood from the heart to the lungs?
    A. Pulmonary arteries
    B. Pulmonary veins
    C. Coronary arteries
    D. Coronary veins

86. The parasympathetic nervous system causes the body to
    A. Increase heart rate
    B. Increase respiration
    C. Decrease adrenaline and heart rate
    D. Decrease excretory processes

87. What nerve innervates the quadriceps?
    A. Femoral
    B. Tibial
    C. Superior gluteal
    D. Obturator

88. Where does the lymphatic system drain?
    A. Aorta
    B. Lymph nodes
    C. Subclavian vein
    D. Kidneys

89. Which stroke encompasses skin rolling?
    A. Kneading
    B. Friction
    C. Vibration
    D. Petrissage

90. How do you stretch the pectoral muscles?
    A. Adduction and medial rotation
    B. Adduction and lateral rotation
    C. Abduction and medial rotation
    D. Abduction and lateral rotation

91. You are gently applying stretch to the leg of a client who is lying supine. This is an example of
    A. Active stretching
    B. Passive stretching
    C. Ballistic stretching
    D. None of the above

92. One example of an endangerment site is
    A. Just below the medial malleolus
    B. The axillary area
    C. The maxilla
    D. The occipital ridge

93. Adhesion reduction may be best achieved by performing which of the following treatments?
    A. Vibration
    B. Percussion
    C. Effleurage
    D. Deep transverse friction

94. Which form does a massage therapist return to the referring physician?
    A. SOAP notes
    B. Progress notes
    C. Insurance notes
    D. Name and address

95. What movements are best used before sports?
    A. Friction and petrissage
    B. Effleurage and friction
    C. Tapotement and effleurage
    D. Friction and tapotement

96. What is the best massage position for a pregnant woman?
    A. Sitting up
    B. On her side
    C. Prone
    D. Supine

97. Deep compressive strokes result in
    A. Increased circulation and hyperemia
    B. Reduction of lactic acid
    C. Stimulation
    D. Tone muscle

98. The purpose of proper draping is
    A. To respect the modesty of the client
    B. To protect the integrity of the therapist
    C. To keep the client warm
    D. All of the above

99. To get the client acclimated to your touch and to warm up the muscle, you should begin bodywork sessions with
    A. Effleurage
    B. Friction

C. Petrissage

D. Tapotement

100. A client who has an area of inflammation because of a torn muscle would benefit from
   A. A heating pad
   B. Cryotherapy
   C. Vigorous friction on the inflamed area
   D. Stretching the muscle

101. The stance in which both feet are placed perpendicular to the edge of the table is called the
   A. Archer
   B. Horse
   C. Moose
   D. Stirrup

102. The cupping technique is best suited for
   A. Acute bronchitis
   B. Cancer of the lungs
   C. Bronchiectasis
   D. Acute tracheitis

103. Which of the following are used when applying massage strokes?
   A. Intension, pressure, excursion
   B. Rhythm and continuity
   C. Speed, duration, sequence
   D. All of the above

104. In body mechanics the horse stance or warrior stance is used
   A. To perform short, transverse strokes, such as petrissage
   B. To perform long effleurage strokes
   C. To perform chair massage
   D. To adjust the massage table to the correct height

105. A system of active, passive, and resisted movements of the body's various joints and muscles, most often the presentation of passive ROM, is called
   A. Active stretching
   B. Table gymnastics
   C. Swedish gymnastics
   D. Passive stretching

106. How should you vary massage treatment time with the age of the patient?
   A. Progressively with increased age
   B. Shorter with increased age
   C. Shorter for very old and very young
   D. The same for any age

107. Which massage technique gives the best information about connective tissue structure in ligaments, tendons, and joints?
   A. Effleurage
   B. Friction
   C. Vibration
   D. Tapotement

108. Joint mobilization techniques are used to help improve
   A. Body alignment
   B. Posture
   C. Reeducating the muscles
   D. All of the above

109. Careful joint movement is important in cases of
   A. Metal hardware at the joint
   B. Hip replacement
   C. The elderly
   D. All of the above

110. Yoga is a form of mediation for
   A. Good appetite
   B. Muscle balance and relaxation
   C. Dancing
   D. Religion

111. Which is the 1st step in beginning massage treatment?
   A. Apply lubricant
   B. Effleurage
   C. Determine contraindications
   D. Diagnose the patient

112. Massage benefits lymph flow best when strokes are
   A. Away from heart
   B. Toward the heart
   C. Heavy in both directions
   D. In certain local areas

113. Which is best to prevent adhesions in muscle tissue?
    A. Friction and effleurage
    B. Friction and petrissage
    C. Friction and tapotement
    D. Friction only

114. To mobilize the hip through its full ROM, bend the leg,
    A. Hold for 30 seconds and abduct
    B. Adduct diagonally, extend, abduct diagonally
    C. Circumduct the flexed hip
    D. B and C

115. The main purpose of deep transverse friction is to
    A. Separate muscle fibers
    B. Lengthen muscle
    C. Shorten muscle fibers
    D. Minimize pain

116. Mild stimulation of the vagus nerve results in
    A. Irregular heartbeat
    B. No change
    C. Increased heartbeat
    D. Decreased heartbeat

117. Deep strokes and kneading techniques can cause an increase in
    A. Vasoconstriction
    B. Blood flow
    C. Diastolic arterial pressure
    D. Systolic arterial pressure

118. Good body mechanics is defined as
    A. Proper use of postural techniques
    B. Biomechanics to decrease fatigue
    C. Making use of the therapist's body weight
    D. All of the above

119. In order to stretch the posterior cervical muscles, use the _____ technique with the neck in forward flexion.
    A. Hyperextension
    B. Horizontal flexion
    C. Cross-arm
    D. Finger push-up

120. Which tendons make up the Achilles tendon?
    A. Gastrocnemius and soleus
    B. Plantaris and semitendinosus
    C. Semitendinosus and soleus
    D. Biceps femoris and gastrocnemius

121. During the interview and health history, the therapist may discover a pain area and find a need to evaluate the _____ before the massage, in order to enhance the therapeutic goals of the client.
    A. Gait
    B. Posture
    C. SOAP
    D. A and B

122. Universal precautions are used when administering first aid because
    A. You have to assume that anyone receiving first aid potentially has infectious diseases
    B. HIV is transmitted by exposure to blood and other body fluids
    C. Hepatitis and other pathogens are transmitted by exposure to blood and other body fluids
    D. All of the above

123. In massaging the body, it is important to
    A. Drape all parts of the body
    B. Expose only the part to be massaged
    C. Cover the entire body with a sheet
    D. Stand still while delivering technique

124. A client comes in and reports that her lower back has been hurting ever since she mowed her lawn yesterday. In which section of the SOAP notes is this information recorded?
    A. S
    B. O
    C. A
    D. P

125. How do you stretch the pectoral muscles?
    A. Adduction and medial rotation
    B. Adduction and lateral rotation
    C. Abduction and medial rotation
    D. Abduction and lateral rotation

Comprehensive Simulated MBLEx Exam

ANSWER KEY

1. B	34. D	67. B
2. B	35. B	68. A
3. C	36. D	69. D
4. B	37. D	70. A
5. D	38. D	71. D
6. D	39. D	72. A
7. D	40. D	73. C
8. B	41. A	74. C
9. D	42. D	75. D
10. B	43. C	76. B
11. A	44. C	77. C
12. A	45. C	78. D
13. C	46. D	79. D
14. C	47. A	80. A
15. A	48. D	81. B
16. C	49. B	82. C
17. D	50. B	83. C
18. C	51. C	84. C
19. C	52. A	85. A
20. C	53. A	86. C
21. D	54. D	87. A
22. A	55. B	88. C
23. B	56. C	89. A
24. A	57. D	90. D
25. C	58. C	91. B
26. A	59. B	92. B
27. A	60. C	93. D
28. B	61. B	94. A
29. C	62. C	95. D
30. B	63. B	96. B
31. A	64. B	97. A
32. A	65. A	98. D
33. D	66. A	99. A

100. B	109. D	118. D
101. B	110. B	119. C
102. C	111. C	120. A
103. D	112. B	121. D
104. A	113. A	122. D
105. C	114. D	123. B
106. C	115. A	124. A
107. B	116. D	125. D
108. D	117. B	

State and Provincial Massage License Laws

The following list contains information about state (U.S.) and provincial (Canada) licensing for massage therapists. It is current up to the time of publication of this text. Please check one of the following websites for more current information: www.amtamassage.org; www.abmp.com; massagemag.com; or your state agency responsible for licensing, or call 800-458-2267.

Education required only lists massage therapy education required. States may also require CPR and other education. Most require graduation from a state-approved or accredited massage school or program. Check state law for most complete information. NCETMB refers to the National Certification Examination for Therapeutic Massage and Bodywork. MBLEx refers to Massage and Bodyworker Licensing Exam. NCCAOM refers to the National Certification Commission for Acupuncture and Oriental Medicine.

UNITED STATES

Alabama Massage Therapy Board
610 S. McDonough St.
Montgomery, AL 36104
(334) 269-9990
www.almtbd.state.al.us
Education required: 650 hours* License
Exam: NCETMB

Alaska
Department of Commerce
PO Box 110806
Juneau, Alaska 99811
(907) 465-2534
www.commerce.state.ak.us

Arizona
(602) 542-8604
www.massageboard.az.gov

Education required: 700 hours* License
Exam: NCETMB, MBLEx

Arkansas State Board of Massage Therapy
103 Airways
Hot Springs, AR 71903
(501) 683-1448
www.arkansasmassagetherapy.com
Education required: 500 hours* License
Exam: MBLEx and state exam

California
(916) 669-5336
www.camtc.org
Education required: 500 hours* CMT
Exam: NCETMB or MBLEx

Colorado
(303) 894-7800
www.dora.state.co.us/massage-therapists
Education required: 500 hours* Certification
Exam: NCETMB or MBLEx

Connecticut—Massage Therapy Licensure
Department of Public Health
410 Capitol Avenue—MS#12APP
P.O. Box 340308
Hartford, CT 06134
(860) 509-7603
www.dph.state.ct.us
Education required: 500 hours*
Exam: NCETMB

Delaware Board of Massage and Bodywork
Cannon Building
861 Silver Lake Blvd., #203
Dover, DE 19904
(302) 744-4500

317

www.professionallicensing.state.de.us/boards/
massagebodyworks
Education required: 500 hours* License
Exam: NCETMB

District of Columbia Massage Therapy Board
Occupational and Professional Licensing
Administration
941 N. Capitol St., N.E., 7th Floor
Washington, DC 20002
(877) 672-2174
www.hpla.doh.dc.gov
Education: 500 hours* License
Exam: NCETMB or MBLEx, NCCA

Florida Board of Massage Therapy
Department of Health
2020 Capitol Circle S.E., Bin #C09
Tallahassee, FL 32399
(850) 488-0595
www.doh.state.fl.us/mqa/massage
Education required: 500 hours* License
Exam: NCETMB, MBLEx, NESL, NCETM

Georgia
(478) 207-2440
www.sos.georgia.gov.plb/massage
Education required: 500 hours* License
Exam: NCETMB, MBLEx

Hawaii
Board of Massage Therapy
P.O. Box 3469
Honolulu, HI 96801
(808) 586-3000
www.state.hi.us/dcca/pvl
Education required: 570 hours* License
Exam: State exam

Idaho—no state regulation
Freedom of Access Law
www.state.id.us

Illinois Department of Professional Regulation
320 West Washington St., 3rd Floor
Springfield, IL 62786
(217) 785-0800
www.ildpr.com
Education required: 500 hours* License
Exam: NCETMB

Indiana
(317) 234-2051
www.in.gov/pla/massage
Education required: 500 hours* Certification
Exam: NCETMB, MBLEx

Iowa Department of Health
Board of Massage Therapy Examiners
Lucas State Office Building, 5th Floor
321 E. 12th St.
Des Moines, IA 50319
(515) 281-6959
www.idph.state.ia.us/licensure
Education required: 500 hours* License
Exam: NCETMB, MBLEx

Kansas—no state regulation

**Kentucky Board of Licensure for Massage
Therapy**
P.O. Box 1360
Frankfort, KY 406021
(502) 564-3296 ext. 240
http://bmt.ky.gov
Education required: 600 hours* License
Exam: NCETMB

Louisiana Board of Massage Therapy
12022 Plank Road
Baton Rouge, LA 70811
(225) 771-4090
www.lsbmt.org/
Education required: 500 hours* License
Exam: NCETMB, MBLEx, NCCAOM

Maine Board of Massage Therapy
Department of Professional and Financial
Regulation
35 State House Station
Augusta, ME 04333
(207) 624-8613
www.maine.gov/professional.licensing
Education required: 500 hours* License
Exam: NCETMB, MBLEx

Maryland Board of Chiropractic Examiners
Massage Therapy Advisory Committee
4201 Patterson Ave., 5th Floor
Baltimore, MD 21215
(410) 764-4738
www.mdmassage.org/

Education required: 500 hours massage*
+ 60 college credits, Registration, License
Exam: NCETMB, NCETM, state law exam

Massachusetts
(617) 727-1747
www.massgov/dpl/boards/mt/index.htm
Education required: 500 hours* License
Exam: NCETMB

Michigan
(517) 241-9288
www.michigan.gov/mdch
Education required: 500 hours* License
Exam: N/A

Minnesota
Freedom of Access Laws in Effect
(651) 201-3728
www.health.state.mn.us/divs/hpsc/hop/ocap/
index.html

Mississippi State Board of Massage Therapy
P.O. Box 12489
Jackson, MS 39236
(601) 732-6038
www.msbmt.state.ms.us
Education required: 700 hours* License
Exam: MBLEx, NESL, state exam

Missouri Massage Therapy Board
3605 Missouri Blvd.
P.O. Box 1335
Jefferson City, MO 65102
(573) 522-6277
http://pr.mo.gov/massage.asp
Education required: 500 hours* License
Exam: NCETMB, MBLEx, NCCAOM,
AMMANCE

Montana
(406) 841-2394
www.massagetherapists.mt.gov
Education required: 500 hours* License
Exam: NCETMB, NCETM, MBLEx

Nebraska Massage Therapy Board
Health and Human Services
Credentialing Division
301 Centennial Mall South, 3rd Floor
Lincoln, NE 68509
(402) 471-2115

www.hhs.state.ne.us/crl/massagerules.htm
Education required: 1000 hours* License
Exam: NCETMB, NCETM, MBLEx, ACE

Nevada
(775) 688-1888
www.massagetherapy.nv.gov/
Education required: 500 hours* License
Exam: NCETMB, MBLEx

New Hampshire
Board of Massage Therapy
Health Facilities Administration
129 Pleasant Street
Concord, NH 03301
(603) 271-0277
www.nhes.state.nh.us/dhhs/Lrs/eligibility/
massagelicense.htm
Education required: 750 hours* License
Exam: NCETMB, MBLEx

New Jersey Board of Nursing
Massage, Bodywork & Somatic Therapy
Examining Committee
P.O. Box 45010
Newark, NJ 07101
(973) 504-6430
www.state.nj.us/lps/ca/
Education required: 500 hours* (License),
Certification
Exam: NCETMB, NCCAOM

New Mexico
Board of Massage Therapy
2055 Pacheco St., #400
Santa Fe, NM 87504
(505) 476-4870
www.rld.state.nm.us/b&c/massage
Education required: 650 hours* License
Exam: NCETMB, MBLEx

New York State Board of Massage Therapy
Cultural Education Center, #3041
Albany, NY 12230
(518) 474-3817 ext. 150
www.op.nysed.gov/massage.htm
Education required: 1000 hours* License/
Registration
Exam: State exam

North Carolina Board of Massage and Bodywork Therapy
P.O. Box 2539
Raleigh, NC 27602
(919) 546-0050
www.bmbt.org
Education required: 500 hours* License
Exam: NCETMB

North Dakota Board of Massage
P.O. Box 218
Beach, ND 58621
(701) 872-4895
www.ndboardofmassage.com
Education required: 750 hours* License
Exam: NCETMB

Ohio Massage Therapy Board
77 South High Street, 17th Floor
Columbus, OH 43266
(614) 466-3934
www.med.ohio.gov
Education required: 750 hours* License
Exam: State exam

Oklahoma—no state regulation

Oregon
State Office Building
3218 Pringle Road S.E., #250
Salem, OR 97302
(503) 365-8657
www.oregon.gov/obmt
Education required: 500 hours* License
Exam: NCETMB, MBLEx + state exam

Pennsylvania—no state regulation

Rhode Island Department of Health
Professional Regulation
3 Capitol Hill, Room 104
Providence, RI 02908
(401) 222-2827
www.health.ri.gov
Education required: 500 hours* License
Exam: NCETMB, MBLEx

South Carolina Department of Labor
Licensing and Regulation
P.O. Box 11329
Columbia, SC 29211
(803) 896-0266

www.llr.state.sc.us/poL/massagetherapy
Education required: 500 hours* License
Exam: NCETMB, MBLEx

South Dakota
(605) 271-7103
www.doh.sd.gov/boards/massage
Education required: 500 hours* License
Exam: NCETMB, NESL, MBLEx, AMMANCE

Tennessee Massage Licensure Board
Cordell Hull Building, 1st Floor
425 Fifth Ave. N.
Nashville, TN 37247
(615) 532-3202
www.state.tn.us/hh.html
Education required: 500 hours* License
Exam: NCETMB, MBLEx

Texas
1100 West 49th St.
Austin, TX 78756
(512) 834-6616
www.dshs.state.tx.us/massage
Education required: 500 hours* License
Exam: NCETMB, MBLEx

Utah
Board of Massage Therapy
P.O. Box 146741
Salt Lake City, UT 84144
(801) 530-6633
www.dopl.utah.gov
Education required: 600 hours* License
Exam: NCETMB, MBLEx

Vermont—no state regulation

Virginia
6606 W. Broadway St., 4th Floor
Richmond, VA 23230
(804) 367-4515
www.dLhp.virginia.gov
Education required: 500 hours* Certification
Exam: NCETMB

State of Washington Department of Health
1300 S.W. Quince St.
P.O. Box 47867
Olympia, WA 98504
(360) 236-4700
www.doh.wa.gov/massage

Education required: 500 hours* License
Exam: NCETMB, MBLEx

State of West Virginia

Board of Massage Therapy
200 Davis St., #1
Princeton, WV 24740
(304) 558-1060
www.wvmassage.org
Education required: 500 hours* License
Exam: NCETMB, MBLEx

Wisconsin Department of Regulation and Licensing

Massage Therapy Board
1400 E. Washington Ave.
Madison, WI 53703
(608) 266-2112
www.drL.wi.gov
Education required: 600 hours* License
Exam: NCETMB, NCCAOM, MBLEx

Wyoming—no state regulation

CANADA

British Columbia

Registered Massage Therapist
(604) 736-3404
Education required: 3,000 hours* Registration
Exam: Written and practical

Newfoundland and Labrador

Registered Massage Therapist
(709) 739-7181
Education required: 2,200 hours* Registration
Exam: NLMTB

Nova Scotia

(902) 429-2190
www.mtans.com
Education: 2,200 hours*
Exam: Written and practical, N/A

Ontario

Massage Therapist
(416) 489-2626
www.cmto.com
Education required: 2-3 year program*
Registration
Exam: OSCE, MSQ and practical

Puerto Rico

(787) 725-8538
Education required: 1,000 hours* License
Exam: TBD

APPENDIX B

Organizations

American Massage Therapy Association (AMTA)
820 Davis Street, Suite 100
Evanston, IL 60201-4444
(847) 864-0123
www.amtamassage.org

AMTA Foundation
820 Davis Street, Suite 100
Evanston, IL 60201-4444
(847) 869-5019
www.amtafoundation.org

American Organization for Bodywork Therapies of Asia (AOBTA)
1010 Haddonfield-Berlin Rd., Suite 408
Voorhees, NJ 08043
(856) 782-1616
www.aobta.org

American Polarity Therapy Association (APTA)
P.O. Box 19858
Boulder, CO 80308
(303) 545-2080
www.polaritytherapy.org

Associated Bodywork & Massage Professionals (ABMP)
1271 Sugarbush Drive
Evergreen, CO 80439-7347
(800) 458-2267
www.abmp.com

Canadian Massage Therapist Alliance (CMTA)
344 Lakeshore Road East, Suite B
Oakville (Ontario)
Canada L6J 1J6
(905) 849-8606
www.cmta.ca

Canadian Touch Research Center
760 Saint-Zotique Street East
Montreal (Quebec)
Canada H2S 1M5
(514) 272-5141
www.ccrt-ctrc.org

Commission on Massage Therapy Accreditation (COMTA)
820 Davis Street, Suite 100
Evanston, IL 60201-4444
(847) 869-5039
www.comta.org

Day-Break Geriatric Massage Institute
7434-A King George Drive
Indianapolis, IN 46240
(317) 722-9896
www.daybreak-massage.com

Dr. Vodder School of North America
P.O. Box 5701
Victoria (British Columbia)
Canada V8R 6S8
(250) 598-9862
www.vodderschool.com

Federation of State Massage Therapy Boards
7111 West 151st St. Suite 356
Overland Park, KS 66223
(913) 681-0380
FSMTB at mblex@fsmtb.org

International Association of Infant Massage Instructors (US)
1891 Goodyear Avenue, Suite 622
Ventura, CA 93003
www.iaim-us.com

International Institute of Reflexology, Inc.
5650 First Avenue North
P.O. Box 12642
St. Petersburg, FL 33733-2642
(727) 343-4811
www.reflexology-usa.net

**International Loving Touch Foundation
(Infant Massage)**
P.O. Box 16374
Portland, OR 97292
(503) 253-8482
www.lovingtouch.com

International Spa Association (ISPA)
2365 Harrodsburg Road, Suite A325
Lexington, KY 40504
(888) 651-4772
www.experienceispa.com

**Jin Shin Do® Foundation for Bodymind
Acupressure™**
P.O. Box 416
Idyllwild, CA 92549
(909) 659-5707
www.jinshindo.org

**National Center for Complementary and
Alternative Medicine**
National Institutes of Health
Bethesda, MD 20892
www.nccam.nih.gov

**National Certification Board for Therapeutic
Massage and Bodywork (NCBTMB)**
Chicago, IL
(800) 296-0664 or (630) 627-8000
www.ncbtmb.com

**National Certification Commission for
Acupuncture and Oriental Medicine
(NCCAOM)**
11 Canal Center Plaza, Suite 300
Alexandria, VA 22314
(703) 548-9004
www.nccaom.org

**National Association of Nurse Massage
Therapists (NANMT)**
P.O. Box 24004
Huber Heights, OH 45424
(800) 262-4017
www.nanmt.org

**Nurse Healers—Professional Associates
International (Therapeutic Touch)**
3760 South Highland Drive Suite 429
Salt Lake City, UT 84106
(801) 273-3399
www.therapeutic-touch.org

Rolf Institute of Structural Integration®
205 Canyon Blvd.
Boulder, CO 80302
(800) 530-8875 or (303) 449-5903
www.rolf.org

**TouchPro Institute
(Professional Chair Massage)**
584 Castro Street, #555
San Francisco, CA 94114
(800) 999-5026
www.TouchPro.com

Touch Research Institutes (TRI)
University of Miami School of Medicine
P.O. Box 016820
Miami, FL 33101
(305) 243-6781
www.miami.edu/touch-research

Glossary

Abdominal—Anterior trunk.

Abductors—Muscle that, when flexed, pulls part of the body away from the center of the body.

Absolute contraindication—Any condition where massage may be harmful and not indicated.

Acetylcholine—A chemical that mediates nerve activity to the skeletal muscles.

Acne vulgaris—An infection of the sebaceous glands and hair follicles, caused by bacteria.

Acquired immunodeficiency syndrome (AIDS)—A disease caused by the human immunodeficiency virus (HIV).

Active assisted stretching—Stretching in which the client contracts the agonist to stretch the antagonist while outside forces assist the lengthening action.

Active resisted stretches or isometric movements—Gentle resistance applied by the therapist while the client is actively engaging in the stretch.

Acupressure—A western term for a form of bodywork based on the meridian theory in which acupuncture points are pressed to stimulate the flow of energy or Chi.

Acupuncture—The Chinese medical practice in which the skin is punctured with needles at specific points along the meridian channels or paths of energy.

Acute—Lasting for a short time.

Addison's disease—Partial or complete failure of adrenal functions, which can result from an autoimmune disease, local or general infection, or adrenal hemorrhage.

Adductor—Muscle that, when flexed, pulls part of the body toward the body.

Adhesion—Fibrous tissue that forms an abnormal union between two previously separate structures.

Agonist—Muscle that is most responsible for causing desired joint action.

Allergies—Hypersensitivity and overreaction to otherwise harmless agents.

All-or-none response—When each individual muscle fiber, once sufficiently stimulated, contracts to its fullest, and in the absence of sufficient stimuli, each muscle fiber relaxes to its fullest.

Amma—A form of traditional Japanese massage using acupressure.

Amphiarthrotic joints—Joints that are slightly movable.

Anatomical position—Standard body position. The body is erect and facing forward, arms are at the side, palms forward while feet are slightly apart, and toes pointing forward.

Anemia—Decrease in red blood cells or decrease in the amount of functional hemoglobin in the blood, which decreases the oxygen-carrying capacity of the blood, causing this condition.

Angina pectoris—Chest pain, often caused by constriction of coronary arteries and myocardial anoxia (lack of oxygen in the heart muscle).

Ankylosing spondylitis—Inflammatory disease causing calcification and fusion of the joints between the vertebrae and sacroiliac joint.

Anterior or ventral—The front of a structure.

Antiseptic—A substance that retards pathogenic growth and removes pathogenic organisms from tissue without destroying the tissue.

Apnea—Spontaneous respiration is temporarily stopped or absent.

Aponeurosis—The attachment of skeletal muscle to bone, to another muscle, or to the skin by a broad, flat tendon.

Arrector pili—The muscles that allow hairs to stand upright.

Arteries—Vessels that move blood away from the heart.

Arteriosclerosis—Narrowing of arteries due to the accumulation of lipid plaques in the walls, reducing blood flow.

Arthritis—Chronic disease characterized by inflammation, swelling, and pain in the joints.

Asthma—A respiratory disorder caused by inflammation of the bronchi, characterized by difficulty in breathing, wheezing, coughing, and thick mucus production.

Atrium—Superior heart chamber that receives blood from the body through large veins.

Autoimmune diseases—A group of diseases characterized by an alteration of immune functions as a result of an attack by the body's own immune system.

Axillary—Armpit, the pyramid-shaped area formed by the underside of the anterior and posterior aspects of the shoulder.

Axon or efferent process—A single cylindrical extension of the neural cell that transmits impulses away from the cell body.

Ball-and-socket joint—Type of joint that permits all movements and offers the greatest range of movement (e.g., the hip [iliofemoral joint] and shoulder [glenohumeral joint]). Also known as a *spheroid* or a *triaxial joint*.

Baroreceptors—Pressure-sensitive receptor cells that affect blood pressure by sending impulses to the cardiac center and to the vasomotor center in the medulla oblongata.

Basement membrane—Attaching surface of epithelial tissue.

Benign—Pertaining to a condition that is not cancerous or life-threatening.

Bindegewebsmassage—A connective tissue massage believed to affect vascular and visceral reflexes.

Blood-brain barrier—A very selective semi-permeable membrane that controls which substances are allowed into the brain.

Blood pressure—The pressure exerted by blood on an arterial wall during the contraction of the left ventricle.

Body mechanics—Biomechanics, the use of proper body techniques to deliver massage therapy with the utmost efficiency and minimum trauma to the therapist.

Bone—The hardest and most solid of all connective tissue. Bone is made of compact tissue, a spongy cancellous tissue, collagenous fibers (for strength), and mineral salts (for hardness).

Bony landmark—Part of a bone that is used for reference to muscles (i.e., trochanter of the femur).

Bow stance—A foot stance used in massage therapy when performing any gliding strokes where length is important. The feet are placed on the floor in a 90-degree angle, one foot pointing straight and the other pointing toward the side.

Brachial—Area in the upper arm, between the shoulder and the elbow.

Bradycardia—Slow heart rate (fewer than 50–60 beats per minute).

Brainstem—The inferior part of the brain that contains three main structures: midbrain, pons, and medulla oblongata.

Bronchioles—Smaller divisions of the bronchi.

Bronchitis—Inflammation of the bronchial mucosa that causes the bronchial tubes to swell and extra mucus to be produced.

Buccal—Pertaining to the cheek area.

Bursa—A saclike structure with a synovial membrane that contains synovial fluid.

Bursitis—Acute or chronic inflammation of the bursa. Infection, trauma, disease, or excessive friction or pressure in the joint causes it.

Business property insurance—A type of insurance that covers the cost of business property, such as a desk, massage table, chairs, and stereo equipment in your business location.

Calcitonin—Substance that decreases blood calcium and phosphorus by stimulating osteoblasts (bone-forming cells) to make bone matrix, causing calcium and phosphorus to be deposited in the bones.

Capillaries—Blood vessels with thin, permeable membranes for efficient gas exchange.

Capillary exchange—The system where nutrients and oxygen are provided to tissues and waste from cells is removed.

Carcinogen—Cancer-causing agent.

Carpal tunnel syndrome—A painful repetitive strain injury of the hand and wrist caused by compression of the median nerve.

Cartilage—An avascular, tough, protective tissue capable of withstanding repeated stress. Since cartilage has no direct blood supply, it is slow to heal.

Cell body, cyton, or soma—Part of the neuron that contains the nucleus and other standard equipment (i.e., organelles) of the cell.

Centering—A mental, emotional, and physical state of the therapist that is calm, yet responsive.

Central nervous system—Part of the nervous system that occupies a central or medial position in the body. Its primary purpose is to interpret incoming sensory information and to issue instructions in the form of motor response. The major components of the CNS include the brain (i.e., cerebrum, cerebellum, diencephalons, brainstem), meninges, cerebrospinal fluid, and spinal cord.

Cerebellum—Part of the brain concerned with muscle tone, coordinating skeletal muscles and balance (posture integration and equilibrium), and controling fine and gross motor movements. It is a cauliflower-shaped structure located posterior and inferior to the cerebrum.

Cerebral palsy—Motor disorder resulting in loss of muscular coordination and muscle control.

Cerebrospinal fluid—A clear, colorless fluid circulating around the brain and spinal cord. It provides a medium for nutrient exchange and waste removal as well as shock absorption.

Cerebrum—The largest part of the brain that governs all higher function (i.e., language, memory, reasoning, and some aspects of personality).

Cervical—Pertaining to the neck area.

Chemoreceptors—Chemical stimuli activated by sensory receptors that detect smells, tastes, and chemistry changes in the blood.

Chi, Ki—Energy along 14 meridians and 365 acupoints located throughout the body.

Chronic—Conditions that have a long duration, sometimes a lifetime.

Cirrhosis—A chronic degenerative disease of the liver in which the hepatic cells are destroyed and replaced with fibrous connective tissue, giving the liver a yellow-orange color.

Code of ethics—A guideline of moral principles that governs one's course of action.

Cold or ice immersion baths—A treatment of immersing the affected area in a container of icy/cold water. This method is convenient for feet and hands.

Collagen—An insoluble, fibrous protein that constitutes about 70% of the dermis and offers support to the nerves, blood vessels, hair follicles, and glands.

Compression massage—Rhythmic pumping on a muscle belly to create a sustained increase in circulation and muscle relaxation.

Connective tissue—The most abundant and ubiquitous tissue of the body. Some connective tissue types serve as nutrient transport systems, some defend the body against disease, some possess clotting mechanisms, and others act as a supportive framework and provide protection for vital organs.

Contamination—Airborne, fluid-borne, direct contact of infectious or causative agents entering an organism. When an organism is contaminated, the next phase is infection.

Contract—A written agreement between two or more parties that is enforceable by law and outlines expectations, duties, and responsibilities.

Contracture—Condition of a joint, which is abnormal and usually permanent, where the muscle is fixed in a flexed position.

Contralateral—Related to the opposite side of the body.

Contusion—An injury resulting from a blow to soft tissue, commonly called a bruise. The discoloration comes from blood escaping from the blood vessels that were broken or damaged from the blow.

Cryotherapy—The application of cold on the body. The methods may include ice, icy water, frozen gel, or chemical cold packs.

Cushing's disease—A metabolic disorder caused by an overproduction of adrenocorticol steroids.

Cyriax, James—An osteopath from England who developed a system to test all joints to isolate lesions in the soft tissue.

Cytoplasmic organelles—Small cellular structures that provide special functions such as reproduction, storage, and metabolism. Types of organelles are the nucleus, ribosomes, endoplasmic reticulum, Golgi apparatus, mitochondria, lysosomes, and centrioles.

Deltoid—Large muscle of the upper arm that forms the curve of the shoulder and upper arm.

Dendrites or afferent processes—Typically short, narrow, and highly-branched neural extensions that receive and transmit stimuli toward the cell body.

Dermis—Tissue under the epidermis that contains adipose tissue, many blood vessels, and nerve endings.

Diabetes mellitus—A group of conditions that lead to elevated blood glucose levels (hyperglycemia).

Diarthrotic joints—Freely movable joints that allow movement in more than one dimension; also known as synovial joints.

Disinfecting—The removal of pathogenic microorganisms from surfaces by a chemical or mechanical agent.

Dislocation—Displacement of bones due to extreme force.

Distal—Away from the point of reference, usually away from the midline or central point.

Diuretic—Any substance that promotes the formation and excretion of urine.

Documentation—Information that is recorded on paper.

Dorsal cavity—Located on the back or posterior.

Draping—Technique of covering the client with a drape during massage to promote warmth and professional atmosphere that satisfies the client's need for privacy and comfort.

Eczema—An acute or chronic superficial inflammation of the skin characterized by redness, watery discharge, crusting, scaling, itching, and burning.

Effleurage—A massage stroke of purposeful, gliding movements that follow the contour of the client's body.

Elastic cartilage—A soft and more pliable cartilage than hyaline or fibrocartilage that gives shape to the external nose and ears and to internal structures, such as the epiglottis and the auditory tubes.

Ellipsoidal joints—Joints that are essentially a reduced ball-and-socket joint and allow flexion, extension, abduction, and adduction, but rotation is not permitted (e.g., radiocarpal joints in the wrist). Also known as *condyloid* or *biaxial joints*.

Embolus—A blood clot, bubble of air, or any piece of debris transported by the bloodstream.

Emphysema—Abnormal condition of the lungs in which there is overinflation of the alveoli, leading to a breakdown of their walls and a decrease in respiratory function.

Endangerment sites—Areas of the body that contain certain anatomical structures that are vulnerable to injury.

Endorphin—Any natural protein in the brain that helps to reduce pain.

Epilepsy—Neurological disorder characterized by convulsive seizures and impaired consciousness.

Epinephrine or adrenaline—An adrenal hormone that increases blood pressure by stimulating vasoconstriction, rather than affecting cardiac output.

Estrogen—Female hormone that promotes the development of secondary sex characteristics in females.

Excursion—The distance traversed on the client's body or the length of a massage stroke.

Expiration or exhalation—A procedure that occurs when the diaphragm relaxes and ascends back up toward the thoracic cavity. Air is forced out of the lungs.

Extensor—A muscle that extends a joint.

External—Nearest the outside of a body cavity.

Femoral or crural—Pertaining to the femur or the thigh area, between the hip and the knee.

Fibrocartilage—Of the three cartilage types the one with the greatest tensile strength. Fibrocartilage is found in the intervertebral disks, in the meniscus of the knee joint, and between the pubic bones (pubic symphysis).

Fibromyalgia—A chronic inflammatory disease that affects muscle and related connective tissue.

Fibrosis or scar formation—A process in which the original tissue type is replaced with a different kind of tissue. Fibrosis occurs when the damage is so severe that there are not enough healthy cells to reproduce the tissue required or when the damaged tissue does not have the ability to readily reproduce itself. The scar tissue formed by fibrosis is usually stronger than the original tissue.

Five elements—In Chinese medicine these are water, fire, wood, earth, and metal, which form a star.

Fixator or stabilizer—Specialized synergist that stabilizes the joint over which the prime mover exerts its action, allowing the prime mover to perform a motion more efficiently.

Flaccid—Pertaining to a condition where a muscle lacks normal tone and appears flattened rather than rounded.

Flexibility—The ability of the muscles, joints, and soft tissues to bend.

Flexor—A muscle that bends a joint.

Foot reflexology—A therapeutic system theory in which the entire body (organs, glands, and body parts) has reflex points located on the feet. By using applied pressure, one can release blockages around the corresponding body part and rebalance the entire body.

Fracture—A disruption in the structure of the bone. Types of fractures include simple, compound, spiral, transverse, commuted, oblique, impacted, complete and incomplete.

Friction—A brisk, often heat-producing compression stroke that may be delivered either superficially to the skin or to deeper tissue layers of muscle, depending upon the intention of the therapist.

Frontal or coronal plane—The plane passing through the body from side to side to create anterior (ventral) and posterior (dorsal) sections.

Fungus—A microorganism that requires an external carbon source; fungi reproduce by spore formation. Fungus growth is promoted by a warm and moist environment and includes molds and yeast.

Furunculus—A boil or an abscess caused by the staphylococcal bacteria resulting in necrosis (death) of a hair follicle.

Gait—The walking pattern.

Ganglion—A cluster of nerve cell bodies located in the peripheral nervous system.

General liability insurance—Insurance that covers liability costs that are a result from bodily injury, property damage, and personal injury. Also referred to as *premise liability*.

Gliding joints—These joints permit movements limited to gliding in flexion, extension, abduction, and adduction (intercarpal and intertarsal joints). Also known as *arthrodia* or *biaxial joints*.

Gluteal—Curve of the buttocks formed by the large gluteal muscles.

Golgi tendon organs—Receptors that are stimulated by both tension and excessive stretch and are located at the musculotendinous boundary of skeletal muscles. These protective mechanisms help to ensure that muscles do not become excessively stretched or do not contract too strongly and damage their tendons.

Gout—A disease in which a defect in uric acid metabolism causes acid and its salts to accumulate in the blood.

Hepatitis—Inflammation of the liver.

Hernia—A protrusion of surrounding connective tissue or cavity wall of an organ or part of an organ.

Hinge joint—Joint that controls movement limited to flexion and extension (elbow and interphalangeal joints). Also known as *ginglymus* or *monoaxial joints*.

Homeostasis—A somewhat stable or balanced condition of the body's internal environment within a limited range.

Horse stance—Positioning of feet during massage therapy when applying strokes that traverse relatively short distances such as petrissage and certain friction strokes. The feet are placed on the floor, parallel, with toes pointing forward, a little more than hip distance apart.

Hot pack—A means of applying moist heat for pain relief. Also known as *hydrocollator packs, fomentation packs, hot compresses*, and *hot dressings*.

Hydrotherapy—Therapeutic use of water and complementary agents (salt and soap) at temperatures no more than 8 degrees from normal body temperature. The water can be either cold or hot.

Hydrotherapy tubs or spas—Immersion baths and whirlpool baths, where the water is treated to remain clean and sanitary for multiple use.

Hygiene—The principles of health maintenance.

Hyperemia—The noticeable reddened skin that results from increased blood flow.

Hypertension—Elevated blood pressure; 140/90 mm Hg is regarded as the threshold of hypertension and 160/95 is classified as serious hypertension.

Hypertrophy—Increase in the size and diameter of muscle fibers without cell division.

Hypoglycemia—A condition of low blood sugar.

Hypoxia—A decrease in the amount of oxygen in the blood.

Ice massage—Circular friction and cryotherapy.

Inferior or caudal—Situated below or toward the tail end.

Inflammation—A protective mechanism with the purpose of stabilization and preparation for damaged tissue repair. It is the body's immediate reaction to soft tissue injury. The primary symptoms are localized heat, swelling, redness, pain, and decreased range of motion.

Insertion—The muscle attachment undergoing the greatest movement.

Insulin—A substance secreted by pancreatic beta cells that decreases blood glucose levels by enhancing the uptake of glucose into the cells.

Interosseous membrane—A tough membrane that connects bones (ulna and radius) by attaching to their periosteum. Also known as interosseous ligament since it connects bone to bone.

Ischemia—A reduction of oxygenated blood to an organ or body part, marked by pain and tissue dysfunction.

Isometric contraction—Increase in muscle contraction without change in muscle length or angle; no movement.

Isotonic or dynamic contractions—A contraction of the muscle where it changes length against resistance and movement occurs.

Jin Shin Do®—A modern version of traditional Chinese acupressure theory based on eight Strange Flows. Iona Teeguarden developed it in 1970.

Kinesiology—The study of the body's muscles, joints, and their movements.

Kyphosis—An abnormal convex curvature of the spine.

Lateral—Located farthest away from the midline of the body.

Law of facilitation—A neurological law that states once an impulse has traveled a certain nerve pathway, it tends to "imprint" or "facilitate" the pathway. Accordingly, it will take the same path on future occasions.

Leukocytes—White blood cells or white corpuscles.

Ling, Henrik (1776–1839)—Swedish physiologist and gymnastics instructor; known as the "Father of Swedish Massage." He developed his own system of medical gymnastics and exercise, known by different names: the Ling System, Swedish Movements, or the Swedish Movement Cure. An important part of the Ling System was a style known as Swedish Massage.

Local twitch response—An involuntary firing or twitching in muscle in response to the sensory stimulation on the trigger point.

Loose connective tissue—The packing material of the body. It attaches the skin to underlying structures, wraps and supports body cells, fills in the spaces between organs and muscles, and stabilizes them in their proper places.

Lordosis—An abnormal concave curvation of the spine.

Lumbar—The area between the thorax and hips of the pelvis.

Lyme disease—Disease caused by the bacterium *Borrelia burgdorferi*, transmitted by a tick bite, and causing a recurrent form of arthritis.

Lymph—The fluid of the lymph system.

Lymph nodes—Structures located along lymph vessels that collect and filter lymph. They protect the body from unwanted invaders.

Malignant—A condition that can worsen and cause death if not treated.

Malignant melanoma—Cancer of the melanocytes of the skin, which begins as raised dark lesions with irregular borders that appear uneven in color.

Massage—A systematic and scientific manipulation of the soft tissue for the purpose of improving and maintaining health. It can also be defined as organized intentional touch or therapeutic touch.

Mastication—Process of chewing.

Mechanoreceptors—Sensory receptors that respond to mechanical stimuli. They are sensitive to touch, pressure, vibration, stretching, muscular contraction, proprioception, sound, and equilibrium.

Medial—Located more toward or near the midline of the body.

Meissner's corpuscles—Receptors for light touch, responding to the actual movement and the length of the movement. They monitor low-frequency vibration and adapt slowly.

Meningitis—An inflammation or infection of the meninges often characterized by a sudden severe headache, vertigo, stiff neck, and severe irritability.

Meridian—Refers to the Chi energy that circulates through 12 channels passing through organs and the extremities.

Metabolic disease—Involves abnormal activities of cells and/or tissues (e.g., diabetes, cardiovascular conditions, and jaundice). Metabolic diseases are not contagious, but may have originated from a contagious disease, such as hepatitis, which can lead to jaundice or vice versa.

Metabolism—Total of all chemical and physical processes that occur in an organism.

Metastasis—The spreading of cancerous cells to distant body parts usually by way of the bloodstream or lymphatic system.

Midsagittal or median plane—The plane that runs longitudinally or vertically, down the body, dividing the body into right and left sections. This plane creates right lateral and left lateral portions of the body.

Modality—A broad term used to denote any technique, procedure, or product used to produce a positive response for the client.

Motor neurons—Neurons responsible for carrying messages to muscles or glands.

Motor unit—A single motor neuron and all its associated skeletal muscle fibers. A single muscle is composed of many motor units.

Multiple sclerosis—The progressive destruction of myelin sheaths in the central nervous system.

Muscle cramp—Acute, painful contraction of a muscle.

Muscle energy techniques (MET)—Techniques of stretching that use neurophysiological muscle reflexes to improve mobility of the joints.

Muscle fatigue—The inability of a muscle to contract even though it is still being stimulated.

Muscle or neuromuscular spindles—Stretch-sensitive receptors that monitor deviations in the length of a muscle and the rate of change.

Muscle spasm—An increase in muscle tension, with or without shortening, causing disability and pain.

Muscular atrophy—Reduction of muscle size due to poor nutrition, lack of use, motor unit dysfunction, or lack of motor nerve impulses.

Muscular dystrophy—An inherited disease of the skeletal muscles that weakens and atrophies, leading to increasing disability.

Myofascial—Pertaining to techniques aimed at restoring mobility in the body's fascia and softening connective tissue.

Myofilament—Bundle of smaller structures called actin and myosin that comprise a myofibril.

Negative feedback system—A method of the endocrine system that triggers the negative (opposite) response.

Nephrons—The filtering system of the kidneys that filters waste products from the blood.

Nerve—Impulse-carrying fiber connecting the brain and the spinal cord with other parts of the body.

Nerve compression—Pressure against the nerve due to contact with hard tissue (bone or cartilage), also known as *impingement*.

Nerve entrapment—Pressure against the nerve due to adjacent soft tissue (muscle, tendon, fascia, and ligaments), also known as *entrapment neuropathy*.

Networking—The development of business relationships with various groups of people with similar views.

Neuroglia or glial cells—Connective tissues that support, nourish, protect, insulate, and organize the neurons.

Neuromuscular or myoneural junction—Fluid-filled space between nerve endings and muscle fibers.

Neuropathy—Decrease or change in sensation in hands and feet.

Neurotransmitters—A collective term for a range of chemicals that facilitate, arouse, or inhibit the transmission of nerve impulses between synapses.

Nociceptor—Receptor for detecting pain; also known as *free nerve ending*.

Norepinephrine or noradrenaline—Hormone that assists the body in maintaining the stress response. Its effects are increased heart rate, blood pressure, and blood glucose levels, as well as dilation of the small passageways of the lungs.

Origin—The tendinous attachment of the muscle that is relatively fixed during the muscle's action.

Osteoarthritis—Arthritis characterized by degeneration of cartilage in joints; more common in the elderly. Symptoms include pain after exercise or use, joint stiffness, and swelling.

Osteoporosis—Decreased bone mass and increased susceptibility to fractures.

Pacinian's or laminated corpuscles—Pressure-sensitive receptors that respond to skin displacement and high-frequency vibration, adapting quickly to all external stimuli.

Palmar—The anterior surface or the palm of the hand.

Palpatory assessment—Assessment through touching.

Papule—A small round, firm, elevated area in the skin, varying in size from a pinpoint to that of a small pea.

Parasympathetic nervous system or craniosacral outflow—An anabolic system that conserves the body's energy properties.

Parietal—Pertaining to the walls of a cavity or an organ.

Parkinson's disease—A neurological disorder that is progressive and degenerative in nature. It is marked by the destruction of certain areas of the brain (specifically, dopamine-producing neurons) and depletion of the neurotransmitter dopamine.

Passive stretching—Form of stretching where the client remains relaxed (passive) and the therapist applies the stretch.

Pathogen or pathogenic agent—A biological agent capable of causing disease.

Pectoral—Pertaining to the thorax or chest area.

Pedal—Referring to the foot.

Percussion or tapotement—A massage stroke that consists of repetitive, striking movements of the hands either simultaneously or alternately, with loose wrists and fingers, in order to stimulate the underlying tissue.

Pericarditis—An inflammation of the parietal pericardium that may be due to trauma or infection.

Periosteum—A fibrous dense vascular connective tissue sheath that surrounds the bone and penetrates the bone, anchoring itself to the bone.

Peripheral—Also referred to as superficial, the outside surface (periphery) or surrounding external area of a structure.

Peripheral nervous system—A portion of the nervous system that is composed of nerves emerging from the central nervous system.

Peritoneum—The largest serous membrane in the body that encompasses the entire abdominal wall. Sections of the peritoneum include the mesenteries, the parietal and visceral peritoneum, and the greater and lesser omentum.

Peritonitis—Acute inflammation of the peritoneum, caused by bacteria or irritating substances entering the abdominal cavity.

Petrissage—A massage stroke that is a rhythmic lifting of the muscle tissue away from the bone or underlying structures, followed by firm kneading or squeezing the muscle followed by a release of tissue.

Phlebitis—An inflammation of a vein accompanied by pain.

Plantar—The bottom surface of the foot.

Plexus—A network of nerves.

Polarity—A form of bodywork that uses simple touch and gentle rocking.

Popliteal—Posterior aspect of the knee.

Posterior or dorsal—Referring to the back of a structure.

Prone—Face-down lying position.

Proprioceptive neuromuscular facilitation (PNF)—A therapy for rehabilitation of soft tissue disorders based on reciprocal inhibition relaxation; also known as *contract-relax technique*.

Protocol—Description of the steps used in the therapy plan.

Proximal—Nearer to the point of reference, usually toward the trunk of the body.

Psoriasis—Red, flaky skin elevations marked by remissions and exacerbations.

Pulmonary edema—A disproportionate amount of blood and interstitial fluid in the lungs.

Range of motion (ROM)—A measurement of joint movement, which can be either active or passive.

Reciprocal inhibition (RI)—Occurs when muscle acting on a joint contracts and the opposite muscle is reflexively inhibited.

Referred pain—Pain elicited at a site distant from the injured or diseased body part.

Reflex arc—The functional component of the nervous system in which sensory and motor neurons innervate a muscle, gland, or organ.

Renal—Pertaining to the kidneys.

Sauna bath—A hot-air bath with temperatures ranging from 160 to 180°F in 6-8% humidity.

Schwann's cells—Cells located in the peripheral nervous system that produce the myelin sheaths for axons.

Sciatica—A condition whereby the sciatic nerve is inflamed with resulting dull pain and tenderness in the buttock region and sharper pain or numbness radiating down the leg.

Scleroderma—An autoimmune disorder affecting blood vessels and connective tissue.

Scoliosis—An abnormal lateral curvature of the spine.

Scope of practice—Defines the working parameters of a particular profession. This may vary from state to state.

Seated position—A massage given to a client while seated; also known as chair position. The client may be seated in an ordinary chair or one that is specially designed for client comfort.

Sebaceous or oil glands—Glands that attach to hair follicles; they possess ducts (exocrine) and secrete sebum.

Senile lentigo—A condition found on older people, especially those who have had excessive exposure to the sun, whereby the skin has tan or brown patches.

Serous membranes—Membranes that line closed body cavities and secrete a thin, fluid between the parietal and visceral layers, which lubricates organs and reduces friction between the organs in the thoracic or abdominopelvic cavities.

Shiatsu—A general term for Japanese bodywork based on traditional meridian theory, in which *tsubo* (acupoints) are pressed to balance the flow of energy or chi.

Shingles—A reactivation of the latent herpes zoster (chickenpox) virus, causing an acute infection of the peripheral nervous system.

Skeletal or voluntary muscle—Muscle that attaches to bones and their membranes, fascia, and other muscles. Nerve impulses must be present in order that these muscles may contract.

Skin pallor—Refers to unnatural paleness or lack of skin color.

Sliding filament theory—Explanation of how muscle filaments slide past each other in order to change muscle length.

Smooth visceral or involuntary muscle—Muscle that lines the walls of hollow organs, adapts to sustain long contractions and use very little energy.

SOAP—An acronym for reporting. **S**ubjective assessment information, **O**bjective assessment information, **A**pplication of massage or therapy, and **P**lan course of action.

Somatic reflex—Reflex responsible for the contraction of skeletal muscle (e.g., knee jerk or patella reflex).

Spasticity—Increased muscle tone and stiffness associated with an increase in tendon reflexes.

Spina bifida—A congenital defect in which there is a malformation in the spine.

Spinal cord—The structure within the vertebral canal that is an extension of the brainstem from the foramen magnum to the region of L2.

Spinal nerves—The nerves that originate from the spinal cord.

Sprain—The stretching or tearing of the ligamentous structure of a joint, with associated pain, swelling, and possible disability.

Squamous cell carcinoma—A type of skin cancer that begins as a scaly pigmented area; can develop into an ulcerated crater.

Static stretching—Slow held stretches with no bouncing.

Steam bath or wet sauna—Hot vapor baths in a specially designed chamber where temperatures are maintained at 105–130°F at 100% humidity.

Sterilization—A technique that uses heat, water, chemicals, or gases to destroy microorganisms.

Strain—A muscle or tendon injury caused by a violent contraction, forced stretching, or synergistic failure.

Stretching—Lengthening or extending the muscle tissue to its full length.

Summation—Occurs when a subthreshold stimulus is repeated in succession and cumulatively creates a nerve impulse.

Superior, cranial, or cephalic—Situated above or toward the head.

Supine—Lying face up.

Sympathetic nervous system or thoracolumbar outflow—A catabolic system that is involved with spending body resources and with preparing the body for emergency situations.

Synaptic transmission—The one-way bridging of the synaptic gap to convey the nerve impulse (from axon to dendrite) to the next neuron.

Synarthrotic joint—Type of joint in which movement is absent or extremely limited.

Synovial fluid—Viscous fluid that provides nutrition and lubrication to joints.

Synovial membrane—Membrane that lines joint cavities of freely moving joints and secrete synovial fluids.

Tachycardia—Rapid heart rate (more than 100 beats per minute).

Temporal mandibular joint (TMJ)—A joint where the jawbone articulates with the temporal bone of the skull; irregularities often cause pain and tenderness.

Tendinitis—Inflammation of the tendon, accompanied by pain and swelling.

Tendon—Tough fibrous connective tissue that attaches muscle to bone, fascia, or other connective tissue structures.

Testosterone—An androgenic hormone that promotes secondary male sex characteristics, as well as libido (sex drive) and sperm production.

Thermoreceptor—Receptor sensitive to temperature changes located immediately under the skin.

Thoracic duct—The lymphatic duct that drains lymph from the parts of the body not drained by the right lymphatic duct.

Thyroxin—A hormone secreted by the thyroid gland that stimulates the metabolic rate of the body.

Tonus—A state of continuous, partial muscle contraction.

Topical—Pertaining to the surface.

Torticollis—Condition in which the head leans to one side because of neck muscle contractions (wry neck).

Touch—Laying the hands on the skin.

Trager, Milton—Founder of a method using gentle shaking to eliminate tension.

Transverse or horizontal plane—The plane that creates the superior and inferior sections.

Travell, Janet—Theorized that trigger points cause myofascial pain.

Treatment record—A journal of treatment or therapy sessions that contains the client's information and SOAP forms for each session.

Trigger point—Hypersensitive area in muscles, fascia, tendons, and ligaments that refer pain to distal regions of the body.

Ulcer—A lesion in a membrane that is exposed to acidic gastric juices, most commonly found in parts of the digestive tract.

Universal donor—A donor with type O blood, which will not react adversely to any other blood types.

Universal precautions—A health-preserving system that includes the following: handwashing; gloves; protective eyewear; nose-face masks; protective clothing; methods for laundering, cleaning, and disinfecting equipment; and proper methods for disposing of used medical and biological material.

Universal recipient—A recipient with type AB blood, which can receive all other blood types.

Urinary incontinence—The inability to control micturition.

Varicose veins—Dilated veins possessing incompetent valves.

Vasodilation—The diameter of a blood vessel becomes wider.

Vein—Blood vessel that drains the tissues and organs and returns blood back to the heart and lungs.

Vibration—A massage stroke that is a rapid shaking, trembling, or oscillating movement applied with full hands, fingertips, to induce relaxation.

Vodder, Emil—The founder of manual lymph drainage, which assists the flow of lymph through the vessels.

Yang—Symbolizes the back of the body, the light, high, hot, outside, active, and excessive of the natural process and complements yin.

Yin—Symbolizes the front of the body, the dark, low, cold, inside, passive, and deficiency of the natural process and complements yang, the opposite.

References

The following reference books have been used by the National Certification Board for Therapeutic Massage and Bodywork (NCBTMB) for development of the Certifying Examination and also in preparation for the review book content areas.

American Red Cross. *Community First Aid and Safety*. St. Louis, MO: Mosby Lifeline, 2002.

*Ashley, Martin. *Massage: A Career at Your Fingertips*. 3rd edition. Barrytown, NY: Station Hill Press, 1999.

Beck, Mark F. *Theory and Practice of Therapeutic Massage*. 5th edition. New York: Thomas Delmar Learning/Cengage Learning, 2010.

Benjamin, Patricia and Frances M. Tappan. *Tappan's Handbook of Healing Massage Techniques*. 4th edition. Upper Saddle River, NJ: Prentice Hall, 2005.

*Beresford-Cooke, Carola. *Shiatsu Theory and Practice: A Comprehensive Text for the Student Professional*. 2nd edition. New York: Churchill Livingstone, 2003.

Biel, Andrew. *Trail Guide to the Body*. 3rd edition. Boulder, CO: Books of Discovery, 2005.

Clemente, Carmine. *Anatomy: A Regional Atlas of the Human Body*. 4th edition. Baltimore, MD: Williams and Wilkins, 1997.

*Fritz, Sandy. *Fundamentals of Therapeutic Massage*. 3rd edition. St. Louis, MD: Mosby, 2004.

Fritz, Sandy, and M. James Grosenbach. *Essential Sciences for Therapeutic Massage: Anatomy, Physiology, Biomechanics and Pathology*. 2nd edition. St. Louis, MD: Mosby, 2004.

Kendall, Florence Peterson, Elizabeth Kendall McCreary, and Patricia Geise Provance. *Muscles: Testing and Function*. 4th edition. Baltimore: Williams and Wilkins, 1993.

Maciocia, Giovanni. *The Foundations of Chinese Medicine*. New York: Churchill Livingstone, 1989.

Salvo, Susan. *Massage Therapy: Principles and Practice*. Philadelphia, PA: W.B. Saunders Company, 1999.

Sohnen-Moe, Cherie M. *Business Mastery*. 3rd edition. Rochester, VT: Healing Arts Press, 1997.

*Tappan, Frances M., and Patricia J. Benjamin. *Handbook of Healing Massage Techniques*. 4th edition. Upper Saddle River, NJ: Prentice Hall, 2005.

Thomas, C.L. ed. *Taber's Cyclopedic Medical Dictionary*. 19th edition. Philadelphia, PA: Davis Co., 2001.

Thompson, Diana L. *Hands Heal, Communication, Documentation, and Insurance Billing for Manual Therapist*. 2nd edition. Self-published, 2002.

Totora, Gerard, and Sandra Reynolds Grabowski. *Principles of Anatomy and Physiology*. 10th edition. New York: Harper and Collins Publishers, 2004.

*Werner, Ruth. *A Massage Therapist's Guide to Pathology*. 2nd edition. Baltimore: Williams and Wilkins, 2002.

*The author recommends these books for both NCTMB and the MBLEx exams as comprehensive resources of massage and bodywork study.

INDEX